9 Update in Intensive Care and Emergency Medicine

Edited by J. L. Vincent

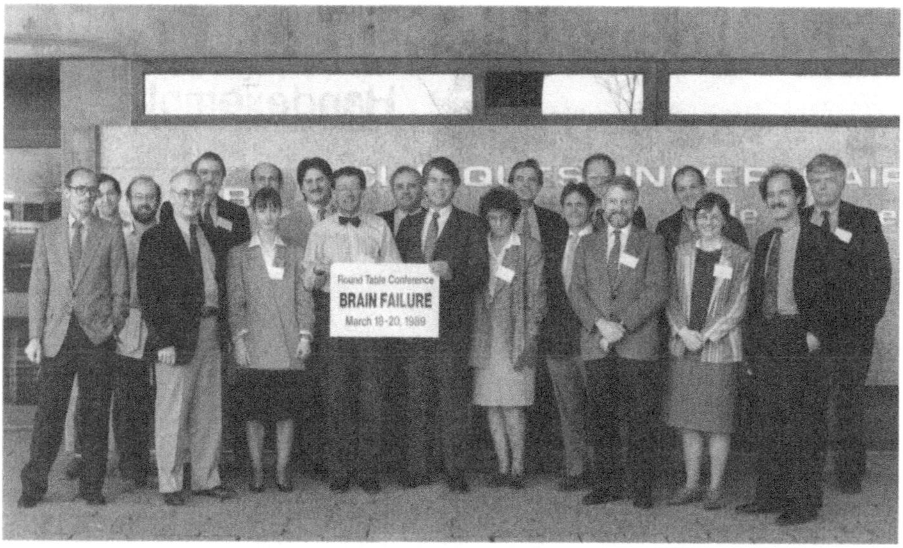

The Research Conference was organized by the European Society of Intensive Care Medicine in conjunction with the Society of Critical Care Medicine in Brussels (Erasme University Hospital) on March 18–20, 1989. Participants to the Research Conference were (from left to right): R. L. Chiolero (Lausanne), J.-F. Hartmann (Paris), D. Zegers de Beyl (Brussels), E. D. Means (Kalamazoo), R. J. Traystman (Baltimore), J. Wendon (London), D. M. Payen (Paris), D. Chyatte (New Haven), D. Bihari (London), G. N. Woodruff (Harlow), J. W. Holaday (Washington DC), M. Hemmer (Luxemburg), J. Cottrell (Brooklyn), D. P. Becker (Los Angeles), M. D. Ginsberg (Miami), J. D. Miller (Edinburgh), A. Forster (Geneva), C. S. Robertson (Houston), A. I. Arieff (San Francisco), M. Fisher (Sydney). P. Demediuk (San Francisco) is not on the photograph.

Brain Failure

Edited by
D. Bihari and J.W. Holaday

With 60 Figures and 31 Tables

Springer-Verlag Berlin Heidelberg New York
London Paris Tokyo Hong Kong

Series Editor

Prof. Dr. Jean Louis Vincent
Clinical Director, Department of
Intensive Care, Erasme Hospital,
Free University of Brussels,
Route de Lennik 808,
1070 Brussels, Belgium

Volume Editors

Dr. David Bihari
Intensive Care Unit, Guy's Hospital,
St. Thomas Street, London SE1 9RT,
United Kingdom

Dr. John W. Holaday
Department of Neuropsychiatry,
Walter Reed Army Institute of
Research, Washington, DC 20307,
USA

ISBN-13: 978-3-540-51655-2 e-ISBN-13: 978-3-642-83929-0
DOI: 10.1007/978-3-642-83929-0

Library of Congress Cataloging-in-Publication Data
Brain failure / edited by D. Bihari and J.W. Holaday
(Update in intensive care and emergency medicine: 9)
(U.S.: alk. paper) 1. Brain--Wounds and injuries--Complications and sequelae. 2. Brain--Pathophysiology. I. Bihari, David, 1954- II. Holaday, John W. III. Series. [DNLM: 1. Brain Diseases. W1 UP66H v. 9 / WL 348 B8143] RD594.B72 1989 616.8′047--dc20 89-21827

Typesetting and printing: Zechnersche Buchdruckerei, Speyer
Bookbinding: J. Schäffer, Grünstadt

2119/3140-543210 - Printed on acid-free paper

Contents

List of Contributors

Arieff, A. I.
Department of Medicine, Veterans Administration Medical Center, 4150 Clement Street, San Francisco, CA 94121, U.S.A.

Becker, D. P.
Department of Neurosurgery, UCLA Medical Center, Rm.74-140 CHS, 10833 Le Conte Avenue, Los Angeles, CA 90024, U.S.A.

Bernton, E. W.
Department of Neuropsychiatry, Walter Reed Army Institute of Research, Washington, DC 20307, U.S.A.

Bihari, D.
Department of Intensive Care, Guy's Hospital, St. Thomas Street, London SE1 9RT, United Kingdom

Braughler, J. M.
The Upjohn Company, Kalamazoo, MI 49001, U.S.A.

Brunko, E.
Unité de Recherche sur le cerveau, Free University of Brussels, Faculté de Medecine, Bld de Waterloo 115, 1000 Brussels, Belgium

Bryant, H. U.
Department of Immunology, Eli Lilly and Co, Lilly Corporate Center, Indianapolis, IN 46285, U.S.A.

Chiolero, R. L.
Department of Anesthesiology, C.H.U.Vaudois, 1011 Lausanne, Switzerland

Chyatte, D.
Department of Neurosurgery, Yale University School of Medicine, 333 Cedar Street, New Haven, CT 06510, U.S.A.

Faden, A. I.
Department of Neurology, Veterans Administration Medical Center, 4150 Clement Street, San Francisco, CA 94121, U.S.A.

Fisher, M.
Intensive Therapy Unit, Royal North Shore Hospital of Sydney, St. Leonards N.S.W. 2065, Australia

Forster, A.
Department of Anesthesiology, Hôpital Cantonal Universitaire, Rue Micheli-du-Crest 24, 1211 Geneve 4, Switzerland

Fraser, C. L.
Department of Geriatrics, Veterans Administration Medical Center, 4150 Clement Street, San Francisco, CA 94121, U.S.A.

Ginsberg, M. D.
Department of Neurology (D4-5), University of Miami School of Medicine, P.O. Box 016960, Miami, FL 33101, U.S.A.

Gunning, K.
Department of Anesthesiology, Hôpital Cantonal Universitaire, Rue Micheli-de-Crest 24, 1211 Genève 4, Switzerland

Hall, E. D.
The Upjohn Company, Kalamazoo, MI 49001, U.S.A.

Hartmann, J.-F.
Department of Intensive Care, Hôpital Robert Debré, 48 Boulevard Sérurier, 75019 Paris, France

Helfaer, M. A.
Department of Anesthesiology, The Johns Hopkins Medical Institutions, 600 N. Wolfe St, Baltimore, MD 21205, U.S.A.

Hemmer, M.
Department of Anesthesiology, Centre Hospitalier, Rue Barblé 4, Luxemburg, Luxemburg

Holaday, J. W.
Department of Neuropsychiatry, Walter Reed Army Institute of Research, Washington, DC 20307, U.S.A.

Iversen, L. L.
Neuroscience Research Centre, Merck Sharp and Dohme Research Lab., Terlings Park, Eastwick Road, Harlow, Essex, CM20 2QR, United Kingdom

Joffe, R.
Department of Neurology, Royal North Shore Hospital
of Sydney, St. Leonards N.S.W. 2065, Australia

Kemp, J.A.
Neuroscience Research Centre, Merck Sharp and Dohme
Research Lab., Terlings Park, Eastwick Road, Harlow,
Essex, CM20 2QR, United Kingdom

Kenner, J.R.
Department of Neuropsychiatry, Walter Reed Army Institute
of Research, Washington, DC 20307, U.S.A.

Kirsch, J.R.
Department of Anesthesiology, The Johns Hopkins Medical
Institutions, 600 N. Wolfe St, Baltimore, MD 21205, U.S.A.

Koehler, R.C.
Department of Anesthesiology, The Johns Hopkins Medical
Institutions, 600 N. Wolfe St, Baltimore, MD 21205, U.S.A.

Lamer, C.
Department of Intensive Care, Lariboisière Hospital,
2 rue Ambroise Paré, 75475 Paris Cédex 10, France

Mavroudakis, N.
Department of Neurology, Erasme University Hospital,
Route de Lennik 808, 1070 Brussels, Belgium

Means, E.D.
The Upjohn Company, Kalamazoo, MI 49001, U.S.A.

Miller, J.D.
Department of Clinical Neurosciences, Western General
Hospital, Edinburgh EH4 2XU, Scotland, United Kingdom

Payen, D.M.
Department of Anesthesiology and Intensive Care, Lariboisière
Hospital, 2 rue Ambroise Paré, 75475 Paris Cédex 10, France

Robertson, C.S.
Department of Neurosurgery, Baylor College of Medicine,
One Baylor Plaza, Houston, TX 77030, U.S.A.

Schutz, Y.
Department of Physiology, C.H.U.Vaudois,
1011 Lausanne, Switzerland

Traystman, R.J.
Department of Anesthesiology, The Johns Hopkins Medical Institutions, 600 N. Wolfe St, Baltimore, MD 21205, U.S.A.

de Tribolet, N.
Department of Neurosurgery, C.H.U.Vaudois, 1011 Lausanne, Switzerland

Vink, R.
Department of Neurology, Veterans Administration Medical Center, 4150 Clement Street, San Francisco, CA 94121, U.S.A.

Wendon, J.
Liver Unit, Kings College Hospital, Denmark Hill, London SE5 8RX, United Kingdom

Williams, R.
Liver Unit, Kings College Hospital, Denmark Hill, London SE5 8RX, United Kingdom

Woodruff, G.N.
Neuroscience Research Centre, Merck Sharp and Dohme Research Lab., Terlings Park, Eastwick Road, Harlow, Essex, CM20 2QR, United Kingdom

Zegers de Beyl, D.
Department of Neurology, Erasme University Hospital, Route de Lennik 808, 1070 Brussels, Belgium

Brain, Endocrine and Immune Interactions: Implications in Intensive Care*

J. W. Holaday, H. U. Bryant, J. R. Kenner, and E. W. Bernton

Introduction

With the trend to specialize in medicine and biomedical research, the body has been studied as a series of individual systems; this has afforded us a wealth of detailed knowledge at the system level, but often at the expense of a functional knowledge of the whole. Within the past few years, important functional links among the brain, endocrine and immune systems have been demonstrated to play a role in the intact organism's adaptive and maladaptive responses to injury and disease. Precise knowledge about the interactions among these networks may allow for exciting new therapeutic strategies with direct relevance to the practice of critical care and emergency medicine.

Chronic responses to the physiological stress of injury or disease include marked changes in the regulation of neuroendocrine function by the brain, pituitary and target glands, and often include a sustained elevation of circulating glucocorticoids and the reduced secretion of gonadotropins, thyroid stimulating hormone, prolactin and growth hormone in the plasma [1-3]. The hormones are known to play important roles in the regulation of growth, reproduction and metabolism, all of which may affect survival. Recent observations by our group and others suggest that regulation of immune host defenses should be included in the list of events mediated by neuroendocrine hormones; thus, changes in neuroendocrine status following critical illnesses or injury may contribute to the coincident immunologic dysfunction which is often observed. Brain/endocrine/immune interactions, however, are not unidirectional, e.g. the release of monokines (interleukin-1 [IL-1]) or tumor necrosis factor (TNF) from macrophages, as part of immunological responses to infection or inflammation, may also affect brain and neuroendocrine function. Furthermore, other cytokines, such as colony stimulating factor (CSF), may act upon macrophages or brain microglial cells ("macrophages of the brain") to release substances that stimulate neuronal growth in vitro. Many of the drugs routinely used for the treatment of critical illnesses or injury have profound effects upon the immune system by actions at

---

* The views of the author(s) do not purport the position of the Department or the Department of Defense, (para 4-3, AR 360-5).
Research was conducted in compliance with the Animal Welfare Act and other Federal statutes and regulations relating to animals and experiments involving animals, and adheres to principles stated in the 'Guide for the Care and Use of Laboratory Animals', NIH publication 86-23, 1985 edition.

various levels of the brain/endocrine/immune axis. The effects of glucocorticoids on immune responses are well recognized [4]; however, the immunological responses to drugs that alter the release of other hormones, including dopamine, metoclopramide, haloperidol, morphine, mucolytics, cyclosporine and other pharmacological agents commonly used in critical care and emergency medicine, have not been appreciated. Below, we will review evidence that pharmacological manipulation of the brain/endocrine/immune axis results in many effects that are of potential relevance to clinicians involved in intensive care or emergency medicine.

These studies emphasize our own work defining:

1. the importance of prolactin (PRL) as an immunopermissive hormone based on studies with hypoprolactinemic animals and on the production of immunoreactive/prolactin (ir-PRL) by cells of the immune system;
2. chronic morphine treatment as a "pharmacologic stressor",
3. the ability of PRL to reverse both morphine and glucocorticoid-induced immunosuppression;
4. the effects of immune cell products (e.g. interleukin-1) on the release of PRL and other pituitary hormones; and
5. the effects of cytokines on nerve cell growth and differentiation.

T-Cell-Dependent Immunity Is Compromised by Hypoprolactinemia

In Vivo Studies

Prolactin is a peptide hormone classically associated with lactation and the reproductive cycle; however, the evolutionary history of prolactin research has revealed that this fascinating molecule subserves many additional physiological functions in vertebrates (for review, see [5]). Although prolactin shares some structural similarity and biological actions with growth hormone (GH) and placental lactogen (PL), prolactin acts upon its own receptors to result in many trophic, metabolic, endocrine and immunologic actions.

The release of prolactin from pituitary lactotrophs in vivo varies according to time of day and is further modulated by behavioral and environmental stimuli, the reproductive cycle, steroid hormones, immunoregulatory cytokines and various drugs (Table 1). Among the primary neuroendocrine processes involved in regulating circulating levels of this hormone, prolactin secretion is tonically inhibited by the release of dopamine from the tuberoinfundibular dopaminergic neurons into the portal bloodstream to act upon dopamine-2 (DA-2) receptors located on lactotroph cells of the anterior pituitary. At the cellular level, DA-2 receptor-mediated inhibition of adenylate cyclase results in decreased cyclic AMP (as well as changes in Ca^{++} flux) and, ultimately, decreased prolactin release [5, 6]. The opposite effect occurs when dopamine antagonists, such as metoclopramide or haloperidol, are used; thus, inhibition of this dopaminergic system by dopamine antagonists results in prompt prolactin secretion. In healthy drug-free individuals, once released into the circulation, prolactin exerts ne-

Table 1. Potential immunological effects of drugs commonly used in critical care and emergency medicine

Drug	Drug type	Endocrine effect	Immunological effect	Site of action
Dopamine Bromocryptine	DA-agonist	↓ Prolactin	Immunosuppression	T-cell
Haloperidol Metoclopramide	DA-antagonist	↑ Prolactin	Immunostimulation	T-cell
Morphine (chronic)	Opioid agonist	↑ Corticosterone ↓ Prolactin	Immunosuppression	Same sites as glucocorticoids
Cysteamine	Mucolytic	↓ Prolactin	Immunosuppression	Reducing agent ↓ prolactin T-cell

gative feedback control to regulate its own release by stimulating these dopaminergic neurons, restoring once again the dopaminergic inhibitory tone [6].

As predicted by the neuroendocrine system described above, the pharmacological administration of DA-2 agonists (e.g. dopamine or bromocryptine) suppresses prolactin release, whereas centrally or peripherally-acting neuroleptic or antiemetic DA-2 antagonists (e.g. haloperidol and metoclopramide respectively) promptly stimulate prolactin release by blocking endogenous dopaminergic tone. In the critical care setting, we suggest that the use of dopamine infusions to maintain hemodynamic and renal function may contribute to the compromised immunological function and anergic status of patients (see conclusions). Conversely, the use of haloperidol or metoclopramide may improve immune function.

Growth hormone may also play an important role in the regulation of host defenses [7, 8]. Pharmacologically, there is a key difference between the regulation of pituitary prolactin and growth hormone secretion. Although prolactin secretion can be totally inhibited by direct actions of dopamine or any drug with dopaminergic actions at pituitary DA-2 receptors, dopamine agonists stimulate secretion of pituitary growth hormone by actions upon the brain's neuroendocrine pathways [6]; thus, certain pharmacologic means of inhibiting prolactin secretion, either experimentally or clinically, have no effect on growth hormone secretion. Both prolactin and growth hormone secretion, however, tend to be increased by estrogens and inhibited by glucocorticoids [5].

Secretion of both hormones is increased acutely by stress in humans, but secretion appears to attenuate rapidly with chronic stress. Sustained stress greatly inhibits prolactin secretion in response to subsequent stimuli acting at a suprapituitary level (e.g. the superimposition of an acute stress or opiates) [9–11]. One key question as yet unresolved is whether primate growth hormone, which binds with high affinity to both growth hormone and prolactin receptors to produce lactation, can or cannot mimic the immunopermissive effects of prolactin described below; this is in contrast to non-primate growth hormone that does not bind to prolactin receptors or produce lactation. Nonetheless, from animal experimentation, we would predict that alterations in prolactin secretion in chronically stressed individuals may, along with stress-induced increases in circulating adrenal corticosteroids, be an important co-determinant of changes in immune function associated with adaptation to chronic stress, such as critical illnesses.

The history of evidence to specifically link prolactin with immune function is relatively recent. In 1983, Nagy et al. reported that the drug bromocryptine, a dopamine agonist which inhibits prolactin secretion, suppressed antibody formation to sheep red blood cells and the delayed hypersensitivity response in rats [12]. The effect was blocked by coincident treatment with prolactin; however, little was known about the precise mechanisms by which prolactin exerted its immunological actions.

We have recently shown that suppression of prolactin secretion in mice with bromocryptine:

1. increases the lethality of an infectious challenge with Listeria monocytogenes,
2. abrogates T-lymphocyte-dependent activation of macrophages, as well as the production of lymphocyte interferon following inoculation with Listeria or mycobacteria (Fig. 1),
3. suppresses T-lymphocyte proliferation without affecting the production of interleukin-2.

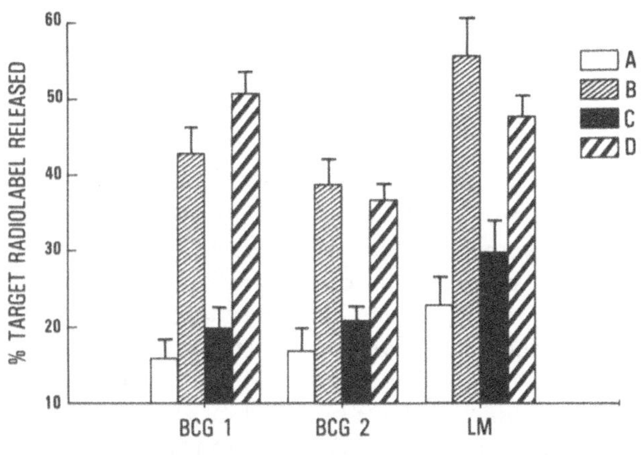

Fig. 1. Effects of bromocryptine on the induction of activated, tumoricidal macrophages during Mycobacterium bovis (BCG) or L. monocytogenes (LM) infection. Adherent peritoneal cells from groups of C3H/HeN male mice, including controls (A-unactivated macrophages from animals that were not inoculated) or from two separate studies of animals inoculated intraperitoneally with viable M. Bovis, strain BCG (BCG 1, BCG 2) or with LM 10 days previously were cultured with radiolabeled TU-5 tumor target cells. Groups of 5 mice each were treated on days 1 to 4 with daily injections of either: (B) vehicle, (C) bromocryptine mesylate (200 micrograms in 0.2 ml vehicle) (D) bromocryptine 200 micrograms and ovine prolactin (100 micrograms in 0.1 ml vehicle). Tumor cytotoxicity was estimated by measurement of radiolabel release in triplicate cultures at 48 h and expressed as percent of total tumor-cell radiolabel. Note that the activation of macrophages by inoculation with either BCG or LM (columns B) above control values (columns A) was blocked by bromocryptine coadministration (columns C) and this was reversed by bromocryptine plus prolactin (columns D). See [8] for details

All of the changes can be prevented by coincident administration of ovine prolactin [13]. Results in experimental animals demonstrate that hypoprolactinemia produced by dopamine agonists compromises host defenses by preventing T-cell production of macrophage activating factors and preventing T-cell proliferation [13].

Cysteamine is a dithiol reducing agent which is used as a mucolytic, as an antidote for acetaminophen overdose and for the treatment of nephropathic cystinosis. Cysteamine inactivates prolactin by cross-linking sulfhydryl bonds, a mechanism distinct from the neuroendocrine inhibition of pituitary prolactin secretion by dopamine agonists described above. As further evidence for the role of prolactin in immune function, cysteamine appears to selectively inactivate prolactin, but not its molecular cousin, growth hormone. We demonstrated that mice made hypoprolactinemic by cysteamine HCI treatment were as immunosuppressed as bromocryptine-treated mice [14]. Measurement of circulating prolactin levels in mice treated with varying doses of cysteamine demonstrated a positive correlation between the level of prolactin and lymphocyte proliferation in response to the mitogen, concanavalin-A (Con-A). As before, immunocompetence was restored by the administration of exogenous prolactin [14]; thus, two separate lines of experimental evidence point to the importance of prolactin in T-cell immunity and indicate that hypoprolactinemia comprises host defenses.

Additional studies have shown that the in vivo administration of exogenous prolactin or dopamine antagonists such as metoclopramide, which stimulate secretion of endogenous prolactin, resulted in significant increases in lymphocyte proliferative responses to mitogens in immunocompromised mice; these treatments were also found to reverse immunosuppression produced by administration of the drug cyclosporine (unpublished observation, Bernton EW, Bryant HU, Holaday, JW). Results from the laboratories of Russell and colleagues [15] have indicated that prolactin and cyclosporine may mutually compete for binding sites on lymphocytes; thus, the immunosuppressive actions of cyclosporine may, in part, be a consequence of its actions to inhibit prolactin's immunostimulatory effects by blockade of the prolactin receptor. As mentioned below, prolactin also reverses immunosuppression due to elevated clycocorticoids or chronic morphine treatment in mice. Although the collective evidence strongly indicates that prolactin stimulates immune function, prolactin cannot be considered to function as an immunostimulant per se, since hyperprolactinemia does not enhance immune function above control levels; instead, it appears to be an important counter-regulatory hormone that can oppose the immunosuppressive actions of stress or of drugs such as cyclosporine, morphine or glucocorticoids.

In Vitro Studies

Several reports indicate that lymphocytes may function as "neuroendocrine systems" in microcosm. Since lymphocytes are themselves capable of producing many of the hormones primarily associated with the anterior pituitary [8], we looked for evidence that lymphocytes may also produce a prolactin-like protein.

Immunocytochemical studies using monoclonal antibodies specific for prolactin (but not growth hormone) demonstrated that, following mitogenic stimulation with Con-A, phytohemagglutinin or antibody to the T3 receptor, a large subpopulation of human or murine lymphocytes accumulate prolactin-immunoreactive (ir-PRL) material within [16]. We and others [17] have also documented the production of ir-PRL using western blots of electrophoretically separated proteins from lymphocyte lysates or supernatants [16, 18]. Ir-PRL appears to play a critical role in lymphocyte proliferation. Specifically, low dilutions of antisera to prolactin-inhibited proliferation of mouse and human lymphocytes, as well as transformed lymphocytic cells responsive to T- and B-cell growth factors. The inhibitory activity could be affinity-adsorbed from the antisera by purified prolactin [19]; thus, prolactin or a prolactin-like protein may be a cytokine produced in an autocrine manner by proliferating cells of lymphoid and possibly other lineages [20]. The studies raise the interesting question as to the immunoregulatory role of pituitary prolactin secretion if a similar protein can be produced to act in an autocrine fashion by immune cells.

Chronic Morphine Treatment and Immunosuppression

It has long been known that heroin addicts are more susceptible to infectious disease, which is at least partially attributable to a compromised immune function in addition to the obvious shared use of paraphernalia [21, 22]. Of course, morphine or similar opiate drugs are extensively used for pain management in critically ill or traumatized patients. The use of morphine for its desired analgesic effects may have undesirable actions, such as immunosuppression, that may contribute to the anergy of critical illnesses.

We observed that chronic administration of morphine to mice, via a pellet implant model classically used to illustrate tolerance to the analgesic effects of morphine, resulted in atrophy of the spleen and thymus and suppressed blastogenic responses of splenocytes to both T- and B-cell mitogens (Fig. 2) [23]. Chronic exposure to morphine in this manner also suppressed macrophage responses [24], interleukin-2 production [25] and antibody formation [26]. Additionally, morphine-pelleted mice demonstrated a decrease in B-cells and a decrease in the ratio of T-helper cells to T-suppressor cells, as shown by flow cytometric analysis [25]. Finally, implantation of a morphine pellet was associated with an increased lethality to bacterial infection with Listeria monocytogenes [24].

Potential Mechanism of Morphine's Immunosuppressant Actions

The battery of immunologic defects produced by morphine bears a striking resemblance to that observed in animals following chronic administration of glucocorticoids or chronic stress. Interestingly, the morphine pellet regimen we used in mice was also associated with adrenal hypertrophy [23] and an elevation of circulating corticosterone [27]; these observations prompted our investigations

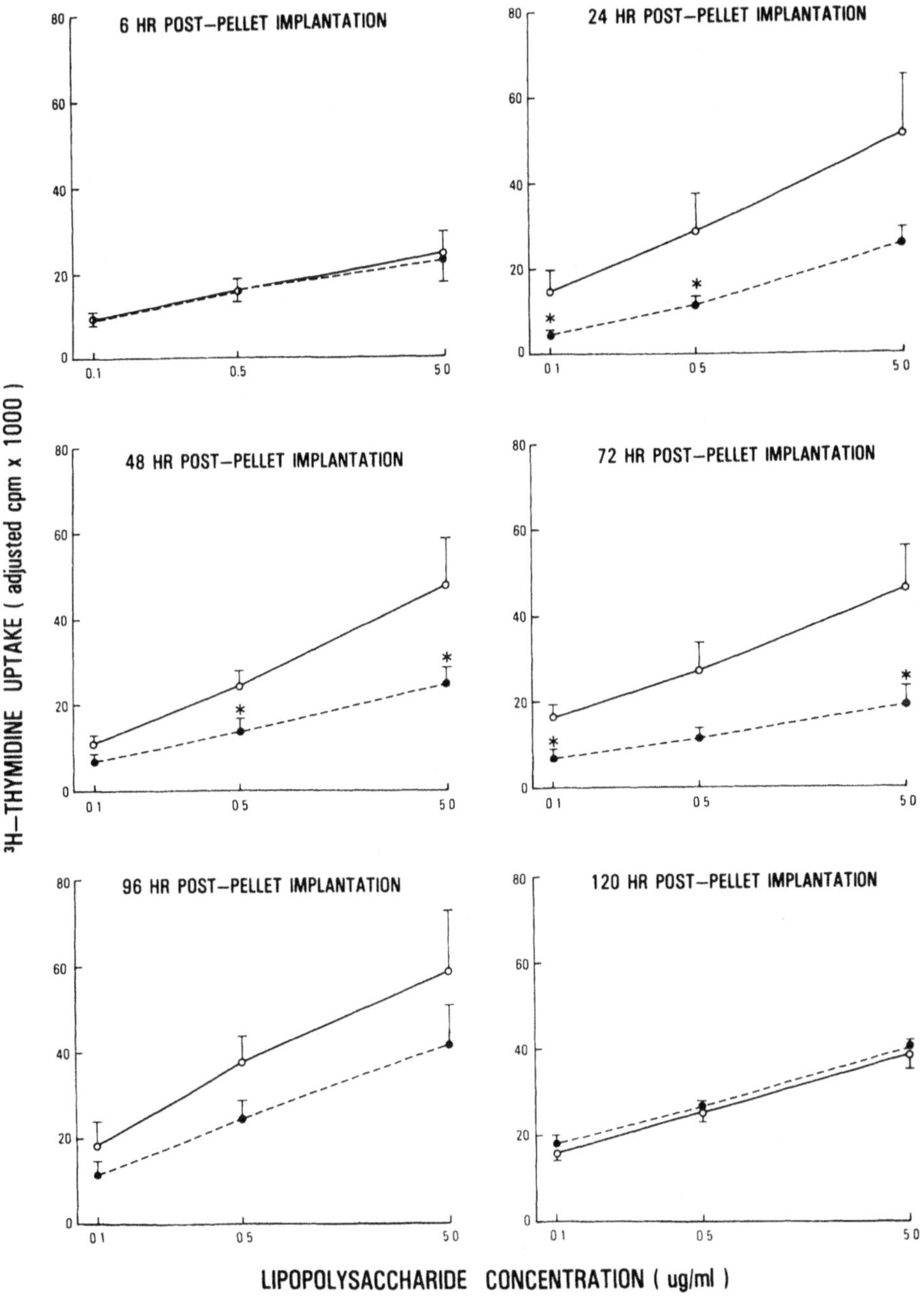

Fig. 2. Suppression of thymidine uptake stimulated by lipopolysaccharide in splenocytes obtained from placebo (open circles, solid line) or morphine-pelleted (closed circles, dashed line) mice at various times following initiation of chronic morphine exposure. See [18] for details

into the role of activation of the hypothalamo/pituitary/adrenal axis in morphine-induced immunosuppression.

We found that adrenalectomy blunted the immunosuppressive actions of chronic morphine. In complementary studies, it was shown that the administration of a glucocorticoid receptor antagonist, RU-486, blocked morphine-induced immunologic deficits [27]. The studies indicated that the immunosuppressive effect of chronic morphine treatment were at least in part due to activation of the hypothalamo/pituitary/adrenal axis, resulting in immunosuppressive effects due to elevated concentrations of adrenal corticosteroids; from these and other studies, we concluded that morphine indeed may be considered to be acting as a "pharmacologic stressor" in this model [27].

Finally, administration of prolactin itself, or drugs which induce the release of endogenous prolactin (e.g. metoclopramide), have been shown to reverse the immunosuppressive effects of chronic morphine treatment [27]. In additional studies, we demonstrated that the suppression of certain immune responses by glucocorticoids can also be reversed by increasing circulating prolactin levels [28]. Collectively, these studies offer further evidence to establish the role of the neuroendocrine system as a modulator of morphine-induced immunosuppression and suggest glucocorticoids and prolactin may have mutual counter-regulatory effects on immune target organs.

Interleukin-1 Directly Affects Anterior Pituitary Hormone Release

Interleukin-1 (IL-1) is rapidly secreted by mononuclear phagocytes (e.g. macrophages) following inflammation, endotoxemia or infectious stimuli; thus, patients suffering from septic shock or traumatic injuries initially have significant elevations in IL-1 and other cytokines [29]. In addition to amplifying T-cell responses to antigens, this monokine has numerous hormone-like systemic effects and pharmacological actions within the brain, e.g. the central injection of IL-1 induces sleep, fever and the synthesis of acute phase proteins by the liver [30]. We were interested in determining whether IL-1, by direct actions on the anterior pituitary, could play a role in orchestrating acute neuroendocrine adaptations to infectious stressors; this research was motivated by the question as to whether IL-1, acting like a hormone, could provide a mechanistic explanation for the past diagnostic use of bacterial pyrogen (endotoxin) as a clinical tool to stimulate the release of anterior pituitary hormones.

Four-hour application of sub-nanomolar concentrations of human recombinant IL-1 beta, or mouse recombinant IL-1 alpha to 72 hour monolayer cultures of dispersed rat pituitary cells, resulted in significant increases in the secretion of adrenocorticotrophic hormone (ACTH), growth hormone (GH), thyroid stimulating hormone (TSH) and luteinizing hormone (LH). By contrast, prolactin secretion was slightly decreased [31]. IL-1 also stimulated increased prostaglandin E2 production in these cultures; however, the cyclo-oxygenase inhibitor indomethacin (at doses that blocked PG-E2 secretion) when given along with IL-1 in the above system, did not affect the observed alterations in hormone release. The data suggest that, although IL-1 stimulates the arachidonic acid cascade, prostaglandins do not serve as intermediaries in the IL-1-induced secretion of pituitary hormones.

More recent work has utilized perifusion of hemipituitaries to study the time course of IL-1 actions and to minimize paracrine interactions by multiple hormones accumulating in static monolayer cultures; these studies showed that human IL-1 beta stimulated almost immediate release of ACTH, GH, TSH and LH into the perifusate. Prolactin release in response to IL-1 differed in that fresh hemipituitary perifusates demonstrated increased prolactin release, whereas prolactin levels were decreased by IL-1 in pituitary sections incubated for 72 h [32]. While other investigators have shown that the stimulation of ACTH release in rats injected with IL-1 seemed to be mediated by stimulation of corticotropin-releasing factor (CRF) via hypothalmic actions [33], our studies suggest that physiologic concentrations of IL-1 may function as a direct and relatively non-specific anterior pituitary secretagogue; these suggestions are reinforced by recent data demonstrating IL-1-immunoreactive innervation of the hypothalamus, including the median eminence [34], as well as by evidence indicating the presence of IL-1 receptors in the brain and pituitary [35]. Growth hormone secretion in response to viral infection or endotoxin injection in humans [36, 37] may also be a consequence of IL-1 release; thus, IL-1 might be another hypophysiotrophic factor and have actions upon the brain or directly on the pituitary to affect responses to infection or injury.

Effects of Macrophage- and Glial-Derived Factors on Neuronal Growth

Injury to the brain or spinal cord by trauma, neurodegenerative disorders or infection results in the loss of nerve cells, usually followed by the invasion of glial cells into the affected tissues; neuronotropic substances would have obvious applications in these pathological conditions, offering the possibility of sustaining neurons or growing new ones.

Several cytokines play a trophic role in immune function, regulating the growth of lymphocytes. Meltzer and Gendleman [38] recently demonstrated that macrophage colony stimulating factor (M-CSF) and granulocyte-macrophage colony stimulating factor (GM-CSF), when added to human monocytes, results in the production of an unknown peptide factor that sustains neuron growth when added to fetal neural cell cultures in vitro. It was previously known that neurons will survive in culture only when co-cultured with the "nursemaid" astrocytes and microglia, perhaps owing to the production of neurotrophic factors by these cells. Since monocytes, astrocytes and microglia share remarkable similarity in morphology and function, we wondered whether fresh fetal brain cultures that contain microglia and astrocytes (as well as neurons) were also capable of generating neurotrophic factors in vitro by the direct addition of M-CSF and GM-CSF [39]. Indeed, when added to fresh fetal brain cultures, M-CSF and GM-CSF sustained the growth of neurons; however, when added to cultures deprived of growth factors for 24 h, M-CSF and GM-CSF did not sustain neuronal growth. Actively proliferating cell types such as astrocytes and microglia most likely would not survive a 24-h delay without adequate growth factors.

Since the cells are known to respond to M-CSF and GM-CSF, it supports our hypothesis that astrocytes and microglia may produce a neurotrophic factor similar to that produced by stimulated monocytes. Neurotrophic activity was not reproduced by known cytokines, including IL-1, IL-2, TNF, and others [39]; thus, the isolation and characterization of neurotrophic factors, such as described above, may ultimately offer the therapeutic potential for minimizing the loss of nervous system function following injury, ischemia, infection or neurodegenerative disorders.

Clinical Relevance and Conclusions

The basic science evidence reviewed above provides a brief review of some important functional interactions among the brain, endocrine and immune systems; these interactions are bi-directional, with the neuroendocrine axis regulating the production of hormones that modify immune function, including adrenocorticotrophic hormone (ACTH) and adrenal glucocorticoids, as well as prolactin. We have demonstrated that the immunosuppressive effects of hypoprolacinemia, morphine and glucocorticoids are reversed by prolactin or by drugs that stimulate endogenous prolactin release. Furthermore, prolactin is synthesized by lymphocytes themselves and plays an autocrine role in their proliferation. In the opposite direction, monokines produced by macrophages as part of the biological responses to inflammation, infection or ischemia can directly affect the release of pituitary hormones. Indeed, monocytes stimulated by M-CSF and GM-CSF produce factors that sustain the growth and development of cultured neurons. Importantly, many of the pathophysiological conditions that are treated by practitioners of critical care and emergency medicine are characterized by derangement of the brain/endocrine/immune axis, e.g. the sick euthyroid condition may result in part from effects of IL-1 or TNF, released by monocytes in response to infection on the hypothalamo/pituitary/thyroid axis. Two reports indicate that the in vivo administration of IL-1 results in decreased TSH levels, possibly explaining the derangement of normal hypothalamic/pituitary/thyroid function in critical illnesses [40, 41]. Additionally, many of the drugs commonly used to treat these patients have heretofore unrecognized effects on the immune system; these drugs, including dopamine, haloperidol, metoclopramide, morphine and others, affect the release of hormones that, in turn, modulate immune function. Interestingly, there is evidence that the use of drugs such as haloperidol or metoclopramide do not interfere with the vasodilatory effects or renal perfusion responses to dopamine when both drugs are given concurrently [42]. One critical and unresolved question is whether growth hormones (particularly human growth hormone, which is active at the classic prolactin receptor, i.e. that in liver, breast and prostate tissue) has the ability to antagonize immunosuppressive effects of administered glucocorticoids and of increased glucocorticoid levels brought about by chronic stress. Hypotensive, critically-ill patients and patients with Parkinson's Disease are commonly treated with dopamine and dopamine agonists, which potently suppress prolactin, but tend to stimulate growth hormone release [43]; thus, if prolactin and human growth hormone have redundant permissive effects on immune target tissue, they would not be expected to contribute to suppressed immune functions in humans, since the loss of prolactin would be opposed by the gain in growth hormone. If, on the other hand, the ligand specificity of immune target tissues is restricted to prolactin, then drugs which modify prolactin secretion can be expected to have clear effects on primate immune host defenses similar to those already demonstrated in rodents. Berczi and Nagy have comprehensively reviewed the work of many investigators on in vivo effects of prolactin and growth hormone on immune function and hematolymphopoesis [12]; however, this issue requires further basic and clinical investigation.

Although much of the evidence reviewed above reflected animal experimentation, there are several clinical correlates of the above to indicate that dopamine agonists do indeed play a role in suppressing human immune responses via suppression of prolactin release, e.g. it was noted by Palestine [44] that the use of bromocryptine for the treatment of Parkinson's Disease also improved autoimmune uveitis in a small population of patients with this coincident condition. The response was attributed to the decrease in circulating prolactin. The combined use of cyclosporine and bromocryptine to prevent rejection of transplanted organs has also been suggested. In collaboration with Chernow et al., we are also testing the hypothesis that commonly-used hemodynamic drugs, such as dopamine, potently suppress prolactin secretion and iatrogenically contribute to the anergy associated with critical illnesses.

The studies reviewed above important evidence that the tendency to compartmentalize biomedical research into separate categories such as neurology, endocrinology, immunology, etc. may obscure a more holistic perspective of the intact organism's responses to injury or infection. It is through the cross fertilization of research in these areas that important basic and clinical observations will be made. As specific examples, the use of many drugs commonly found in the intensive care setting may have been beneficial or detrimental actions well beyond their intended purpose. Future clinical research based upon animal and in vitro studies, such as those reviewed above, may reveal that therapy with prolactin, growth hormone, or drugs such as metoclopramide, might reconstitute immune host defenses. Additionally, the use of prolactin or prolactin-stimulating drugs concomitantly with glucocorticoids may allow for the chronic use of glucocorticoids as anti-inflammatory agents without the adverse consequence of immunosuppression. There are clear indications that brain/endocrine/immune responses will become increasingly relevant to the practice of critical care and emergency medicine.

Acknowledgements: We thank Drs. Fein, Smallridge, Beach, Meltzer and Gendleman for their collaborative efforts in the studies. We are grateful to Jean Paige and Linda Daugherty for their assistance in preparing the manuscript.

References

1. Tache Y, Du Ruisseau P, Tache J, Selye H, Collu R (1976) Shift in adenohypophyseal activity during chronic intermittent immobilization of rats. Neuroendocrinology 22:325–336
2. Ross LH, Grant J (1988) Parenteral nutrition. In: Chernow B, Holaday JW, Zaloga GP, Zaritsky AL (eds) The pharmacologic approach to the critically ill patient, 2nd edn. Williams & Wilkins, Baltimore, pp 818–847
3. Burnham KD (1988) Thyroid hormones. In: Chernow B, Holaday JW, Zaloga GP, Zaritsky AL (eds) The pharmacologic approach to the critically ill patient, 2nd edn. Williams & Wilkins, Baltimore, pp 818–847
4. Parrillo JE, Fauci AS (1979) Mechanisms of glucocorticoid action on immune processes. Ann Rev Pharmacol Toxicol 19:129–201
5. MacLeod RM, Scapagnini U, Thorner MO (1985) Prolactin – basic and clinical correlates. Springer, Berlin Heidelberg New York Tokyo
6. Demarest KT, Riegle GD, Moore KE (1985) The interrelationship between the rapid "tonic" and the delayed „induction" components of the prolactin-induced activation of tuberoinfundibular dopamine neurons. In: MacLeod RF, Scapagnini U, Thorner MO (eds) Prolactin – basic and clinical correlates. Springer, Berlin Heidelberg New York Tokyo, pp 533–542
7. Snow ED, Feldbush TL, Oakes JA (1981) The effect of growth hormone and insulin upon MLC responses and the generation of cytotoxic leukocytes. J Immunol 125:161–164
8. Weigent DA, Blalock JE (1987) Interactions between the neuroendocrine and immune systems: Common hormones and receptors. Immunol Rev 100:79–86
9. Tache Y, Du Ruisseau P, Tache J, Selye H, Collu R (1976) Shift in adenohypophyseal activity during chronic intermittent immobilization of rats. Neuroendocrinology 22:325–336
10. Tache Y, Du Ruisseau P, Ducharme JR, Collu R (1978) Pattern of adenohypophyseal hormone changes in male rats following chronic stress. Neuroendocrinology 26:208–219
11. Yelvington DB, Weiss GK, Ratner A (1984) Effect of corticosterone on the prolactin response to psychological and physical stress in rats. Life Sci 35:1705–1711
12. Nagy E, Berczi I, Wren GE, Asa SL, Kovacs K (1983) Immunomodulation by bromocryptine. Immunopharmacology 6:231–243
13. Bernton EW, Meltzer MS, Holaday JW (1988) Suppression of macrophage activation and T-lymphocyte function in hypoprolactinemic mice. Science 239:401–403
14. Bryant HU, Bernton EW, Shakarjian TK, Holaday JW (1988) Cysteamine produces dose-related bidirectional immunomodulatory effects in mice. J Pharmacol Exp Ther (in press)
15. Russell DH, Matrisian L, Kibler R, Larson DF, Poulos B, Magun BE (1984) Prolactin receptors on human lymphocytes and their modulation by cyclosporine. Biochem Biophys Res Commun 121:899–906
16. Kenner JR, Smith PF, Bernton EW, Hartmann D, Holaday JW (1988) Murine splenic lymphocytes demonstrate Con-A inducible prolactin-like immunoreactivity as determined by immunocytochemistry (ICC). Soc Neurosci Abs 14:756
17. Montgomery DW, Zukoski CF, Shah GN, et al (1987) Concanavalin-A-stimulated murine splenocytes produce a factor with prolactin-like bioactivity and immunoreactivity. Biochem Biophys Res Commun 145:692–698
18. Hartmann DP, Holaday JW, Bernton EW (1988) Inhibition of lymphocyte proliferation by antibodies to prolactin (submitted)
19. Bernton E, Hartmann D, Holaday J (1987) Antibody to mouse prolactin inhibits murine lymphocytes responses to T-cell growth factors. J Leukocyte Biol 42:335
20. Holaday JW, Bryant HU, Kenner JR, Bernton EW (1988) Pharmacologic manipulations of the endocrine/immune axis. Progress in Neuroendocrinimmunology 1:6–8
21. Louria DB, Hensle T, Rose J (1967) The major medical complications of heroin addiction. Ann Intern Med 67:1–22
22. Donahoe RM, Nicholson JKA, Madden JJ, et al (1986) Coordinate and independent effects of heroin, cocaine and alcohol abuse on T-cell E-rosette formation and antigenic marker expression. Clin Immunol Immunopathol 41:254–260
23. Bryant HU, Bernton EW, Holaday JW (1988) Morphine pellet-induced immunomodulation in mice: Temporal relationships. J Pharmacol Exp Ther 245:913–920

24. Bryant HU, Bernton EW, Kenner JR, Shakarjian TK, Holaday JW (1988) Suppression of macrophage function and increased lethality to bacterial infection in mice given morphine pellet implants. FASEB J 2:A1260
25. Peritt D, Jerrells TR, Holaday JW, Bryant HU (1988) Suppression of interleukin-2 production with chronic morphine treatment. FASEB J 2:A485
26. Weber RJ, Ikejiri B, Rice KC, Pert A, Hagan AA (1987) Opiate receptor-mediated regulation of the immune response in vivo. In: Problems of drug dependence. Proceedings of the 48th Annual Scientific Meeting, the Committee on Problems of Drug Dependence, NIDA Res Monogr 76:341-350
27. Bryant HU, Bernton EW, Holaday JW (1988) Morphine-induced immunosuppression: Involvement of glucocorticoids and prolactin. In: Problems of drug dependence. Proceedings of the 50th Annual Scientific Meeting, the Committee on the Problems of Drug Dependence, NIDA Res Monogr (in press)
28. Bernton EW, Bryant HU, Woldeyesus J, Holaday JW (1988) Suppression of lymphocyte and adrenal cortical function by corticosterone: In vivo antagonism by prolactin. Pharmacologist (in press)
29. Luger A, Graf H, Schwartz H-P, Stummvoll H-K, Luger TA (1986) Decreased serum interleukin 1 activity and monocyte interleukin 1 production in patients with fatal sepsis. Crit Care Med 14:458-461
30. Meltzer MS, Nacy CA (1987) Cell-cell interactions during inflammation: The role of the macrophage. In: Cerra FB, Shoemaker WC (eds) Critical care state-of-the-art, vol 8. Society of Critical Care Med, Fullerton CA, pp 119-132
31. Bernton E, Beach J, Holaday JW, Smallridge R, Fein H (1987) Release of multiple hormones by a direct action of interleukin-l on pituitary cells. Science 238:519-521
32. Beach JE, Smallridge RC, Kinzer CA, Bernton EW, Holaday JW, Fein HG (1989) Interleukin-1 releases multiple hormones from perifused rat pituitaries. Life Sci 44:1-8
33. Berkenbosch F, van Oert J, Del Ray A, Tilders F, Besedovsky H (1987) CRF-producing neurons in the rat are activated by interleukin-1. Science 238:524-526
34. Breder C, Dinarello C, Saper C (1988) Interleukin-1 immunoreactive innervation of the human hypothalamus. Science 240:321-323
35. Tracey DE, Webster EL, Grigoriadis DE, De Souza EB (1988) Corticotropin-releasing factor (CRF) and interleukin-1 (IL-1) receptors in the brain/pituitary/immune axis. Abstracts, American College of Neuropsychopharmacology, 27th ann meeting. San Juan, PR
36. Bunner D, Morris E, Smallridge C (1984) Circadian growth hormone and prolactin blood concentrations during selflimited viral infection in man. Metabolism 4:337-346
37. Kohler P, O'Malley B, Rayford P, Lipsett M, Odell W (1967) Effect of pyrogen on blood levels of pituitary trophic hormones. Observations of the usefulness of the growth hormone response in the detection of pituitary disease. J Clin Endocrinol Metab 27:219-225
38. Meltzer MS, Gendelman HE (1988) Effects of colony stimulating factors on the interaction of monocytes and the human immunodeficiency virus. Immunol Letters 19:193-198
39. Bryant HU, Holaday JW, Gendelman HE, Meltzer MS, Bernton EW (1989) Neuronotrophic effects of granulocyte and macrophage colony-stimulating factors. In: Hendrie HC et al (eds) Neuronal control of bodily function (in press)
40. Rettori V, Jurcovicova J, McCann SM (1987) Central action of interleukin-1 in altering the release of TSH, growth hormone and prolactin in the male rat. J Neurosci Res 18:179-183
41. Dubuis JM, Dayer JM, Siegris-Kaiser CA, Burger AG (1988) Human recombinant interleukin-1 beta decreases plasma thyroid hormone and thyroid-stimulating hormone levels in rats. Endocrinol 123:2175-2181
42. Dasta JF, Armstrong DK, Reilley TE, Frolicher DA, Tallman RD (1985) A re-evaluation of haloperidol's reported antagonism of dopamine-induced renal vasodilation. Crit Care Med 13:348
43. Rao MR, Bartke A, Parkening TA, Collins TJ (1984) Effect of treatment with different doses of bromocryptine on plasma profiles of gonadotrophins, prolactin and testosterone in mature male rats and mice. Int J Andrology 7:258-268
44. Palestine AG, Nussenblatt RB (1988) The effect of bromocriptine on anterior uveitis. Am J Ophtalmol 104(4):488-489

Chemical Pathobiology of CNS Trauma

A. I. Faden and R. Vink

Introduction

Mechanisms by which traumatic brain injury (TBI) or traumatic spinal cord injury (TSCI) lead to irreversible tissue damage remain speculative. In addition to the direct mechanical damage produced by trauma, there is also a more delayed form of injury resulting from release of various autodestructive biochemical substance [1, 2]; these may contribute to secondary tissue damage through effects on cerebral blood flow, cerebral metabolism, and/or through disruption of cellular membranes. Potentially important biochemical factors include changes in tissue cations (particularly calcium and magnesium), and release of such substances as endogenous opioids, excitotoxins, free radicals, eicosanoids, and biogenic amines, among others. Of potential clinical relevance is the fact that many of these delayed biochemical changes can be modified by administration of specific pharmacological agents, with limitation of secondary injury and tissue damage, leading to improved behavioral outcome [3].

Magnetic resonance spectroscopy (MRS) and microdialysis represent techniques that have recently been applied to delineate the temporal profile and magnitude of various biochemical and metabolic changes after CNS trauma, as well as to assess the effects of potential drug therapies. Such studies, as well as more classical biochemical assays, suggest that secondary biochemical injury after CNS trauma is a multifactorial process, which includes changes in tissue cations, hydrolysis of membrane lipids with generation of free radicals and eicosanoids, and release of endogenous opioids and excitotoxins. A variety of experimental pharmacotherapies, including opiate-receptor antagonists, excitotoxin antagonists, thyrotropin-releasing hormone (TRH) analogs, inhibitors of arachidonate metabolism, free radical scavengers, and magnesium supplementation are all capable of limiting tissue damage and improving neurological recovery following experimental CNS trauma [3].

Magnetic Resonance Spectroscopy (MRS) Studies

^{31}P MRS permits the non-invasive evaluation of changes in high energy phosphates, intracellular pH and intracellular free magnesium. Vink et al. showed that traumatic brain injury causes rapid changes in ^{31}P spectra that are related to severity of injury [4]. Following fluid-percussion induced TBI in rats, they observed a fall in intracellular pH (from 7.09±0.07 at baseline, to 6.88±0.09 at 40 min postinjury), which occurred in animals subjected to moderate (1.5–2.2 atmospheres [atm]) and high (2.5–3.3 atm) but not low level (0.1–1.2 atm) injury; intracellular pH returned to baseline by 90 min postinjury. Transient elevations in brain lactate level (shown using ^1H MRS) were observed that temporally paralleled the pH changes and were significantly correlated with them for all injury levels [5]. With moderate levels of injury, the ratio of phosphocreatine to inorganic phosphate (PCr/Pi) showed a biphasic decline: the first occurred at 40 min with recovery by 100 min; the second decline occurred by 2 h and persisted for the remaining 6 h observation period. The first but not the second decrease in PCr/Pi was associated with tissue acidosis. With moderate injury no changes in ATP occurred at any time during the injury observation period of 8 h. These findings indicate altered mitochondrial energy production following brain injury that any account, in part, for the reduced capacity of the cell to recovery from traumatic injury. Alterations in ATP occurred only in the most several injured animals, and such changes were associated with marked tissue acidosis and a 100% mortality rate. At 4 h posttrauma the PCr/Pi ratio correlated linearly with the severity of injury.

^{31}P MRS also showed that traumatic brain injury was associated with a severe depletion of free intracellular magnesium, which was proportional to injury severity [6, 7]. This was associated with a less profound, but nonetheless significant, decline in total tissue magnesium. Changes in magnesium were associated with marked calculated changes in cellular bioenergetic state, including shifts in the equilibrium constants of the creatine-kinase, adenylate kinase, and ATPase reactions resulting in alterations of [ADP], [AMP], cytosolic phosphorylation potential, free energy of ATP hydrolysis, and energy charge [8]. Alterations in cytosolic phosphorylation potential following trauma were linearly correlated with changes in intracellular free magnesium concentration. Moreover, there was an association between cytosolic phosphorylation potential and reversibility of injury. Taken together, these results suggest that reductions in cellular bioenergetic state following traumatic brain injury occur through a posttraumatic decrease in the cell's capacity for oxidative phosphorylation, which itself may be directly related to the intracellular free magnesium concentration change [8].

Application of ^{31}P MRS to experimental spinal cord injury has revealed certain similarities to TBI but also notable differences. At very low levels of impact trauma in rabbits, there is a substantial decline in intracellular free magnesium, followed by a delayed loss of ATP and tissue acidosis [9]. After moderate or severe injury, there is rapid loss of ATP and tissue acidosis, associated with lactate accumulation [10]. PCr/Pi progressively declines over a 3–4-h period posttrauma [11].

Taken together, MRS studies of TBI and TSCI clearly demonstrate the development of delayed biochemical and metabolic changes that are associated with irreversible tissue damage. They also reveal a profound alteration in intracellular magnesium levels, which may partially underlie changes in cellular bioenergetic state and subsequent cell death.

Microdialysis Methods

Microdialysis thechniques are still in early development. Depending upon the characteristics of specific probes, this technique can be utilized to repeatedly monitor changes in extracellular fluid chemistry in relation to a specific CNS insult [12]. Early application has been to monitor changes in biogenic amines, ascorbate, cations and amino acids. Although the technique is invasive and the probe itself does cause damage, it can be effectively used to measure and correlate posttraumatic changes over time in the same animal. For example, we have found marked increases in the excitatory amino acids glutamate and asparate within the extracellular space after both experimental TBI and TSCI; changes are maximal by 10 minutes posttrauma and are related to injury severity (unpublished observation). Another group has reported preliminary findings in TBI that show similar changes [13].

Biochemical Pathobiology

Endogenous Opioids

The endogenous opioid dynorphin has been found to increase at the trauma site after experimental TSCI in cats; levels were significantly correlated to injury severity whereas changes in other opioids such as β-endorphin and leucine-enkephalin were not related to degree of trauma [14].

That dynorphin may contribute to secondary injury after TSCI is indicated by a recent study showing that treatment with specific antibodies to dynorphin, but not antibodies to leucine-enkephalin, limit posttraumatic neurological deficits [15].

Dynorphin is an endogenous ligand for the kappa opiata receptor [16]. A variety of opiate receptor antagonists have been shown to limit pathophysiological consequences of TSCI, with beneficial effects on blood flow, somatosensory-evoked responses, histopathology and neurological outcome [17–20]. Recent experiments utilizing kappa-active or kappa-selective opiate antagonists suggest that the kappa receptor does mediate certain of the pathophysiological consequences of TSCI [21, 22].

Following traumatic brain injury in cats, there is also accumulation of dynorphin A-immunoreactivity but not leucine-enkephalin-like immunoreactivity in injury regions [23]. The dynorphin increases occur predominantly in those areas showing significant decrease in regional cerebral blood flow [23]. Similarly, following severe fluid-percussion-induced brain trauma in rats, but not at low levels of injury, there is a significant increase in dynorphin levels (but not leucine-enkephalin or β-endorphin) in the striatum, frontal cortex, parietal cortex, pons, and medulla (unpublished observations). Pathological damage to brain tissue after injury is most pronounced in those regions showing significant increases in dynorphin levels [23]. Taken together, these results indicate that dynorphin but not leucine-enkephalin or β-endorphin-like immunoreactivity may accumulate at injury sites following traumatic brain injury, suggesting a potential role for dynorphin ligand in the injury process.

Fatty Acids and Eicosanoids

Traumatic injury to the spinal cord results in the activation of phospholipases with the subsequent release of free fatty acids (FFA), including arachidonic acid [24]. Polyunsaturated fatty acids (including arachidonic acid) produce tissue edema and inhibit membrane-dependent enzymes such as (Na^+, K^+)-ATPase [25]. Arachidonic acid may produce its detrimental effects either through direct disruption of cell membranes of through actions of certain eicosanoid metabolites including prostaglandins, thromboxanes, and leukotrienes [24]. Thromboxanes and the peptide-leukotrienes are potent vasoconstrictor agents that have been implicates in secondary brain ischemia [26]. Large increases in arachidonic acid are found within minutes following experimental traumatic spinal cord injury [24]; a later release of arachidonic acid also occurs that is associated with spinal cord edema and inhibition of (Na^+, K^+)-ATPase at 24 h following injury [27]. Several groups have demonstrated accumulation of cyclooxygenase products (i.e., thromboxanes and prostaglandins) of arachidonic acid metabolism in spinal cord following experimental traumatic injury [24, 28–30]. Although lipoxygenase products of arachidonic acid metabolism (e.g., leukotrienes) have been found to increase after experimental brain ischemia and trauma [31], there has been only one report of an increase in the lipoxygenase product leukotriene C_4 after experimental spinal cord injury [32]. Hallenbeck et al. demonstrated that combination therapy with indomethacin (a cyclooxygenase inhibitor to block thromboxane), prostacyclin (the vasodilator prostaglandin I_2), and heparin significantly improved outcome following traumatic cervical spinal cord injury in cats [33]. Hall and Wolf have found that pretreatment with cyclooxygenase inhibitors or a combinatin of thromboxane synthetase inhibitor and a stable prostacyclin analog limits the posttraumatic decline in spinal cord blood flow in cats [34]. We have recently shown that the mixed cyclooxygenase-lipoxygenase inhibitor BW-755C improves outcome after TSCI in rats [35].

Traumatic brain injury in rats is associated with small increases in FFA levels at 10 min and 4 h posttrauma and much larger increases at 24 h. Amongst the FFA, the largest increases were observed in stearate, arachidonate, and docosahexaenoate [38]. Thromboxane levels are markedly elevated (30-fold) at 10 min after injury with substantial reductions by 4 h and with return to near baseline levels by 24 h [36]. These results are consistent with the hypothesis that changes in lipid metabolism occur after injury and may, through the effects of their metabolites, contribute to secondary damage. The relative role of specific lipoxygenase or cyclooxygenase pathways of arachidonic acid metabolism in secondary injury remains to be established.

Free Radicals

Traumatic spinal cord injury causes early central hemorrhagic necrosis in spinal cord gray matter. Such hemorrhagic change may act as a catalyst for the generation of toxic free radicals [37]. Free radicals may contribute to the pathophysiology of secondary spinal cord injury in several ways; through lipid peroxidation of membrane phospholipids, with subsequent effects on lipid-dependent enzymes such as (Na^+, K^+)-ATPase [37, 38], and possibly through the activation of lipoxygenase. There is experimental evidence in traumatic spinal cord injury [34, 37] that prophylactic treatment with antioxidants may limit secondary injury. Recently, 21-aminosteroids, which are potent inhibitors of lipid peroxidation, have been shown to limit neurological dysfunction after TSCI, even when administered after trauma [39].

Cations

Following spinal cord injury, there appears to be a rapid and profound decrease in extracellular calcium, presumably resulting from the movement of calcium intracellularly [40, 41]. These increases in intracellular calcium are toxic to cells and may be a final common mechanism of cell death following injury to the CNS [42].

Perhaps surprisingly, calcium channel antagonists have not proved beneficial in improving neurologic outcome following spinal trauma [43, 44] or ischemia [45, 46]. Faden et al. found that nimodipine, at doses that had proved effective in the treatment of experimental cerebral ischemia, failed to improve outcome following ischemic spinal cord injury in rabbits, whether the drug was administered before or after the induction of ischemia; indeed, there was a trend toward worsened outcome following such treatment [45]. A similar observation has been made by Cheng et al. using verapamil in a related spinal cord ischemia model [46]. Ford and Malm found no beneficial effects for nimodipine following traumatic spinal cord injury in cats [44]. The lack of beneficial effects on neurological outcome with calcium channel antagonists in experimental spinal cord injury might relate to the time of treatment, drug dosage used, or treatment induced hypotension.

Tissue levels of sodium increase and potassium levels decrease after TSCI [47, 48] but these changes do not appear to be highly correlated with injury severity, suggesting that these changes may not critically relate to secondary injury [49].

Intracellular free magnesium levels and total tissue levels of magnesium decrease after TBI and TSCI in relation to injury severity [6, 7, 9, 50]. That such changes may critically relate to secondary injury is suggested by several findings. Animals made magnesium-deficient through dietary restriction show worsened outcome after TBI [51] and enhanced lipid membrane breakdown after TSCI (unpublished finding). Moreover, magnesium supplementation attenuates posttraumatic neurological deficits after TBI [52]. Finally, treatments that improve outcome after TBI are associated with significant recovery of intracellular free magnesium and/or total tissue magnesium levels [53, 54].

Excitotoxins

Recent studies suggest the hypothesis that excitatory amino acids are released after CNS trauma and contribute to delayed injury through actions at N-methyl-

D-aspartate (NMDA) receptors [54, 55]. As indicated in the Microdialysis Section, glutamate and aspartate levels in the extracellular increases in excitatory amino acids after TSCI have also been found utilizing ^{1}H MRS in rabbits (unpublished observation). Changes in glutamate and aspartate levels in tissue are also correlated to injury severity after TSCI and TBI. NMDA administered intrathecally exacerbates TSCI in rats, whereas the stereoisomer NMLA, which is less active at NMDA receptors, does not affect injury severity [56]. A variety of competitive and non-competitive NMDA antagonists have now been found to limit neurological, histological and/or biochemical changes after CNS trauma; these include MK-801, dextrorphan and CPP [55, 56]. The mechanism by which these excitotoxins may produce injury remains speculative, although changes in sodium, calcium and magnesium have been implicated.

Other Factors

A variety of other biochemical changes occur after CNS trauma that may contribute to secondary injury [3]; these include among others: acetylcholine, biogenic amines, kinins and proteases. Considerable experimental work is required to clarify the interactions of these and other biochemical changes and the mechanisms by which such factors, singly or in combination, contribute to delayed tissue damage after CNS trauma.

References

1. Siesjo BK, Wieloch T (1985) In: Becker DP, Povlishock (eds) Central nervous system trauma status report. NIH Publications. NINCDS, Bethesda, MD pp 513–532
2. Faden AI (1983) Recent pharmacological advances in experimental spinal injury: theoretical and methodological considerations. Trends Neurosci 6:375–377
3. Faden AI (1987) Pharmacotherapy in spinal cord injury: A critical review of recent developments. Clin Neuropharmacol 10 (3):195–201
4. Vink R, McIntosh TK, Weiner MW, Faden AI (1987) Effects of traumatic brain injury on cerebral high-energy phosphates and pH: A ^{31}P NMR study. J Cereb Blood Flow Metab 7:563–571
5. Vink R, McIntosh TK, Yamakami I, Faden AI (1988) ^{31}P NMR characterization of graded traumatic brain injury in rats. Magn Res Med 6:37–48
6. Vink R, McIntosh TK, Demediuk P, Faden AI (1987) Decrease in total and free magnesium concentration following traumatic brain injury in rats. Biochem Biophys Res Commun 149:594–599
7. Vink R, McIntosh TK, Demediuk P, Weiner M, Faden AI (1988) Decline in intracellular free Mg^{2+} may lead to irreversible tissue damage following brain injury. J Biol Chem 15:757–761
8. Vink R, Faden AI, McIntosh TK (1989) Changes in cellular bioenergetic state following graded traumatic brain injury in rats: determination by ^{21}Phosphorus NMR. J Neurotrauma (in press)
9. Vink R, Yum SW, Lemke M, Demediuk P, Faden AI: Traumatic spinal cord injury in rabbits decreases intracellular free magnesium concentration as measured by ^{31}P MRS. (Submitted)
10. Vink R, Knobloch SM, Faden AI (1987) ^{31}P magnetic resonance spectroscopy of traumatic spinal injury. Magn Res Med 5:390–394

11. Vink R, Noble LJ, Knoblach SM, Bendall MR, Faden AI (1989) Metabolic changes in rabbit spinal cord after trauma: NMR spectroscopy studies. Ann Neurol (in press)
12. Ungerstedt B (1984) In: Marsden GA (ed) Measurement of neutrotransmitter release in vivo. Wiley, Chichester, pp 81–105
13. Katayama Y, Cheng MK, Gorman L, Tamura T, Becker DP (1988) Increase in extracellular glutamate and associated massive ion fluxes following concussive brain injury. Soc Neurosci Abstr 14:1154
14. Faden AI, Molineaux CJ, Rosenberger JG, Jacobs TP, Cox BM (1985) Endogenous opioid immunoreactivity in rat spinal cord following traumatic injury. Ann Neurol 17:386–390
15. Faden AI (1988) Role of dynorphin and k-opiate receptors in the pathophysiology of secondary spinal cord injury. Neurology 38 (Suppl): 158
16. Cox BM (1982) Endogenous opioid peptides: a guide to structures and terminology. Life Sci 31:1645–1658
17. Faden AI, Jacobs TP, Holaday JW (1980) Endorphin-parasympathetic interaction in spinal shock. J Auton Nerv Syst 2:295–304
18. Young W, Flamm ES, Demopoulos HB, Tomasula JJ, DeCrescito V (1981) Naloxone ameliorates posttraumatic ischemia in experimental spinal contusion. J Neurosurg 55:209–219
19. Inoue Y (1986) Evoked spinal potentials in the Wistar rat: Effect of cord compression and drugs. J Japan Orthop Assoc 60:777–785
20. Arias MJ (1985) Effect of naloxone on functional recovery after experimental spinal cord injury in the rat. Surg Neurol 23:440–442
21. Faden AI, Sacksen I, Noble LJ (1988) Opiate-receptor antagonist nalmefene improves neurological recovery after traumatic spinal cord injury in rats. J Pharmac Exp Ther 245:742–748
22. Faden AI, Takemori AE, Portoghese TS (1987) k-selective opiate antagonist nor-binaltorphimine improves outcome after traumatic spinal cord injury in rats. CNS Trauma 4:227–237
23. McIntosh TK, Hayes RC, DeWitt DS, Augra V, Faden AI (1987) Endogenous opioids may mediate secondary damage after experimental brain injury. Am J Physiol 253:E565–E574
24. Demediuk P, Saunders RD, Clendenon NR, Means ED, Anderson DK, Horrocks LA (1985) Changes in lipid metabolism in traumatized spinal cord. Prog Brain Res 63:1–16
25. Chan PH, Fishman RA (1984) The role of arachidonic acid in vasogenic brain edema. Fed Proc 43:210–213
26. Chen ST, Hsu CY, Hogan EL, Halushka PV, Linet OI, Yatsu FM (1986) Thromboxane, prostacyclin, and leukotrienes in cerebral ischemia. Neurology 36:466–470
27. Faden AI, Chan PH, Longar S (1987) Alterations in lipid metabolism, Na^+, K^+-ATPase activity, and tissues water content of spinal cord following experimental traumatic injury. J Neurochem 48:1809–1816
28. Hsu CY, Halushka PV, Hogan EL, Banik NL, Lee WA, Perot LP (1985) Alteration of thromboxane and prostacyclin levels in experimental spinal cord injury. Neurology 35:1003–1009
29. Jacobs TP, Feuerstein GZ, Faden AI (1985) Thromboxane of prostacyclin ratio changes following experimental spinal cord trauma in the rabbit. Neurosci Abstr 11:4
30. Demediuk P, Faden AI (1988) Traumatic spinal cord injury in rats causes increases in tissue thromboxane but not peptidoleukotrines. J Neurosci Res 20:115–121
31. Kiwak KJ, Moskowitz MA, Levine L (1985) Leukotriene production in gerbil brain after ischemic insult, subarachnoid hemorrhage, and concussive injury. J Neurosurg 62:865–869
32. Saunders RD, Dugan LL, Demediuk P, Means ED, Horrocks LA, Anderson DK (1987) Effects of methylprednisolone and the combination of α-tocopherol and selenium on arachidonic acid metabolism and lipid peroxidation in traumatized spinal cord tissue. J Neurochem 49:24–31
33. Hellenbeck JM, Jacobs TP, Faden AI (1983) Combined PGI_2 indomethacin, and heparin improves neurological recovery after spinal trauma in cats. J Neurosurg 58:749–754
34. Hall ED, Wolf DL (1986) A pharmacological analysis of the pathophysiological mechanisms of posttraumatic spinal cord ischemia. J Neurosurg 64:951–961
35. Faden AI, Lemke M, Demediuk P (1988) Effects of BW755C, a mixed cyclo-oxygenase-lipoxygenase inhibitor, following traumatic spinal cord injury in rats. Brain Res 463:63–68

36. Demediuk P, Faden AI, Romhanyi R, Vink R, McIntosh TK (1988) Traumatic brain injury in the rat: Effects on lipid metabolism, tissue magnesium and water content. J Neurotrauma (in press)
37. Anderson DK, Means ED (1984) Lipid peroxidation in spinal cord: $FeCl_2$ induction and protection with antioxidants. Neurochem Path 1:249-264
38. Demopoulos HB, Flamm ES, Pietronigro DD, et al (1980) The free radical pathology and the microcirculation in the major central nervous system disorders. Acta Physiol Scand [Suppl] 492:91-119
39. Hall ED, McCall JM, Chase RL, Yonkers PA, Braughler JM (1987) A nonglucocorticoid steroid analog of methylprednisolone duplicates its high dose pharmacology in models of central nervous system trauma and neuronal membrane damage. J Pharmacol Exp Ther 242:137-142
40. Stokes BT, Fox P, Hollinden G (1983) Extracellular calcium activity in the injured spinal cord. Exp Neurol 80:561-572
41. Young W, Flamm ES (1982) Effect of high-dose corticosteroid therapy on blood flow, evoked potentials and extracellular calcium in experimental spinal injury. J Neurosurg 57:667-673
42. Harris RJ, Branston NM, Symon L, Bayhan M, Watson A (1982) The effects of a calcium antagonist, nimodipine, upon physiological responses of the cerebral vasculative and its possible influence upon focal cerebral ischemia. Stroke 13:759-766
43. Faden AI, Jacobs TP (1984) Nimodipine in experimental ischemia. J Neurosurg 61:802-803
44. Ford WJ, Malm DN (1985) Failure of nimodipine to reverse acute experimental spinal cord injury. CNS-Trauma 2:9-17
45. Faden AI, Jacobs TP, Smith MT (1984) Evaluation of the calcium channel antagonist nimodipine in experimental spinal cord ischemia. J Neurosurg 60:796-799
46. Cheng MK, Robertson C, Grossman RG, et al (1984) Neurological outcome correlated with spinal evoked potentials in a spinal cord ischemia model. J Neurosurg 60:786-795
47. Beranek R, Fantis A, Kunc Z (1952) Posttraumatic spinal cord oedema. Cs Fysiol 1:51-54
48. Lewin MG, Hansehout RH, Pappius HM (1974) Chemical characteristics of traumatic spinal cord edema in cats. J Neurosurg 40:65-75
49. Demediuk P, Lemke M, Faden AI (1989) Spinal cord edema and changes in tissue content of sodium, potassium, and magnesium following impact trauma in rats. Proceedings of the Sixth International Symposium on Brain Edema (in press)
50. Lemke M, Demediuk P, McIntosh TK, Vink R, Faden AI (1987) Alterations in tissue Mg^{2+}, Na^{+} and spinal cord edema following impact trauma in rats. Biochem Biophys Res Commun 147:1170-1175
51. McIntosh TK, Faden AI, Yamakami I, Vink R (1988) Magnesium deficiency exacerbates and pretreatment improves outcome following traumatic brain injury in rats: ^{31}P magnetic resonance spectroscopy and behavioral studies. J Neurotrauma 5:17-31
52. McIntosh TK, Vink R, Yamakami I, Faden AI: $MgCl_2$ but not ATP-$MgCl_2$ protects against neurological deficit after brain injury. Brain Res
53. Vink R, McIntosh TK, Faden AI (1988) Treatment with the thyroptrophin-releasing hormone analog CG3703 restores magnesium homeostasis following traumatic brain injury in rats. Brain Res 460:184-188
54. Faden AI, Lemke M, Simon RP, Noble J (1988) N-methyl-D-aspartate antagonist MK-801 improves outcome following traumatic spinal cord injury in rats: behavioral, anatomical, and neurochemical studies. J Neurotrauma 5:27-37
55. Faden AI, Simon RP (1988) A potential role for excitotoxins in the pathophysiology of spinal cord injury. Ann Neurol 23:623-626
56. Demediuk P, Faden AI (1988) Excitatory amino acids in experimental spinal cord trauma: injury-induced changes in total tissue levels and pharmacological intervention with the competitive antagonist CPP. Soc Neurosci (Abstr) 14:419

Pathophysiology and Treatment of Stroke

M. D. Ginsberg

Introduction

A truly comprehensive exegesis of stroke pathophysiology and therapy would require an entire monograph. Indeed, several clinically oriented volumes are available, which can be strongly recommended [1, 2]. The goal of the present chapter, which of necessity must be more modest, will be to focus upon the topic of completed stroke of ischemic origin and to emphasize primarily

a) recent advances in our understanding of how ischemia results in tissue injury and
b) emerging therapeutic strategies directed at intervention in these pathomechanisms.

Some Basic Observations Regarding Cerebral Vulnerability

It is common knowledge that the brain is an abundantly nourished organ with a high and incessant level of metabolic activity, receiving approximately 15% of the body's cardiac output and accounting for 20% of the body's oxygen consumption [3]. Further, its sole normal substrate is glucose, which must be delivered to it continuously if it is to function normally. These factors help to determine the brain's unique vulnerability to injury in ischemia, hypoglycemia, and hypoxia.

Central to the issue of ischemic injury is the notion of tissue thresholds, which have become well defined through experimental investigations [4, 5]. As cerebral blood flow is reduced progressively from normal levels, evidence of incipient tissue energy failure may be observed at cerebral blood flow (CBF) levels approximately 45% of normal [6], but more severe reductions, to approximately 35–40% of normal, are required to suppress brain electrical function and produce failure of evoked responses [5]. At still lower CBF levels, electrical failure is complete and intracellular potassium ion is massively released into the brain's extracellular space, to levels that may exceed 50 mM. Unless circulation is promptly restored, the tissue proceeds inexorably to cell death. Other workers have emphasized the time-dependence of ischemic thresholds: CBF levels of 0.14 ml/gm/min or less, for example, lead to cell death by 45 min, whereas higher levels of residual blood flow necessitate longer times to produce cerebral injury [7].

Positron-emission tomographic studies have helped to define metabolism-blood flow interrelationships during hemodynamic compromise of the brain. In a series of patients with unilateral or bilateral carotid artery occlusions, elevations of local cerebral blood volume were commonly observed, signifying vasodilatation in response to diminished cerebral perfusion. Reductions of the cerebral blood flow/cerebral blood volume (CBF/CBV) ratio were found to be a sensitive index of compromised "perfusion reserve" [8]. Elevations of the oxygen extraction fraction (OER) denote the brain's attempt to maintain normal cerebral oxygen consumption in the face of diminished perfusion. Once ischemic stroke has occurred, the normally coupled relationship between cerebral blood flow and cerebral oxygen utilization is disturbed. Early in an ischemic stroke (approximately the first four days), local CBF may be decreased but OER elevated - the condition of so-called "misery perfusion" - an attempt of the affected tissue to continue to metabolize in the face of restricted oxygen supply [9]. Alternatively, OER may be decreased, signifying "luxury perfusion" in relation to the metabolic needs of the tissue. In patients studied later in their course, however, both CBF and oxygen utilization ($CMRO_2$) tend to be focally reduced and OER typically low [10]. Local $CMRO_2$ levels greater than 1.25 ml/100 g/min tend to be observed in patients with good clinical outcome, whereas $CMRO_2$ levels less than 1.25 ml/100 g/min tend to be associated with a poor outcome in most patients [11]. Baron has stated this $CMRO_2$ threshold to be approximately 1.6 ml/100 g/min [9].

PET has also provided solid evidence for remote metabolic depression in the form of "crossed cerebellar diaschisis" contralateral to a hemispheral infarct [12].

Overview of Traditional Management of Completed Ischemic Stroke

General management principles have been well summarized in clinical texts [1]:

a) The airway must be kept patent and ventilation properly maintained.
b) Proper blood pressure should be maintained, and overzealous reductions of blood pressure in hypertensive patients with acute ischemic stroke should be avoided.
c) Hypoglycemia should be excluded.
d) Seizures should be treated promptly.
e) Sources of underlying fever should be identified and treated.
f) Electrolyte and water imbalances should be attended to.
g) Deep venous thrombosis and consequent pulmonary embolism should be prevented by frequent turning, use of support-stockins, and early mobilization from bed; low-dose heparin therapy is often employed. Other systemic complications should be quickly identified; pneumonia, urinary tract infections, decubitus ulcers, underlying myocardial infarction, heart failure, or arrhythmia, and coexistent failure of other organ systems.

More specific traditional therapeutic measures depend upon the etiology of the underlying stroke.

Thus, anticoagulation is employed

a) in cases of embolic stroke, not in order to treat the stroke itself but to prevent recurrent embolization; and
b) in stroke-in-evolution, when intracranial hemorrhage has been excluded and progressing vascular occlusion is suspected, in an effort to abort this progression [13].

The efficacy of the latter, however, has not been well established. Cerebral edema is infrequently of serious clinical concern in ischemic stroke but may occasionally dominate the clinical picture in large hemispheric infarctions and may give rise to transtentorial herniation; it must be aggressively managed but is often rather refractory to treatment [14]. No consistent benefit has been shown to result from the use of corticosteroids in ischemic stroke.

Several forms of therapy have shown initial promise in at least certain experimental studies, yet have not proven beneficial in the clinical setting. These include barbiturate therapy; prostacyclin therapy [15]; and the use of pentoxyfilline [16]. Recent trials of hemodilution in acute stroke have also shown a lack of benefit [17]. Vasodilator therapy may be associated with an "intracerebral steal", i.e., a shunting of blood flow away from ischemic tissue into the normal cerebrovascular bed, and is therefore not recommended.

Molecular Pathophysiology: Role of Calcium Ion

A rather large body of experimental literature has tended to implicate increases in intracellular cytosolic calcium ion as central to the pathophysiology of ischemic brain injury [18, 19]. The critical facts are that ionized calcium functions as a ubiquitous intracellular messenger and regulator, and is held at intracellular levels approximately one ten-thousandth of those of the extracellular space by energy-requiring ionic pumps as well as by intracellular binding and complexing [20]. As CBF falls in the ischemic brain to approximately 10 ml/100 g/min, extracellular calcium ion declines precipitously, presumably owing to its intracellular entry [21]. A putative scenario has been put forth [18, 22], according to which, with the onset of ischemia, energy failure and the decline in cell membrane potential favor the intracellular entry of calcium ion via voltage-dependent channels, as well as the release of calcium from storage sites in mitochondrial and endoplasmic reticulum. Increased cytosolic calcium ion activates phospholipases, with a consequent breakdown of membrane lipids and the release of free fatty acids, whose subsequent metabolism may be deleterious to cell function. Indeed, at sites of intracellular injury, tissue calcium deposition is common [23].

A Therapeutic Question: Is There a Role for Calcium Channel Blockers in Ischemia?

Considerable effort has been expended to evaluate whether pharmacologic agents which block the entry of calcium ion through voltage-dependent channels might confer neuroprotection in cerebral ischemia. Many calcium channel blockers are known to be potent vasodilators of the normal cerebral circulation. The dihydropyridines, which have been particularly well studied, produce marked increases in CBF without affecting cerebral oxygen or glucose metabolism [24, 25], suggesting the possibility that any anti-ischemic efficacy of these agents might occur in part via hemodynamic mechanisms. In experimental studies of temporary global ischemia, impressive partial amelioration of postischemic hypoperfusion has been shown with pre-ischemic or early postischemic administration of the dihydropyridine nomodipine, but without improvement of postischemic hypometabolism [26, 27]. Nonetheless, improvement of clinical outcome following global ischemia has been only inconsistently observed. A benefit has been shown with preischemic nimodipine therapy [26], but improvement is only equivocal if therapy is delayed to the early postischemic period [27, 28]. Nicardipine has been shown to confer impressive histological protection if therapy is begun prior to ischemia [29].

Other classes of calcium channel blockers have also shown limited success in experimental studies. In one investigation, flunarizine administered either pre- or postischemia led to large reductions in histological injury in both hippocampus and basal ganglia without affecting CBF [30]. However, still other studies of flunarizine, lidoflazine and verapamil have yielded negative results.

Numerous studies of the calcium channel blockers in *focal* ischemia have also been carried out. When nimodipine was assessed in a rat model of MCA occlusion, the extent of infarction was mildly reduced when therapy was begun prior to ischemia [31] but not if delayed until five minutes following vascular occlusion [32]. In other laboratories, positive results were reported with postischemic therapy, but these could not be subsequently confirmed.

Clinical Studies of Calcium Channel Blockers in Brain Ischemia

A recent randomized double-blinded trial in patients with acute ischemic stroke assessed oral nimodipine (120 mg/day for 4 weeks) when added to a "standard" regimen consisting of low-molecular weight dextran and subcutaneous heparin. The nimodipine-treated group showed a nearly 60% reduction of mortality at 4 weeks though this appeared attributable to reductions in systemic, non-neurologic causes; a beneficial effect of therapy was seen on neurological clinical score of patients having an intermediate range of neurological disability [33].

Promising Results with a Calcium Channel Blocker – Serotonin Antagonist

We have recently achieved a remarkable reduction of infarct volume in rats treated the novel phenylalkylamine-class calcium channel blocker (S)-emopamil [34]. Treated rats exhibited a 50–60% reduction of cortical infarct volume compared to controls, when treatment was either initiated prior to ischemia or was deferred up to 1 hour following permanent MCA occlusion [34]. Interestingly, this agent differs from its congener verapamil

a) in exhibiting extraordinarily high blood-brain barrier penetrability,
b) in being a potent serotonin S_2 antagonist.

Since the efficacy of this agent in focal ischemia far exceeds that of conventional calcium channel blockers, we suspect that these latter properties may be crucial to its efficacy.

Neurotransmitter Mediation of Ischemic Neuronal Injury

Accumulating observations now offer convincing evidence that excitatory neurotransmitters may serve as key mediators of ischemic brain injury. As a result, a new arena of therapeutics is emerging. Early observations suggested that the excitatory neurotransmitters glutamate and aspartate had the potential of being neurotoxic, and more recent data suggest an injurious role not only in ischemia but in diverse neurological conditions such as Huntington's disease and brain injury from epilepsy [35]. Of the three receptor subtypes mediating the action of the excitatory amino acids glutamate and aspartate, particular attention has focused on the *N*-methyl-D-aspartate (NMDA) receptor-subtype, whose associated ion-channel is unique in that it is permeable to both sodium and calcium ions, and its current is both agonist- and voltage-dependent and relatively long-lived. NMDA-mediated synaptic transmission is thought to be involved in long-term potentiation and synaptic plasticity [36].

The concept of exitotoxicity in brain ischemia has ben extensively reviewed [37]. Rothman [38] provided relevant early observations in cultured hippocampal neurons that mature but not immature, undifferentiated cells became injured when exposed to anoxia or cyanide, and that magnesium treatment prevented this injury; these data suggested that the damage was mediated by synaptic activity. A non-specific excitatory amino acid antagonist protected both against anoxia- and glutamate-induced cytotoxicity [39]. Kirino observed in both the gerbil and the rat that CAl pyramidal neurons of the hippocampus underwent *delayed* cell death following short periods of ischemia, with light-microscopic neuropathology first appearing only 2–3 days following the insult [40, 41]. Large early increases in the metabolic rate of affected cells [42] and increased synaptic activity with subsequent electrical failure preceded morphologic evidence of injury. That the delayed death of hippocampal neurons is exitotoxic has been bolstered by the observation that glutamate is massively released into the extracellular space during anoxia/ischemia [43]; and that this injury may be averted by deafferentation of excitatory afferent circuits to the hippocampus [44, 45] or by drugs which antagonize exitotoxic neurotransmission [37].

Two mechanisms of glutamate neurotoxicity have been emphasized:

a) a rapid or early form involving increased sodium permeability, leading to intracellular entry of chloride ion and water and resulting in cell swelling and osmotic lysis; and
b) a delayed form, dependent upon calcium entry via agonist- or voltage-sensitive channels [46–48].

The relevance of excitotoxicity to human ischemic disease has been underscored by the recent observation that patients dying 18 h or less following cardiac arrest show minimal hippocampal injury whereas injury is severe in patients dying after 24 h [49]. Thus, human ischemic hippocampal injury may occur in a delayed manner and, as such, may be potentially amenable to postischemic therapeutic intervention.

Non-Glutamate Neurotransmission in Ischemic Vulnerability

The possibility that dopaminergic neurotransmission might contribute to vulnerability of the striatum during ischemia was indirectly suggested by our observation, in a model of graded hemispheral ischemia, that the striatum was the predominant locus of neuropathological alterations and that this was preceded by a unique, disproportionate resumption of local striatal glucose metabolism relative to blood flow in the early post-ischemic period [50]. Unilateral substantia nigra lesion carried out two weeks prior to reversible forebrain ischemia suppressed the degree of postischemic metabolism/flow uncoupling [51]; abolished the massive release of dopamine into the striatal extracellular space (which would otherwise occur) [52]; and markedly attenuated the degree of ipsilateral ischemic neuronal death [53] - thus establishing the participatory role of dopamine in striatal ischemic injury. Other evidence suggests that both dopamine and glutamate may be required to produce striatal injury [52]. Striatal vulnerability preferentially affects neurons bearing the dopamine D_1-receptor [54].

Other neurotransmitter systems in the brain may confer protection from ischemia. These include the noradrenergic system originating in the locus ceruleus; adenosine; and GABA.

Therapeutic Strategies Directed at Neurotransmission

The implication of neurotransmitter mechanisms in ischemic vulnerability has led to the extensive development and evaluation of a variety of putative antagonists of excitatory neurotransmission. Meldrum has comprehensively reviewed this topic [37]. Certain glutamate analogs are potent and selective competitive antagonists of the NMDA receptor; these include D(−)amino-5-phosphonovalerate (AP5), D(−)2-amino-7-phosphono-heptanoate (AP7), and other cyclic phosphonate compounds. Other agents are *non*competitive antagonists acting at sites that served to modify the function of the NMDA receptor/ionophore complex. Magnesium ion and zinc ion represent simple endogenous antagonists. Kynurenate, a nonspecific noncompetitive NMDA antagonist, may act at the glycine receptor site (glycine itself acting endogenously to enhance the excitatory action of glutamate).

The therapeutically most important class of NMDA antagonists are agents which compete for binding at the sigma opiate/phencyclidine (PCP) receptor. These include the dissociative agents PCP and ketamine; various morphinans; and the agent MK-801 [37]. Several of these compounds have already been shown to confer cerebral protection in ischemia. Intra-hippocampal injections of a noncompetitive NMDA antagonist protected hippocampal neurons from early injury in transient forebrain ischemia in the rat [55].

MK-801 has been rather extensively evaluated in animal models of both focal and global ischemia, and these results have been recently summarized [56]. Among the most impressive results are the findings of the Glasgow group [57]. In the cat MCA occlusion model, MK-801 reduced cortical infarct volume by 57% when infused in a dose of 5 mg/kg intravenously 30 min prior to vascular occlusion; and by 65% when administration was deferred to 2 h following vascular occlusion [57]. No protection was seen in the striatum. MK-801 has also been observed to be protective in rat middle cerebral artery occlusion when given either pre- or post-occlusion [57]. Positive results were obtained, as well, in rabbit cerebral embolism and spinal cord ischemia models [58]. Several studies of this agent in global cerebral ischemia also support a protective action [56], although not all investigations have yielded positive results. Further, our laboratory has shown evidence of a long-lasting perturbation of cerebral metabolism following a single injection of MK-801 [59]. It remains bo be seen whether MK-801 will prove suitable for clinical application.

The dextrorotatory morphinans dextrorphan and the related compound dextromethorphan, a commonly used antitussive agent, have been noted to be powerful antagonists of NMDA in brain slice preparations. Dextromethorphan has been found to protect against cerebral infarction in both the modified rat Levine preparation of hypoxia-ischemia [60] and in a rabbit model of focal ischemia produced by unilateral internal carotid and anterior cerebral artery occlusions [61]. Even when first administered at the end of a one-hour period of vascular occlusion in that model, dextromethorphan or dextrorphan therapy were associated with approximately 90% reduction in the extent of severe neuronal change [62]. These drugs would appear to have great promise for stroke therapy.

Selective Reduction of Brain Temperature – A Promising Therapeutic Strategy?

It has long been appreciated that large reductions of whole-body temperature offer protection against cerebral ischemia [63], but logistic difficulties as well as the potential for systemic complications of marked hypothermia have limited the applicability of this strategy in treating brain ischemia. Our laboratory first suspected several years ago, however, that rather *small* fluctuations of *brain* temperature might account for the variability noted in the outcome of various animal ischemia experiments. This led to a formal series of experiments in which brain temperature was directly measured in the course of a transient forebrain ischemic insult and was allowed to vary independently of rectal temperature, which was held constant at 37 °C [64]. We observed that, when no effort was made to control brain temperature, it tended to fall gradually by 5–6 °C during high-grade forebrain ischemia. The histological consequences of this insult proved to be markedly influenced by intra-ischemic brain temperature. For example, hippocampal CAl neurons showed moderate-to-severe damage in all brains held at 36 °C during ischemia but in only 20% of hemispheres held at 34° and in none held at 33 or 30 °C. Injury to the dorsolateral striatum was reduced by 80% at 33–34 °C and was eliminated at 30 °C [64]. This effect was shown not to be due to differential affection of CBF, energy metabolism, or fatty acids in ischemia [65]. However, when intra-ischemic brain temperature was reduced to 33 °C, the (expected) 7-fold elevation of extracellular glutamate during ischemia was almost totally abolished, and dopamine release was reduced by 60% [52]. Further studies have shown that this protective effect is also present if the reduction of brain temperature is delayed until five minutes following resumption of circulation (R. Busto et al., submitted). These results offer strong encouragement of the implementation of strategies for selective brain cooling for eventual clinical trial in ischemic stroke.

Relevance of Plasma Glucose Level in Ischemic Stroke

Twelve years ago, Myers and Yamaguchi first reported their serendipitous observation that Rhesus monkeys administered a glucose load prior to a 15-min period of cardiac arrest developed profound neurological abnormalities with brain edema and widespread necrosis of cerebral gray matter, whereas food-deprived animals exhibited minimal signs and restricted neuropathological abnormalities [66]. This deleterious effect of hyperglycemia in ischemia appears to be mediated via an elevation of brain glucose levels. The anaerobic metabolism of these increased glucose stores during ischemia eventuates in a marked tissue lactic acidosis, which tends to be more severe when the degree of ischemia is incomplete, owing to the continued delivery of glucose to the ischemic brain [67–69]. Concomitants of this process include marked accentuation of postischemic hypoperfusion and deterioration of brain energy metabolites [67–70]. Even moderate elevations of blood glucose are sufficient to worsen outcome [71].We have shown in focal vascular occlusion that hyperglycemia tends to increase infarct volume in tissue receiving collateral circulation (e.g., cerebral cortex) but has no deleterious effect in regions of end-arterial perfusion (e.g., striatum) [72]. Paradoxically, however, hyperglycemia appears to protect neurons at the periphery of an infarcted focus from sporadic ischemic change [73].

Microelectrode studies have shown a step-transition of brain interstitial pH from normal levels to approximately 6.2 as tissue lactate rises from about 13 to 17–18 mmol/kg; from these and other data, it has been inferred that hydrogen ion buffering is compartmentalized in ischemia and that glial cells may serve this function [74, 75]. It is speculated that the transition from isolated ischemic neuronal pathology to frank tissue necrosis (such as occurs in focal ischemic stroke) is mediated by the exhaustion of glial buffering capacity and subsequent cell membrane rupture [76].

The relevance of these observations to ischemic stroke in the human clinical setting, unfortunately, remains uncertain. This stems in large measure from the confounding observations that

a) diabetics in general tend to have a worse prognosis in stroke; and
b) stress-induced hyperglycemia may occur in acute stroke patients, complicating the interpretation of elevated blood glucose in that setting.

Whereas one small prospective analysis concluded that neurologic outcome was worsened by admission plasma glucose levels greater than 120 mg/dl [77], another group was unable to substantiate this in an analysis of data-bank information [78]. Nonetheless, the compelling nature of the evidence in experimental animal models would urge us, as clinicians, to be cautious in subjecting acute stroke patients to high glucose levels.

Oxygen Radical Processes in Brain Ischemia

Oxygen free radicals are unstable, short-lived molecules containing an unpaired electron in their outer orbital. They arise during normal metabolism as partially reduced redox intermediates in the course of mitochondrial oxidative phosphorylation, but their influence is normally counteracted by radical-scavenging systems. When these defenses are inadequate, these highly reactive species may cause cellular injury. Indeed, free radicals have been implicated in a wide spectrum of disease states [79].

Kontos [80] has summarized the possible sources of the superoxide radical in the context of ischemia and reperfusion:

a) in mitochondria, when oxygen is readmitted during tissue reperfusion;
b) as a reaction product of the enzyme xanthine oxidase (which is converted from xanthine dehydrogenase in ischemia);
c) in the course of unsaturated fatty acid metabolism via an enzymatic mechanism involving PGH synthase and radical intermediates of NAD or NADP;
d) by autooxidation of various compounds such as hemoglobin or catecholamines, often in metal-catalyzed reactions; and
e) in phagocytic cells such as polymorphonuclear leukocytes and macrophages.

Though often touted as a mechanism of ischemic injury [18], the direct demonstration of oxygen radical-mediated lipid peroxidation in ischemic or postischemic brain parenchyma has proven extremely elusive. Indirect indices such as consumption of endogenous antioxidants, or levels of unsaturated fatty acids, have resisted unambiguous interpretation [81, 82]. Conjugated diene, a direct tissue fingerprint of lipid peroxidation, is detected only inconsistently and in a highly focal and unpredictable manner during and following global brain ischemia [83]. Searches for tissue conjugated diene in the setting of middle cerebral artery occlusion have also been unrewarding [84]. These data, taken together, would suggest that oxygen radical reactions are not an important cause of injury to brain *parenchyma* in ischemia.

In contrast, positive evidence has recently emerged that in a model of *complete* (but not incomplete) cerebral ischemia followed by reperfusion, superoxide anion is demonstrable on the pial surface [85], apparently derived from the cerebral blood vessel wall [80]. Topical application of superoxide dismutase (SOD) and catalase reverses the vascular abnormalities observed on the pial surface following complete ischemia [30].

Therapeutic Efficacy of Superoxide Dismutase in Brain Ischemia

In gerbils subjected to bilateral common carotid artery occlusion for 40 min, pretreatment with polyethylene glycol (PEG)-conjugated SOD more than doubled the animal survival rate [86]. Similarly, in focal ischemia in rats, infarct volume was reduced by 30% in animals receiving the active form of PEG-SOD and PEG-catalase [86]. (The covalent coupling of SOD or catalase to PEG serves markedly to prolong the circulating half-life of these enzymes and reduces their antigenicity.) Because SOD given intravenously does not cross the blood-brain barrier significantly, the effect observed in these studies is assumed to have been intravascular. Intravenous SOD has also been reported to improve hypoperfusion and recovery of evoked potentials in cats with focal cerebral ischemia [87]. Human copper-zinc SOD and human manganese SOD can now be produced by recombinant DNA technology [80]. Thus, it is likely that clinical trials in cerebral ischemia will soon be proposed.

Remote Consequences of Ischemic Infarction

Corresponding to von Monakow's older notion of suppression of nervous function at a site remote from a primary lesion [88], the notion of diaschisis has attracted recent notice as a factor having possible relevance to clinical impairment and recovery of function in stroke [89]. Controlled animal studies using autoradiographic strategies leave little doubt that both local cerebral blood flow (lCBF) and glucose metabolism (lCMRgl) may be depressed remotely by a focal lesion [90, 91]; recent observations suggest that this may be mediated, at least in part, by serotoninergic systems [92]. In a recent work, we have discovered that the presence of an acute infarct diminishes the capacity of an ipsilateral somatosensory system spared by the lesion to undergo its normal activation of metabolism and blood-flow in response to physiological stimulation [93]. It is also of interest that, following transient forebrain ischemia of a degree insufficient to produce light-microscopic injury, the capacity for metabolic activation of cortex via a physiological stimulus is nonetheless altered for 5–10 days [94].

Pharmacologic Promotion of Recovery of Function in Stroke

The above observations, perhaps, take on greater relevance in the context of findings in experimental models of brain injury that d-amphetamine, combined with behavioral experience, accelerates the course of clinical recovery [95, 96] and, in one study, eventuates in a level of recovery never obtained in the absence of such treatment [97]. These findings have prompted a small clinical trial of d-amphetamine plus physical therapy in stroke patients, whose results are encouraging [98]. Other laboratories have provided evidence that the GABA/benzodiazepine receptor complex may be capable of retarding functional recovery [99].

To summarize, efforts involving pharmacological manipulation of the recuperating brain may have the potential for promoting synaptic plasticity in the clinical context. This general area is deserving of serious continued research.

Thrombolytic Therapy in Cerebral Infarction

The concept of therapeutic clot lysis in ischemic stroke is not new. In several clinical trials in the 1960s and 1970s, often carried out without controls, improvement was described but cerebral hemorrhage emerged as a significant complication [100]. More recent studies have employed local intra-arterial infusion of urokinase or streptokinase in an effort to diminish systemic complications. In one recent retrospective report in patients with acute vertebrobasilar occlusive disease, it was found that recanalization occurred in 19 of 43 patients given intra-arterial thrombolytic therapy. Of these 19, 14 patients survived, 10 with a favorable outcome, whereas only 14% of a comparable group receiving conventional therapy survived, all of whom were moderately disabled [101].

Much current interest centers on tissue-type plasminogen activator, a serine protease now produced by recombinant DNA technology (rt-PA). rt-PA shows marked enhancement of its fibrinolytic activity when bound to fibrin; this property greatly diminishes the potential of systemic fibrinolytic complications [102]. rt-PA, which has been extensively evaluated in the setting of coronary artery thrombosis, is now receiving attention in ischemic stroke. On the background of successful reports of thrombolysis in animal ischemia studies (e.g., [103]), at least two first-phase clinical studies are now under way. An interim report of a study of ischemic stroke patients treated within 90 min suggests that rt-PA appears to be well tolerated; probably does not increase the likelihood of cerebral hemorrhage; and seems to be associated with a higher incidence of clinical improvement than would be expected on the basis of natural history statistics [104]. The next several years will determine whether thrombolytic therapy achieves a routine place in the clinical stroke armamentarium [105].

Acknowledgments: Dr. Ginsberg is the recipient of a Jacob Javits Neuroscience Investigator Award and receives support from USPHS Grants NS-05820 and NS-22603. He is indebted to Mrs. Helen Valkowitz for preparing the typescript.

References

1. Hachinski V, Norris JW (1985) The acute stroke. FA Davis, Phildadelphia
2. Barnett HJM, Stein BM, Mohr JP, Yatsu FM (1986) Stroke. Pathophysiology, diagnosis, and management. Churchill Livingstone, New York
3. Sokoloff L (1976) Circulation and energy metabolism of the brain. In: Siegel GJ, Albers RW, Katzman R, Agranoff BW (eds) Basic neurochemistry. Little, Brown & Co, Boston, pp 388–413
4. Heiss W-D (1983) Flow thresholds of functional and morphological damage of brain tissue. Stroke 14:329–331
5. Astrup J, Symon L, Branston NM, Lassen NA (1977) Cortical evoked potential and extracellular K^+ and H^+ at critical levels of brain ischemia. Stroke 8:51–57
6. Siesjö BK (1978) Brain energy metabolism. Wiley & Sons, Chichester
7. Heiss W-D, Rosner G (1983) Functional recovery of cortical neurons as related to degree and duration of ischemia. Ann Neurol 14:294–301
8. Gibbs JM, Leenders KL, Wise RJS, Jones T (1984) Evulation of cerebral perfusion reserve in patients with carotid-artery occlusion. Lancet 1:182–186
9. Baron JC (1985) Positron tomography in cerebral ischemia. A review. Neuroradiology 27:509–516
10. Wise RJS, Bernardi S, Frackowiak RSJ, Legg NJ, Jones T (1983) Serial observations on the pathophysiology of acute stroke. Brain 106:197–222
11. Lenzi GL, Frackowiak RSJ, Jones T (1982) Cerebral oxygen metabolism and blood flow in human cerebral ischaemic infarction. J Cereb Blood Flow Metab 2:321–335
12. Pantano P, Baron JC, Samson Y, Bousser MG, Derouesne C, Comar D (1986) Crossed cerebellar diaschisis. Further studies. Brain 109:677–694
13. Genton E, Barnett HJM, Fields WS, Gent M, Hoak JC (1977) Cerebral ischemia: the role of thrombosis and of antithrombotic therapy. Stroke 8:148–175
14. Katzman R, Clasen R, Klatzo I, Meyer JS, Pappius HM, Waltz AG (1977) Report of joint committee for stroke resources. Brain edema in stroke. Stroke 8:512–540
15. Hsu CY, Faught RE, Furlan AJ, Coull BM, Huang DC, Hogan EL, Linet OI, Yatsu FM (1987) Intravenous prostacyclin in acute nonhemorrhagic stroke, a placebo- controlled double-blind trial. Stroke 18:352–358
16. Hsu CY, Norris JW, Hogan EL, et al (1988) Pentoxifylline in acute nonhemorrhagic stroke. A randomized, placebo-controlled double-blind trial. Stroke 19:716–722
17. Scandinavian Stroke Study Group (1988) Multicenter trial of hemodilution in acute ischemic stroke. Stroke 19:464–471
18. Siesjö BK (1981) Review. Cell damage in the brain: A speculative synthesis. J Cereb Blood Flow Metab 1:155–185
19. Raichle ME (1983) The pathophysiology of brain ischemia. Ann Neurol 13:2–10
20. Carafoli E (1987) Intracellular calcium homeostasis. Ann Rev Biochem 56:395–433
21. Harris RJ, Symon L (1984) Extracellular pH, potassium, and calcium activities in progressive ischaemia of rat cortex. J Cereb Blood Flow Metab 4:178–186
22. Hass WK (1981) Beyond cerebral blood flow, metabolism, and ischemic thresholds: an examination of the role of calcium in the initiation of cerebral infarction. In: Meyer JS, Lechner H, Reivich M, et al (eds) Cerebral vascular disease 3. Proceedings of the 10th International Salzburg Conference, Excerpta Medica, Amsterdam, pp 3–17
23. Dienel GA (1984) Regional accumulation of calcium in postischemic rat brain. J Neurochem 43:913–925

24. Harper AM, Craigen L, Kazda S (1981) Effect of the calcium antagonist, nimodipine, on cerebral blood flow and metabolism in the primate. J Cereb Blood Flow Metab 1:349–356
25. Mohamed AA, Mendelow AD, Teasdale GM, Harper AM, McCulloch J (1985) Effect of the calcium antagonist nimodipine on local cerebral blood flow and metabolic coupling. J Cereb Blood Flow Metab 5:26–33
26. Steen PA, Newberg LA, Milde JH, Michenfelder JD (1983) Nimodipine improves cerebral blood flow and neurologic recovery after complete cerebral ischemia in the dog. J Cereb Blood Flow Metab 3:38–43
27. Steen PS, Newberg LA, Milde JH, Michenfelder JD (1984) Cerebral blood flow and neurologic outcome when nimodipine is given after complete cerebral ischemia in the dog. J Cereb Blood Flow Metab 4:82–87
28. Vibulsresth S, Dietrich WD, Busto R, Ginsberg MD (1987) Failure of nimodipine to prevent ischemic neuronal damage in rats. Stroke 18:210–216
29. Alps BJ, Hass WK (1987) The potential benefit of nicardipine in a rat model of transient forebrain ischemia. Neurology 37:809–814
30. Deshpande JK, Wieloch T (1986) Flunarizine, a calcium entry blocker, ameliorates ischemic brain damage in the rat. Anesthesiology 64:215–224
31. Mohamed AA, Gotoh O, Graham DI, et al (1985) Effect of pretreatment with the calcium antagonist nimodipine on local cerebral blood flow and histopathology after middle cerebral artery occlusion. Ann Neurol 18:705–711
32. Gotoh O, Mohamed AA, McCulloch J, Graham DI, Harper AM, Teasdale GM (1986) Nimodipine and the haemodynamic and histopathological consequences of middle cerebral artery occlusion in the rat. J Cereb Blood Flow Metab 6:321–331
33. Gelmers HJ, Gorter K, de Weerdt CJ, Wiezer HJA (1988) A controlled trial of nimodipine in acute ischemic stroke. N Engl J Med 318:203–207
34. Nakayama H, Ginsberg MD, Dietrich WD (1988) (S)-emopamil, a novel calcium channel blocker and serotonin S_2 antagonist, markedly reduces infarct size following middle cerebral artery occlusion in the rat. Neurology 38:1667–1673
35. Schwarcz R, Meldrum B (1985) Excitatory amino acid antagonists provide a therapeutic approach to neurological disorders. Lancet II:140–143
36. Cotman CW, Iversen LL (1987) Excitatory amino acids in the brain – focus on NMDA receptors. Trends Neurosci 10:263–265
37. Meldrum B (1989) Excitotoxicity in ischemia: An overview. In: Ginsberg MD, Dietrich WD (eds) Cerebrovascular diseases – Sixteenth Research (Princeton) Conference. Raven Press, New York, pp 47–60
38. Rothman SM (1983) Synaptic activity mediates death of hypoxic neurons. Science 220:536–537
39. Rothman S (1984) Synaptic release of excitatory amino acid neurotransmitter mediates anoxic neuronal death. J Neurosci 4:1884–1891
40. Kirino T (1982) Delayed neuronal death in the gerbil hippocampus following ischemia. Brain Res 239:57–69
41. Kirino T, Tamura A, Sano K (1984) Delayed neuronal death in the rat hippocampus following transient forebrain ischemia. Acta Neuropathol (Berl) 64:139–147
42. Suzuki R, Yamaguchi T, Kirino T, Orzi F, Klatzo I (1983) The effects of 5-minute ischemia in Mongolian gerbils: I. Blood-brain barrier, cerebral blood flow, and local cerebral glucose utilization changes. Acta Neuropathol (Berl) 60:207–216
43. Drejer J, Benveniste H, Diemer NH, Schousboe A (1985) Cellular origin of ischemia-induced glutamate release from brain tissue in vivo and in vitro. J Neurochem 45:145–151
44. Jorgensen MB, Johansen FF, Diemer NH (1987) Removal of the entorhinal cortex protects hippocampal CA1 neurons from ischemic damage. Acta Neuropathol (Berl) 73:189–194
45. Wieloch T, Lindval O, Blomqvist P, Gage FH (1985) Evidence for amelioration of ischemic neuronal damage in the hippocampal formation by lesion of the perforant path. Neurol Res 7:24–26
46. Choi DW (1985) Glutamate neurotoxicity in cortical cell culture is calcium dependent. Neurosci Lett 58:293–297

47. Rothman SM, Olney JW (1986) Glutamate and the pathophysiology of hypoxic-ischemic brain damage. Ann Neurol 19:105–111
48. Rothman SM, Olney JW (1987) Excitotoxicity and the NMDA receptor. Trends Neurosci 10:299–302
49. Petito CK, Feldmann E, Pulsinelli WA, Plum F (1987) Delayed hippocampal damage in humans following cardiorespiratory arrest. Neurology 37:1281–1286
50. Ginsberg MD, Graham DI, Busto R (1985) Regional glucose utilization and blood flow following graded forebrain ischemia in the rat: correlation with neuropathology. Ann Neurol 18:470–481
51. Globus MY-T, Ginsberg MD, Harik SI, Busto R, Dietrich WD (1987) Role of dopamine in ischemic striatal injury: metabolic evidence. Neurology 37:1712–1719
52. Globus MY-T, Busto R, Dietrich WD, Martinez E, Valdes I, Ginsberg MD (1988) Intra-ischemic extracellular release of dopamine and glutamate is associated with striatal vulnerability to ischemia. Neurosci Lett 91:36–40
53. Globus MY-T, Ginsberg MD, Dietrich WD, Busto R, Scheinberg P (1987) Substantia nigra lesion protects against ischemic damage in the striatum. Neurosci Lett 80:251–256
54. Globus MY-T, Mash DC, Dietrich WD, Busto R, Valdes I, Ginsberg MD (1988) Dopamine D-1 but not D-2 receptors are selectively vulnerable to transient ischemia in the rat striatum. Soc Neurosci Abstr 14:501
55. Simon RP, Swan JH, Griffiths T, Meldrum BS (1984) Blockade of *N*-methyl-D- aspartate receptors may protect against ischemic damage in the brain. Science 226:850–852
56. Shearman GT (1989) Effect of the NMDA antagonist MK-801 in animal models of focal and global cerebral ischemia. In: Ginsberg MD, Dietrich WD (eds) Cerebrovascular diseases – Sixteenth Research (Princeton) Conference. Raven Press, New York, pp 73–77
57. Graham DI, Ozyurt E, Park CK, Nehls DG, Teasdale GM, McCulloch J (1989) Protective effects of the NMDA antagonist, MK-801, on focal ischemic brain damage. In: Ginsberg MD, Dietrich WD (eds) Cerebrovascular diseases – Sixteenth Research (Princeton) Conference. Raven Press, New York, pp 65–72
58. Kochhar A, Zivin JA, Lyden PD, Mazzarella V (1988) Glutamate antagonist therapy reduces neurologic deficits produced by focal central nervous system ischemia. Arch Neurol 45:148–153
59. Dietrich WD, Ginsberg MD, Busto R, Globus MY-T (1989) Influence of MK-801 on functional brain activation. In: Ginsberg MD, Dietrich WD (eds) Cerebrovascular diseases – Sixteenth Research (Princeton) Conference. Raven Press, New York, pp 79–85
60. Prince DA, Feeser HR (1988) Dextromethorphan protects against cerebral infarction in a rat model of hypoxia-ischemia. Neurosci Lett 85:291–296
61. George CP, Goldberg MP, Choi DW, Steinberg GK (1988) Dextromethorphan reduces neocortical ischemic neuronal damage in vivo. Brain Res 440:375–379
62. Steinberg GK, Saleh J, Kunis D (1988) Delayed treatment with dextromethorphan and dextrorphan reduces cerebral damage after transient focal ischemia. Neurosci Lett 89:193–197
63. Rosomoff HL (1957) Hypothermia and cerebral vascular lesions. Experimental interruption followed by inductions of hypothermia. Arch Neurol Psychiat 78:454–464
64. Busto R, Dietrich WD, Globus MY-T, Valdes I, Scheinberg P, Ginsberg MD (1987) Small differences in intraischemic brain temperature critically determine the extent of ischemic neuronal injury. J Cereb Blood Flow Metab 7:729–738
65. Busto R, Globus MY-T, Dietrich WD, Martinez E, Valdes I, Ginsberg MD (1989) Ischemia-induced release of neurotransmitters and free fatty acids in the rat brain: effect of mild intraischemic hypothermia. Stroke 20 (in review)
66. Myers RE, Yamaguchi S (1977) Nervous system effects of cardiac arrest in monkeys. Preservation of vision. Arch Neurol 34:65–74
67. Welsh FA, Ginsberg MD, Rieder W, Budd WW (1980) Deleterious effect of glucose pretreatment on recovery from diffuse cerebral ischemia in the cat. Regional metabolite levels. Stroke 11:355–363
68. Rehncrona S, Rosen I, Siesjö BK (1981) Brain lactic acidosis and ischemic cell damage: 1. Biochemistry and neurophysiology. J Cereb Blood Flow Metab 1:297–311

69. Kalimo H, Rehncrona S, Söderfeldt B, Olsson Y, Siesjö BK (1981) Brain lactic acidosis and ischemic cell damage: 2. Histopathology. J Cereb Blood Flow Metab 1:313–327
70. Ginsberg MD, Welsh FA, Budd WW (1980) Deleterious effect of glucose pretreatment on recovery from diffuse cerebral ischemia in the cat. Local cerebral blood flow and glucose utilization. Stroke 11:347–354
71. Pulsinelli WA, Waldman S, Rawlinson D, Plum F (1982) Moderate hyperglycemia augments ischemic brain damage: a neuropathologic study in the rat. Neurology 32:1239–1246
72. Prado R, Ginsberg MD, Dietrich WD, Watson BD, Busto R (1988) Hyperglycemia increases infarct size in collaterally perfused but not end-arterial vascular territories. J Cereb Blood Flow Metab 8:186–192
73. Nedergaard M, Diemer NH (1987) Focal ischemia of the rat brain, with special reference to the influence of plasma glucose concentration. Acta Neuropathol (Berl) 73:131–137
74. Kraig RP, Pulsinelli WA, Plum F (1985) Hydrogen ion buffering during complete brain ischemia. Brain Res 342:281–290
75. Kraig RP, Pulsinelli WA, Plum F (1986) Carbonic acid buffer changes during complete brain ischemia. Am J Physiol 250:R348–R357
76. Plum F (1983) What causes infarction in the ischemic brain?: The Robert Wartenberg Lecture. Neurology 33:222–233
77. Pulsinelli WA, Levy DE, Sigsbee B, Scherer P, Plum F (1983) Increased damage after ischemic stroke in patients with hyperglycemia with or without established diabetes mellitus. Am J Med 74:540–544
78. Mohr JP, Rubenstein L, Edelstein SZ, et al (1985) Approaches to pathophysiology of stroke through the NINCDS data bank. In: Plum F, Pulsinelli WA (eds) Cerebrovascular diseases. Fourteenth Research (Princeton-Williamsburg) Conference. Raven Press, New York, pp 63-68
79. Cross CE, Halliwell B, Borish ET, et al (1987) Oxygen radicals and human disease. Ann Intern Med 107:526–545
80. Kontos HA (1989) Oxygen radicals in cerebral ischemia. In: Ginsberg MD, Dietrich WD (eds) Cerebrovascular diseases - Sixteenth Research (Princeton) Conference. Raven Press, New York, pp 365–371
81. Yoshida S, Abe K, Busto R, Watson BD, Kogure K, Ginsberg MD (1982) Influence of transient ischemia on lipid-soluble antioxidants, free fatty acids and energy metabolites in rat brain. Brain Res 245:307–316
82. Watson BD, Ginsberg MD (1988) Mechanisms of lipid peroxidation potentiated by ischemia in brain. In: Halliwell B (ed) Oxygen radicals and tissue injury. Proceedings of a Brook Lodge Symposium, FASEB, Bethesda, pp 81-91
83. Watson BD, Busto R, Goldberg WJ, Santiso M, Yoshida S, Ginsberg MD (1984) Lipid peroxidation *in vivo* induced by reversible global ischemia in rat brain. J Neurochem 42:268–274
84. Ginsberg MD, Watson BD, Busto R, et al (1989) Peroxidative damage to cell membranes following cerebral ischemia - a cause of ischemic brain injury? Neurochem Pathol (in press)
85. Wei EP, Kontos HA (1987) Oxygen radicals in cerebral ischemia. Physiologist 30:122
86. Beckman JS, Liu TH, Hogan EL, Lindsay SL, Freeman BA, Hsu CY (1989) Evidence for a role of oxygen radicals in cerebral ischemic injury. In: Ginsberg MD, Dietrich WD (eds) Cerebrovascular diseases - Sixteenth Research (Princeton) Conference. Raven Press, New York, pp 373–380
87. Davis RJ, Bulkley GB, Traystman RJ (1987) Role of oxygen-free radicals in focal brain ischemia. J Cereb Blood Flow Metab 7:S10
88. von Monakow C (1914) Die Lokalisation im Grosshirn und der Abbau der Funktion durch kortikale Herde. JF Bergmann, Wiesbaden
89. Feeney DM, Baron J-C (1986) Diaschisis. Stroke 17:817–830
90. Dietrich WD, Ginsberg MD, Busto R, Watson BD (1986) Photochemically induced cortical infarction in the rat. Time course of hemodynamic consequences. J Cereb Blood Flow Metab 6:184–194

91. Dietrich WD, Ginsberg MD, Busto R, Watson BD (1986) Photochemically induced cortical infarction in the rat. Acute and subacute alterations in local glucose utilization. J Cereb Blood Flow Metab 6:195–202
92. Dietrich WD, Busto R, Ginsberg MD (1989) The serotonin antagonist ketanserin inhibits the early remote hemodynamic consequences of photochemically induced cortical infarction. In: Krieglstein J (ed) Pharmacology of cerebral ischemia. Elsevier, Amsterdam (in press)
93. Ginsberg MD, Castella Y, Dietrich WD, Watson BD, Busto R (1989) Acute thrombotic infarction suppresses metabolic activation of ipsilateral somatosensory cortex: Evidence for functional diaschisis. J Cereb Blood Flow Metab 9 (in press)
94. Dietrich WD, Ginsberg MD, Busto R (1986) Effect of transient cerebral ischemia on metabolic activation of a somatosensory circuit. J Cereb Blood Flow Metab 6:405–413
95. Feeney DM, Gonzales A, Law WA (1982) Amphetamine, haloperidol and experience interact to affect rate of recovery after motor cortex injury. Science 217:855–857
96. Hovda DA, Fenney DM (1984) Amphetamine with experience promotes recovery of locomotor function after unilateral frontal cortex injury in the cat. Brain Res 298:358–361
97. Feeney DM, Hovda DA (1985) Reinstatement of binocular depth perception by amphetamine and visual experience after visual cortex ablation. Brain Res 342:352–356
98. Crisostomo EA, Duncan PW, Propst M, Dawson DV, Davis JN (1988) Evidence that amphetamine with physical therapy promotes recovery of motor function in stroke patients. Ann Neurol 23:94–97
99. Hernandez TD, Kiefel J, Barth TM, Grant ML, Schallert T (1989) Disruption and faciliation of recovery of behavioral function: Implication of the gamma-aminobutyric acid/benzodiazepine receptor complex. In: Ginsberg MD, Dietrich WD (eds) Cerebrovascular diseases – Sixteenth Research (Princeton) Conference. Raven Press, New York, pp 327–334
100. Del Zoppo GJ, Zeumer H, Harker LA (1986) Thrombolytic therapy in stroke: possibilities and hazards. Stroke 17:595–607
101. Hacke W, Zeumer H, Ferbert A, Brückmann H, del Zoppo GJ (1988) Intra-arterial thrombolytic therapy improves outcome in patients with acute vertebrobasilar occlusive disease. Stroke 19:1216–1222
102. Verstraete M, Collen D (1986) Thrombolytic therapy in the eighties. Blood 67:1529–1541
103. Papadopoulos SM, Chandler WF, Salamat MS, Topol EJ, Sackellares JC (1987) Recombinant human tissue-type plasminogen activator therapy in acute thromboembolic stroke. J Neurosurg 67:394–398
104. Levy DE, Brott T, Haley EC, Barsan WG, Olinger CP, Reed RL, Marler JR (1989) A safety study of tissue plasminogen activator (rt-PA) in the hyperacute phase of ischemic stroke. In: Ginsberg MD, Dietrich WD (eds) Cerebrovascular diseases – Sixteenth Research (Princeton) Conference. Raven Press, New York, pp 21–27
105. Zivin JA (1989) A perspective on the future of thrombolytic stroke therapy. In: Ginsberg MD, Dietrich WD (eds) Cerebrovascular diseases – Sixteenth Research (Princeton) Conference. Raven Press, New York, pp 33–37

Neurotoxic Amino Acids and Amino Acid Antagonists as Neuroprotective Agents

G. N. Woodruff, L. L. Iversen, and J. A. Kemp

Introduction

Ischemia of the brain may occur following a range of pathological conditions. The mechanisms which underlie the central nervous system (CNS) neuropathology arising from the ischemic insult are complex and a number have been considered. Over the past few years evidence has accumulated to suggest a fundamental involvement of excitatory amino acids. Glutamate and aspartate are widely acknowledged as the major excitatory transmitters in the mammalian CNS [1]. Their effects are mediated by an action of specific excitatory amino acid receptor and there are at least three receptor sub-types, the N-methyl-D-aspartate (NMDA), quisqualate and kainate receptors [2]. Some neurones, for example the hippocampal cells, are selectively vulnerable to ischemic damage. The „excitotoxin theory" suggests that the neurodegeneration which results from periods of anoxia, ischemia or hypoglycemia is caused in part by an excess release of glutamate, leading to over-activity at synapses utilizing excitatory amino acid transmitters [3, 4]. Glutamate antagonists able to penetrate CNS might, thus, have considerable therapeutic potential. In particular, the NMDA receptor subtype [5, 6] seems to be a key target, as competitive NMDA antagonist such as D-AP5 and D-AP7 have been found to exert neuroprotective effects in animal studies [7, 8].

Dizocilpine (MK-801)

Recently there has been much interest in dizocilpine maleate (MK-801) ((+)-5-methyl-10,11-dihydro-5H-dibenzo[a,d]cyclohepten-5,10-imine maleate), (Fig. 1), a potent NMDA antagonist which penetrates readily into CNS. The compound was described originally by Clineschmidt et al. [9, 10] as a potent anticonvulsant agent with anxiolytic and central sympathomimetic properties, but with an unknown mechanism of action.

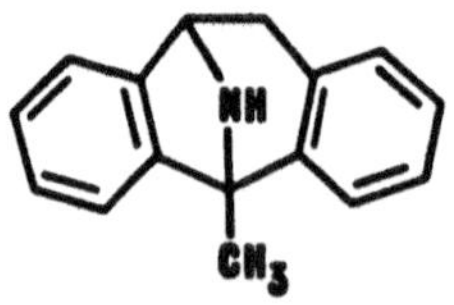

Fig. 1. The structure of dizocilipine (MK-801)

We were able to show that dizocilipine is a potent NMDA antagonist, acting at the level of the associated ion channel. Out neurochemical studies showed that in rat brain membranes, radiolabelled ^{3}H-MK-801 bound to specific sites which appear to be associated with glutamate receptors of the NMDA type [11, 12]. In neurophysiological studies, using rat cerebral cortex slices *in vitro*, MK-801 antagonized the depolarizing actions of NMDA. The selectivity of MK-801 was demonstrated by showing that it had no effect on responses to quisqualic acid of kainic acid [13]. These findings were confirmed by Aram et al. [14] who also showed that iontophoretically applied MK-801 could antagonise NMDA effects on rat spinal cord neurones *in vivo*. The antagonist effects of MK-801 are noncompetitive and agonist-dependent in character.

Further evidence that the action of MK-801 was mediated at the NMDA receptor complex was obtained in a study of the regional distribution of ^{3}H-MK-801 binding sites using quantitative autoradiographic techniques. The results showed an uneven distribution of MK-801 binding sites in rat brain [15]. The highest densities of ^{3}H-MK-801 binding sites were detected in the hippocampus and in superficial layers of cerebral cortex. Moderate levels of binding were observed in the caudate putamen and thalamic medial and lateral geniculate nuclei. Very low levels were present in the cerebellum, substantia nigra, corpus callosum, superior colliculus and medulla pons. This pattern of binding is similar to that previously shown for NMDA sites labelled with ^{3}H-glutamate [16].

The action of MK-801 on NMDA receptors in brain are similar to the effects described for the dissociative anesthetics phencyclidine and ketamine, which also acts as noncompetitive antagonists at these sites as described by Lodge et al. [17]. Like ketamine and PCP, MK-801 sites associated with NMDA receptors may correspond to the high affinity PCP sites previously recognized in brain. PCP is also recognized with moderate affinity by sigma receptors, which have a different anatomical distribution in CNS, being most heavily concentrated in hind brain and spinal cord [18]. Unlike PCP, MK-801 and its (−)enantiomer displace the specific sigma ligand ^{3}H-(+)SKF-10,047 only weakly from its binding sites in rat brain stem [19].

Neuroprotective Effects of MK-801

Neurotoxins

The ability of systemically administered MK-801 to protect against neuronal degeneration in rat brain after intracerebral injections of NMDA agonists has been demonstrated in several studies [20–22]. Treatment with 10 mg/kg (i.p.) MK-801 1 h prior to injection of NMDA into rat hippocampus caused almost complete protection against the extensive histological damage normally caused by such injections. A quantitative assessment of the neuroprotective effects of MK-801 was made by measuring the activity of marker enzymes for intrinsic neurones, using choline acetyltransferase (CAT) as a marker for cholinergic neurones and glutamic acid decarboxylase (GAD) as a marker for GABAergic neurones. MK-801 given at 10 mg/kg 1 h before injection of NMDA or the NMDA agonist quinolinic acid into rat striatum afforded a complete protection against the loss of GAD and CAT normally evoked by excitotoxin injections. The specificity of MK-801 was indicated by the observation that kainic acid-induced decrements in striatal CAT were not protected by MK-801 at doses up to 10 mg/kg. The biochemical measurements were made 7 days after excitotoxin administration. In more recent experiments Foster et al. [23] observed that MK-801 remained remarkably effective as a neuroprotective against NMDA- or quinolinic acid-induced damage in rat striatum even when the drug was administered at intervals up to five hours after the excitotoxin injection. Olney and his colleagues have confirmed the neuroprotective effects of MK-801 in a variety of models. The damage to rat arcuate nucleus caused by systemic administration of NMDA (50 mg/kg. s. c.) was completely prevented by pretreatment with MK-801 (1 mg/kg) [24]. Using chick embryo retina *in vitro*, MK-801 was found to be the most potent compound in protecting against NMDA-induced damage [25]. A similar conclusion was reached in studies demonstrating the ability of MK-801 to protect mouse cortical neurons in primary culture from damage following exposure

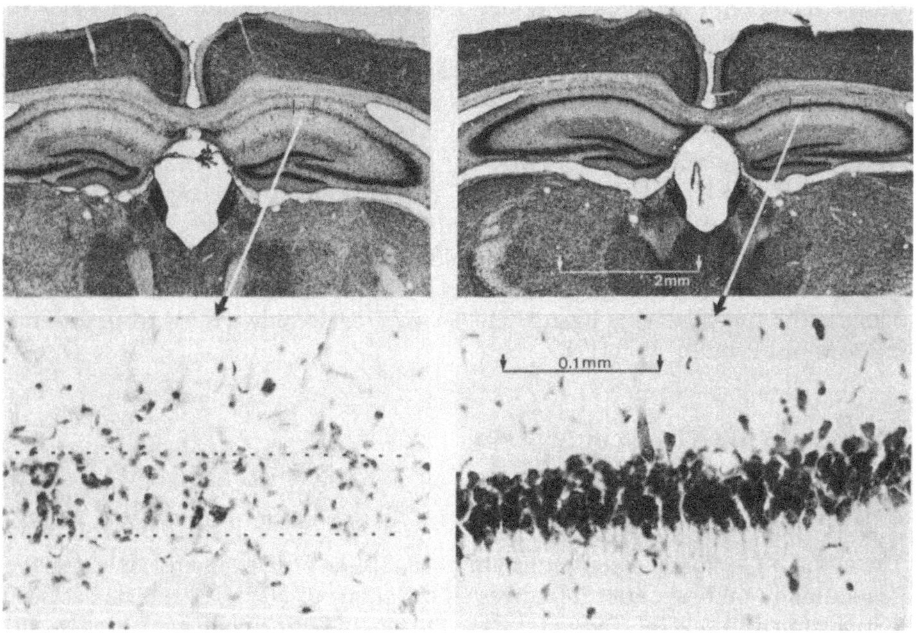

Fig. 2. Systemic administration of MK-801 protects against ischemia-induced hippocampal neurodegeneration in the gerbil. Light micrographs of 40 µm coronal sections of the cresyl violet-stained right hippocampus from a typical untreated gerbil subjected to 5 min of bilateral ischemia. Solid line and arrows illustrate the area of neuronal degeneration that was measured in the 3 coronal sections corresponding to 1.5 (A), 1.7 (B), and 1.9 (C) mm caudal to bregma. The line drawn encircles the degenerating CA1 and CA2 pyramidal neurons, including cell bodies and dendrites, i. e. the total area of neurodegeneration from the hippocampal fissure to the alveus

to NMDA [26]. These authors also found that low concentrations of MK-801 (EC_{50} = 0.1 μm) could prevent neuronal damage caused by transient exposure of tissue cultures to hypoxia [26], a finding we have been able to confirm in our own laboratory (Fig. 2).

Global Ischemia

MK-801 is also effective in various animal models of global ischemia (Table 2). We found that peripheral administered MK-801 protected against neuronal degeneration produced by complete forebrain ischemia in gerbils [27]. Female Mongolian gerbils (60–70 g) were anesthetized with a mixture of 2% halothane, 70% nitrous oxide, 30% oxygen. Cerebral ischemia was induced by occlusion of the common carotid arteries for 5 min. MK-801 was administered at various doses 1 h before the ischemic insult (0.03–10 mg/kg i.p.). This brief period of global ischemia led to no obvious neurological abnormalities or mortality. However, consistent neuronal damage and cell loss were observed histologically 4 days later, particularly in the population of large hippocampal pyramidal cells in the CA1 region. Measurements of neuronal damage in this region were made from both hippocampi in cresyl violet stained coronal sections (Fig. 3). Pretreatment of gerbils 1 h prior to ischemia with MK-801 produced a dose-dependent decrease in the area of CA1 neuronal degeneration, with an ED_{50} of 0.3 mg/kg (i.p.). After pretreatment with higher doses (1–10 mg/kg) the majority of animals

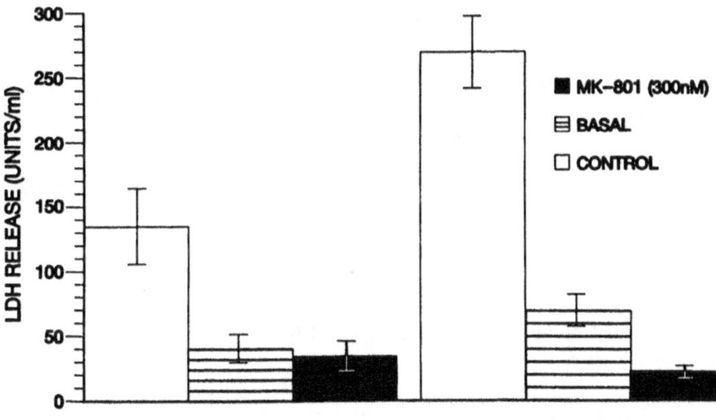

Fig. 3. Protection of cortical neurones from hypoxia-induced injury by MK-801. Lactate dehydrogenase LDH efflux was measured 24 h after a 5 h exposure of sister cultures to hypoxia in the presence or absence of MK-801 (300 nM). Cells were bathed in either normal minimal essential medium (MEM) or MEM lacking glucose and Mg^{2+}-ions. Basal LDH release was measured from cells bathed in the same media for 24 h but not exposed to hypoxia. In MEM MK-801 completely protected against hypoxia-induced injury, reducing LDH release to basal levels. In MEM lacking glucose and MG^{2}-ions the hypoxia-induced injury was exacerbated. However, MK-801 still provided complete protection reducing LDH release to below basal levels, indicating a further protective action against hypoglycemic-induced injury

were completely protected. Most surprisingly, MK-801 remained fully effective in protecting hippocampal neurones when administered 30 min after the ischemic insult, and partial neuroprotection was observed even when a single dose of MK-801 (10 mg/kg) was given 15 or 24 h after the artery occlusion (Table 2) [28].

The neuroprotective effects of MK-801 in the gerbil have been confirmed by Lawrence et al. [29], who found an ED_{50} of approx. 1 mg/kg (i.p. 15 min before) for protection of CA1 hippocampal neurones following a more severe (10 min) bilateral artery occlusion.

MK-801 was also tested in global forebrain ischemia models in the rat, using the methods described by Simon et al. [8] and by Smith et al [30]. In this model, ischemia was induced by bilateral occlusion of the carotid arteries following reduction of blood pressure to less than 50 mmHg. In an acute ischemia model, MK-801 was administered 1 h prior to a 30 min ischemic insult. Following 2 h of reperfusion, the animals were perfusion-fixed and ischemic cell changes in the hippocampus were assessed in Cresyl violet stained coronal (40μm) sections. The percentage of neurones showing early histological signs of ischemic damage was assessed in pyramidal areas CA1, CA2, CA3 and CA4 for each animal. In these, and in all other histological assessment studies, the raters were blind to the experimental history of the tissue. In the acute model, pyknotic pyramidal neurones were observed in the hippocampi of all control animals. Pretreatment with MK-801 (10 mg/kg) significantly reduced the percentage of pyknotik neurones in all areas of hippocampus (Table 1) [31]. In a chronic recovery model, after a 10 min ischemic insult animals survived for 7 days before histological assessment. Control animals showed marked degeneration of hippocampal CA1 and CA2 area pyramidal neurones. Pretreatment with MK-801 1 h prior to the ischemic insult significantly protected the animals against ischemic neurodegeneration, with significant effects at doses as low as 0.3 mg/kg. It was also possible to detect protection against cortical degenerative damage following pretreatment with MK-801 at 1 mg/kg.

Similar results have recently been reported from two other laboratories [32,

Table 1. Effect of MK-801 (10 mg/kg) (1 h before) in acute rat ischemia model. (From [31])

	% of ischemic cells in hippocampal areas (mean ± SEM)			
	CA1	CA2	CA3	CA4
Control (n = 5)	40 ± 15.8	72 ± 16.7	92 ± 5.5	76 ± 4.5
MK-801 (n = 5)	0*	4 ± 4.5**	20 ± 12.3**	28 ± 5.5**

* $p<0.05$; ** $p<0.01$ (unpaired t-test)

Table 2. MK-801 – Summary of neuroprotective studies in global ischemia

Investigator	Species	Insult	MK-801 treatment	Neurological outcome	Neurohistological outcome	Reference
In-house	Gerbil	Bilateral occlusion carotid (5–20 min)	0.1–10.0 mg/kg i.p. 1 h before–24 h after (ED_{50}=0.3 mg/kg)	Improved 4 days survival	Reduced cell loss hippocampus at 4 days	[27, 28]
Lawrence, Washington Univ.	Gerbil	Bilateral occlusion carotid	ED_{50}=1.0 mg/kg, 15 min before	—	Reduced cell loss hippocampus at 4 days	[29]
In-house	Rat	10 min bilateral occlusion carotid + temporary lowering blood pressure	0.2–3.0 mg/kg i.p. 1 h before (ED_{50}=0.5 mg/kg)	—	Reduced cell loss cortex and hippocampus at 3 h and 7 days	[31]
Lodge, Univ. of London	Rat	10 min bilateral occlusion carotid + temporary lowering blood pressure	0.25 + 0.5 mg/kg i.v. 15 min before	—	Reduced cell loss hippocampus at 7 days	[32]
Auer, Univ. of Calgary	Rat	10 min bilateral occlusion carotid + temporary lowering blood pressure	1.0 mg/kg i.v. 20 min before or 20 min after	—	Reduced cell loss hippocampus striatum and cortex at 7 days	[33]
Johnson, Univ. of Michigan	Rat	Unilateral occlusion carotid + 3 h hypoxia in 7-day old pups	1.0 mg/kg s.c. 1 h before –1.25 h post occlusion	—	Greatly reduced loss of cortical tissue at 5 days	[34]
Drummond, Univ. of S. California	Cat	17 min cardiac arrest	0.33 mg/kg 5 min after then 0.075 mg/kg/h for 10 h	No improvement at 2,4 & 7 days	—	[35]
Michenfelder, Mayo Clinic	Dog	11 min aortic occlusion	0.15 mg/kg i.v. 5 min after, then 0.075 mg/kg/h for 8 h	No improvement at 1,2 or 3 days	No reduction in hippocampal damage	[36]
Safar, Univ. of Pittsburgh	Dog	17 min cardiac arrest	0.3 mg/kg i.v. 5 min after, then 0.075 mg/kg/h for 12 h	No improvement at up to 4 days	—	[37]

33] (Table 2). In these models, however, MK-801 was ineffective when administered more than 20 min after the ischemic insult [33].

Dramatic protective effects of MK-801 have been reported in neonatal rat brain [34]. Seven day old rats subjected to unilateral carotid artery occlusion and subsequent hypoxia exhibited severe unilateral hemisphere damage, which could be completely prevented by MK-801 (1 mg/kg i.p.) given up to 1.25 h after the start of hypoxia. MK-801 was ineffective, however, in a number of large animal models which aimed to simulate prolonged cardiopulmonary arrest followed by resuscitation. Thus MK-801 failed to improve neurological or histological outcome in various cat or dog models involving global cerebral ischemia lasting from 10–17 min [35–37]. This may reflect in part the severity of such models and the highly variable outcome observed in the control groups.

Focal Ischemia

MK-801 has been assessed in a variety of animal models of focal ischemia (Table 3). In a study carried out by McCulloch and colleagues at the University of Glasgow [38, 39], early signs of ischemic damage were estimated in the cat cerebral cortex and caudate nucleus 4 h after ligation of the middle cerebral artery (mca). In control animals this procedure leads to a massive involvement of cortical tissue, with more than half of the total cerebral cortex showing signs of ischemic damage. MK-801 (5 mg/kg i.v.) given either 30 min before or 2 h after the ischemic insult provided a remarkable degree of neuroprotection, with the volume of cortical tissue damage reduced in each case by approximately half. In caudate nucleus, where there is no possibility of alternative blood supply from collateral vessels, MK-801 was unable to offer any significant degree of neuroprotection. Similar results were obtained in an acute cat mca model by Reivich et al. (unpublished) who administered MK-801 (1.0 mg/kg) 30 min post-occlusion. McCulloch and colleagues reported similarly large reductions in acute cortical damage in a rat mca model when MK-801 (0.5 mg/kg) was given either 30 min before or 30 min after artery occlusion [40]. Tamura et al. who developed this rodent model, have also reported a large (50%) reduction in cortical damage when MK-801 (10 mg/kg) was given 30 min prior to mca occlusion [41]; although Simon et al. (unpublished) were unable to demonstrate any protective effect of MK-801 in a similar study. The compound was, however, potent and effective in a recently development mouse mca occlusion model (ED_{50} = 0.2 mg/kg) [42]. This suggests that the use of NMDA antagonists may also be valuable in focal ischemia models, including human stroke. The mechanism is likely to involve the rescue of tissue in the „penumbra“ region of an infarct, to protect against damage caused by excess activation of glutamate mechanisms.

An alternative multi-infarct model of focal cerebral ischemia was used by Zivin and colleagues at the University of California [43]. In this model, irreversible occlusions of small cerebral blood vessels in rabbit brain were induced by injecting 50 μm diameter plastic microspheres into the internal carotid artery. A curve was generated showing the relationship between brain damage and the amount of radiolabelled microspheres trapped in the brain. The amount of mi-

Table 3. MK-801 – Summary of neuroprotective studies in focal ischemia

Investigator	Species	Insult	MK-801 treatment	Neurological outcome	Neurohistological outcome	Reference
Tamura, Tokyo	Rat	Permanent MCA occlusion	10.0 mg/kg i.p. 30 min before	—	Reduced volume of cortical infarct at 24 h	[41]
McCulloch, Univ. of Glasgow	Rat	6 h MCA occlusion	0.5 mg/kg i.p. 30 min before *or* 30 min after	—	Ca. 50% reduction in volume of cortical damage at 6 h	[40]
Zivin, UCSD	Rabbit	Carotid infusion 50 m microspheres	0.5 mg/kg s.c. immediately after	Significant improvement at 24 h	—	[43]
Zivin, UCSD	Rabbit	Abdominal aortic occlusion	1.0 mg/kg i.p. 5 min after	Treated animals required longer periods of occlusion to cause spinal motor deficits at 3 days	—	[43]
Reivich, Univ. of Pennsylvania	Cat	2 h MCA occlusion with reperfusion	1.0 mg/kg i.v. immediately after	—	Ca. 50% reduction in volume of cortical damage at 6 h	[Unpublished]
McCulloch, Univ. of Glasgow	Cat	6 h MCA occlusion	5.0 mg/kg i.v. 30 min before *or* 2 h after	—	Ca. 50% reduction in volume of cortical damage at 6 h	[38, 39]
Simon, UCSF	Rat	Spinal cord trauma	1.0 mg/kg i.v. 15 min after	Improved outcome at 4 weeks	—	[44]
Mackenzie, Paris	Mouse	Permanent MCA occlusion, 7 day	$ED_{50}=0.2$ mg/kg i.p. 30 min post	—	Reduced size of lesion	[42]

(MCA = middle cerebral artery)

crospheres producing neurological abnormalities in 50% of control animals was 335.5 ± 54 µg (n = 27). When animals were treated with MK-801 (0.5 mg/kg i.p.) 5 min after embolisation, the dose response curve was shifted significantly to the right, and 534 ± 41 µg (n = 17) microspheres were required to produce similar neurological abnormalities in 50% of the animals ($p < 0.01$). The results showed that MK-801 was effective in reducing CNS damage when given after the onset of ischemic injury in this micro-emboli multi-infarct model.

A role for NMDA receptors mediating spinal cord damage is also suggested by recent reports that MK-801 offers significant protection against both ischemia and mechanical injury-induced spinal deficits [43, 44].

Further studies of the neuroprotective effects of MK-801 are currently underway in a number of other animal models of focal cerebral ischemia.

The results already obtained support the hypothesis that NMDA receptors play an important role in ischemia-induced neuronal degeneration. The ability of peripherally administered MK-801 to prevent neuronal loss even when given many hours after the ischemic episode suggests a potential use of this compound in the treatment of human ischemic neuropathologies. It also indicates that the process of neuronal degeneration triggered by the initial ischemic insult involves a process with a relatively long time course, involving excess activation of NMDA receptors.

References

1. Fagg GE, Foster AC (1983) Amino acid transmitters and their pathways in the mammalian central nervous system. Neurosci 9:701–709
2. Fagg GE, Foster AC, Granang AH (1986) Excitatory amino acid synaptic mechanisms and neurological function. Trends Pharmacol Sci 7:357–363
3. Olney J (1985) Excitatory transmitters and epilepsy-related brain damage. Int Rev Neurobiol 27:337–362
4. Rothman S (1984) Synaptic release of excitatory amino acid neurotransmitter mediates anoxic neuronal death. J Neuroscience 4:1884–1891
5. Foster AC, Fagg GE (1984) Acidic amino acid binding sites in mammalian neuronal membranes: their characteristics and relationship to synaptic receptors. Brain Res Rev 7:103–164
6. Watkins JC, Evans RH (1981) Excitatory amino acid transmitters. Ann Rev Pharmac Toxic 21:165–204
7. Schwarcz R, Meldrum B (1985) Excitatory amino acid antagonists provide a therapeutic approach to neurological disorders. Lancet 2:140–143
8. Simon RP, Swan JH, Griffiths T, Meldrum BS (1984) Blockade of N-methyl-D-aspartate receptors may protect against ischaemic damage in the brain. Science 226:850–852
9. Clineschmidt BV, Martin GE, Bunting PR (1982) Anticonvulsant activity of (+)-5-Methyl-10,11-dihydro-5H-dibenzo[a,d]cyclohepten-5,10-imine (MK-801), a substance with potent anticonvulsant, central sympathomimetic, and apparent anxiolytic properties. Drug Dev Res 2:123–134
10. Clineschmidt BV, Martin GE, Bunting PR, Papp NL (1982) Central sympathomimetic activity of (+)-5 – Methyl-10,11-dihydro-5H-dibenzo[a,d]-cyclohepten-5,10-imine (MK-801), a substance with potent anticonvulsant, central sympathomimetic, and apparent anxiolytic properties. Drug Dev Res 2:135–145
11. Foster AC, Wong EHF (1987) The novel anticonvulsant MK-801 binds to the activated state of the N-methyl-D-aspartate receptor in rat brain. Br J Pharmac 91:403–409

12. Wong EHF, Kemp JA, Priestley T, Knight AR, Woodruff GN, Iversen LL (1986) The anticonvulsant MK-801 is a potent N-methyl-D-aspartate antagonist. Proc Natl Acad Sci 83:7104–7108
13. Kemp JA, Priestley T, Woodruff GN (1986) MK-801, a novel orally-active anticonvulsant, is a potent non-competitive N-methyl-D-aspartate receptor antagonist. Br J Pharmacol 89:535P
14. Aram J, Church J, Davies SN, Martin D, Lodge D (1987) Comparison of phencyclidine thienylcyclohexylpiperidine and MK-801 as NMDA antagonists on rat spinal and cortical neurones. Br J Pharmac 89:778P
15. Bowery NG, Wong EHF, Hudson AL (1988) Quantitative autoradiography of ^{3}H-MK-801 binding sites in mammalian brain. Br J Phamac 93:944–954
16. Monaghan DJ, Cotman CW (1985) Distribution of N-methyl-D-aspartate-sensitive L-[^{3}H]Glutamate binding sites in rat brain. J Neuroscience 5:2909–2919
17. Lodge DR, Aram JA, Church J, et al (1987) Excitatory amino acids and phencyclidine-like drugs. In: Hicks TP, Lodge D, Mc Lennan H (eds) Excitatory amino acid transmission. Alan R Liss, New York, pp 83–90
18. Largent BL, Gundlach AL, Snyder SH (1986) Pharmacological and autoradiographic discrimination of sigma and phencyclidine receptor binding sites in brain with (+)-[^{3}H]-SKF 10,047, (+)-[^{3}H]-3-[3-hydroxyphenyl]-N-(1-propyl) piperidine and [^{3}H]-1-(2-thienyl) cyclohexyl piperidine. J Pharmacol Exp Ther 238:739–748
19. Wong EHF, Knight AR, Woodruff GN (1988) [^{3}H]-MK-801 labels a site on the N-methyl-D-aspartate receptor channel complex in rat brain membranes. J Neurochem 50:274–281
20. Foster AC, Gill R, Kemp JA (1986) Protection of N-methyl-D-aspartate-induced neuronal degeneration by systemic administration of MK-801. Br J Pharmacol 89:870P
21. Foster AC, Gill R, Kemp JA, Woodruff GN (1987) Systemic administration of MK-801 prevents N-methyl-D-aspartate-induced neuronal degeneration in rat brain. Neurosci Lett 76:307–311
22. Foster AC, Gill R, Woodruff GN (1987) MK-801 prevents degeneration of striatal neurons caused by intrastriatal injection of quinolinic acid. Br J Pharmac 90:7P
23. Foster AC, Gill R, Woodruff GN (1988) Neuroprotective effects of MK-801 *in vivo:* selectivity and evidence for delayed degeneration mediated by NMDA receptor activation. J Neuroscience 8:4745–4754
24. Fuller TA, Lawrence JJ, Olney JW (1987) Blockade of N-methyl-aspartate-induced arcuate nucleus damage by PCP, MK-801 and related compounds. Neurosci Abstr 13:412.11
25. Olney JW, Price MT, Salles KS, Labruyere J, Friedrich G (1987) MK-801 powerfully protects against N-methyl aspartate neurotoxicity. Eur J Pharmac 141:357–361
26. Goldberg MP, Visekul V, Choi DW (1988) Phencyclidine receptor ligands attenuate cortical neuronal injury after N-methyl-D-aspartate or hypoxia. J Pharm Exp Ther 245:1081–1092
27. Gill R, Foster AC, Woodruff GN (1987) Systemic administration of MK-801 protects against ischemia-induced hippocampal neurodegeneration in the gerbil. J Neurosci 7:3343–3349
28. Gill R, Foster AC, Woodruff GN (1988) MK-801 is neuroprotective in gerbils when administered during the post-ischemic period. Neuroscience 25:847–855
29. Lawrence JJ, Fuller TA, Olney JW (1987) MK-801 and PCP protect against ischemic neuronal degeneration in the gerbil hippocampus. Soc Neurosci Abstr 13:300.12
30. Smith ML, Bendek G, Dahlgren N, Rosen I, Wieloch T, Seisjö BK (1984) Models for studying long-term recovery following forebrain ischaemia in the rat. A 2-vessel occlusion model. Acta Neurol Scand 69:385–401
31. Gill R, Foster AC, Woodruff GN (1987) Systemic administration of MK-801 protects against ischaemic neuropathology in rats. Br J Pharmac Proc Suppl 91:311P
32. Church J, Zeman S, Lodge D (1988) The neuroprotective action of ketamine and MK-801 after transient cerebral ischaemia in rats. Anesthesiology 69:702–709
33. Rod MR, Auer RN (1989) Pre- and post-ischemic administration of the NMDA receptor antagonist dizocilpine maleate (MK-801) reduces ischemic brain necrosis in the rat. Can J Neurol Sci (in press)
34. McDonals JW, Silverstein FS, Johnston MV (1987) MK-801 protects the neonatal brain from hypoxic-ischemic damage. Eur J Pharmac 140:359–361

35. Fleischer JE, Tateislin A, Drummond JC, et al (1988) Effects of MK-801 upon neurological outcome following cardiac arrest in cats. Soc Neurosurg Anaesthesia and Critical Care, San Francisco (abstract)
36. Michenfelder JD, Lanier WL, Scheithaner BW, Perkins WJ, Shearman GT, Milde JH (1989) Evaluation of the glutamate antagonist dizocilpine maleate (MK-801) on neurologic outcome in a canine model of complete cerebral ischemia: correlation with hippocampal histopathology. Brain Res (in press)
37. Sterz F, Leonov Y, Safar P, Shearman GT, Stezoski SW, Perch H (1989) Effect of excitatory amino acid blocker MK-801 on overall and neurologic outcome after prolonged cardiac arrest in dogs. Stroke (in press)
38. Park CK, Nehls DG, Graham DT, Teasdale GM, McCulloch J (1988) Focal cerebral ischemia in the cat: treatment with the glutamate antagonist MK-801 after induction of ischemia. J Cerebral Blood Flow Met 8:757–762
39. Ozyurt E, Graham DI, Woodruff GN, McCulloch J (1988) Protective effect of the glutamate antagonist MK-801 in focal cerebral ischemia in the cat. J Cerebr Blood Flow Met 8:138–143
40. Park C, Nehls DG, Graham DI, McCulloch J (1988) The glutamate antagonist MK-801 reduces focal ischemic damage in the rat. Ann Neurol 24:543–551
41. Tamura A, Kirino T, Samo K (1989) The effects of a blocker of amino acid neurotransmitter on focal cerebral ischemia. J Clin Exp Med (in press)
42. Gotti B, Benavides J, Mackenzie ET, Scatton B (1989) Activité protectrice des antagonistes du récepteur N-methyl-D-aspartate (NMDA) dans un modèle d'ischémie cérebrale focale chez la souris. Société de Circulation et Métabolisme du cerveau (abstract) (in press)
43. Kochlar A, Zivin J, Lyden P, Mazzarella V (1988) Glutamate antagonist therapy reduces neurological deficits produced by focal central nervous system ischemia. Arch Neurol 45:148–153
44. Faden AI, Simon RP (1988) A potential role for excitotoxins in the pathophysiology of spinal cord injury. Ann Neurol 23:623–626

The Role of Lipid Peroxidation in Ischemic Central Nervous System Injury

E. D. Means, J. M. Braughler, and E. D. Hall

Introduction

The role of lipid peroxidation as a key pathophysiological factor in tissue injury *in vivo* remains in dispute. Particularly contentious issues concern the initiation of lipid peroxidation and the role of iron in this event. An answer to these issues will depend on the advent of more precise and improved methods of measurement. Until then, evidence to support lipid peroxidation as a mediator of tissue injury will rely largely on current methods of detection and experimental observations that pharmacologic antagonism of oxygen radical generation and/or lipid peroxidation results in a therapeutic effect.

Central nervous system (CNS) trauma and ischemia have been particularly implicated as diseases where free radicals and lipid peroxidation may be an important factor in the cascade of secondary events leading to cellular injury [1–5]. This chapter will discuss the basic biochemical and molecular mechanisms involved in lipid peroxidation and also experimental evidence to support the role of lipid peroxidation as a key pathophysiological factor in CNS ischemia. Also discussed will be the results of preclinical experiments in models of experimental CNS trauma and ischemia with a novel 21-aminosteroid.

Free Radical Chemistry and Lipid Peroxidation

General Comments

Molecular oxygen is indisputably essential for life. Nevertheless, oxygen can also precipitate the destruction of tissue and/or impair its ability to function normally. The destructive properties of oxygen are generally thought to be mediated through the formation of reactive oxygen metabolites that can indiscriminately attack cellular lipids, proteins and nucleic acids. Reactive oxygen metabolites, or free radicals, are products of normal cellular metabolism and are usually kept in check by a complex array of cellular defenses. Tissue injury, however, either physical or ischemic, can result in the disruption of normal cellular function to such a degree that oxygen radical production may be substantially increased and cellular defenses overwhelmed. The CNS is particularly sensitive to oxygen radical damage because of the high levels of polyunsaturated lipids that comprise neuronal cell membranes.

Superoxide Radical

Oxygen radical production may occur via a number of pathways (Table 1). The primary radical for initial consideration is the superoxide ion (O_2^-). Superoxide is formed by the single electron reduction of molecular oxygen. While, O_2^- itself is reactive and can, for example, reduce Fe^{III} to Fe^{II} or catalyze the release of Fe^{II} from ferritin [6], it is characteristically unreactive toward biological substrates in aqueous environments [2]. Hydrogen peroxide may be formed as O_2^- undergoes spontaneous dismutation (equation 1) in a reaction that is catalytically accelerated by the enzyme superoxide dismutase (SOD) [7].

$$O_2 + O_2 + 2H^+ \rightarrow H_2O_2 + O_2 \quad (1)$$

In solution, O_2 exists in equilibrium with the hydroperoxyl radical ($HO_2.$).

$$O_2 + H^+ \rightarrow HO_2. \quad (2)$$

Changes in solution pH will obviously affect the relative concentrations of O_2^- and $HO_2.$ as the pKa of this reaction is 4.8. Therefore, at pH around 6.8, the ratio of $O_2^-/HO_2.$ is 100/1 whereas at a pH of 5.8 the ratio is only 10/1.

The $HO_2.$ radical is considerably more lipid soluble than O_2^- and is a far more powerful oxidizing or reducing agent [2]. Therefore, as pH falls and the equilibrium between O_2^- and $HO_2.$ shifts in favor of $HO_2.$, superoxide becomes more reactive, particularly toward lipid. In addition, while the spontaneous dismutation of O_2^- to H_2O_2 is exceedingly slow at neutral pH, $HO_2.$ dismutation to H_2O_2 is on the order of 10^8 times greater than for O_2^-. Thus, in an acidic environment, O_2^- is:

1) converted to the more reactive, more lipid soluble $HO_2.$ and,
2) its rate of dismutation to H_2O_2 is greatly increased.

Finally, it should be considered that the relatively low reactivity of O_2^- enables

Table 1. Sources of oxygen radicals in mammalian systems

Enzymatic - produced by a number of oxidases at subcellular sites.

Examples include:
- Cell cytoplasm - xanthine oxidase
- Mitochondria - Monomine oxidase
- Peroxisomes - D-Amino Acid oxidase
- Plasma membrane - NADPH oxidase (neutrophils)

Non-Enzymatic - produced by the autoxidation of cellular components by molecular oxygen
- Quinones
- Catechols
- Thiols
- Hydropterins
- Flavins
- Hemoglobin

this radical to diffuse some distance before being converted to a more reactive species. Hence, once formed, O_2^- may mediate damage at loci that are distant from its site of origin.

Iron

The involvement of iron in free radical and lipid peroxidation reactions has been studied extensively in recent years and the prime role that it plays is unquestioned. Free iron or iron chelates participate in free radical reactions at several levels. The autoxidation of Fe^{II} results in the formation of O_2^- (reaction 3).

$$Fe^{II} + O_2 \rightarrow Fe^{III} + O_2^- \quad (3)$$

The reverse reaction or reduction of Fe^{III} to Fe^{II} by O_2^- also occurs and competes with the dismutation of O_2^- for available O_2^-. Fe^{II} is also oxidized in the presence of H_2O_2 (Fenton's reagent) to form hydroxyl radical ($OH\cdot$) or perhaps a ferryl ion (Fe^{III}-OH) as in reactions 4 and 5.

$$Fe^{II} + H_2O_2 \rightarrow Fe^{III} + OH\cdot + OH^- \quad (4)$$

$$Fe^{II} + H_2O_2 \rightarrow Fe^{III}OH + OH^- \quad (5)$$

Either $OH\cdot$ or $Fe^{III}OH$ are extremely strong oxidants and can react with an overwhelming array of biological substrates including lipid, DNA, and protein.

Another potential source of $OH\cdot$ is through the Haber-Weiss reaction (reaction 6). While this reaction has a second-order rate constant in aqueous solution of nearly zero, it may be catalyzed in biological systems by the presence of trace amounts of iron or other transition metals. This more likely pathway for $OH\cdot$ formation is known as the iron-catalyzed Haber-Weiss reaction (reactions 7 and 4).

$$H_2O_2 + O_2^- \rightarrow O_2 + OH^- + OH\cdot \quad (6)$$

$$Fe^{III} + O_2^- \rightarrow Fe^{II} + O_2 \quad (7)$$

$$Fe^{II} + H_2O_2 \rightarrow Fe^{III} + OH\cdot + OH^- \quad (4)$$

Thus, iron may participate in the generation of oxygen radicals via several possible routes.

Lipid Peroxidation

Lipid peroxidation is the process whereby unsaturated fatty acids participate in a free radical chain reaction that results in the fragmentation and physiochemical disruption of the membrane environment. Lipid peroxidation is profoundly affected by iron. The role of iron in the initiation of lipid peroxidation through the generation of either OH·, ferryl iron or some other iron-oxygen complex has been a subject of considerable interest. While there is no question that iron catalyzes the formation of various radicals as described above, the identity of the radical or radicals responsible for the initiation of lipid peroxidation is unclear [8–10]. Initiation of lipid peroxidation occurs when a radical species attacks and removes an allylic hydrogen from an unsaturated fatty acid (LH) forming the carbon centered alkyl radical (L·). The alkyl radical readily combines with molecular O_2 to form a peroxyl radical (LOO·) which in turn, can attack another unsaturated fatty acid resulting in the initiating of a radical chain reaction process (reactions 8–10). The rate and extent of lipid peroxidation is dependent upon the degree of fatty acid saturation with more highly unsaturated lipid being most susceptible to radical attack. Radical attack of unsaturated fatty acid also results in the conversion of the normal cis double bond configuration of the fatty acid to the trans configuration. This bond conversion causes fatty acid chains to straighten and leads to physical changes within the membrane.

$$LH + R\cdot \rightarrow L\cdot + RH \qquad (8)$$

$$L\cdot + O_2 \rightarrow LOO\cdot \qquad (9)$$

$$LOO\cdot + LH \rightarrow LOOH + L\cdot \qquad (10)$$

Once lipid peroxidation begins, iron may participate in driving the process as lipid hydroperoxides (LOOH) formed through initiation are decomposed by reactions with either Fe^{II}, Fe^{III} or their chelates (reactions 11–12).

$$LOOH + Fe^{II} \rightarrow LO\cdot + OH^- + Fe^{III} \qquad (11)$$

$$LOOH + Fe^{III} \rightarrow LOO\cdot + Fe^{II} \qquad (12)$$

Both the reactions of LOOH with iron have acidic pH optima [11]. During *in vitro* lipid peroxidation, the major pathway for oxidation of Fe^{II} appears to be through decomposition of LOOH [12, 13]. Either alkoxyl (LO·) or peroxyl (LOO·) radicals arising from LOOH decomposition by iron can initiate so called lipid hydroperoxide dependent lipid peroxidation (reactions 10 and 13) resulting in chain branching reactions.

$$LOO\cdot + LH \rightarrow LOOH + L\cdot \qquad (10)$$

$$LO\cdot + LH \rightarrow LOH + L\cdot \qquad (13)$$

The presence of pre-existing LOOH within normal healthy cell membranes is a subject for consideration. It is obvious that cells would not have evolved defense mechanisms against radical damage and lipid peroxidation (e.g. superoxide dismutase, catalase, glutathione reductase) unless a need existed. During normal cellular energy metabolism, oxygen radicals and H_2O_2 are produced. In addition, oxygen radicals or H_2O_2 and lipid hydroperoxides are produced during processes such as catechol metabolism by monoamine oxidase [14], arachidonic acid metabolism [15], and phagocytosis [16]. Thus, unless cellular defenses against radical production and damage are 100% efficient, a certain fraction of radicals would be expected to escape cellular scavenging processes and result in lipid peroxidation. It has in fact, been proposed by Sevanian and co-workers that oxidation of fatty acids within membranes and their hydrolysis by phospholipases is involved in the normal turnover of membrane lipid [17, 18]. Thus, provided that a source of iron exists, lipid hydroperoxide dependent lipid peroxidation may be initiated since sufficient LOOH may pre-exist in normal membranes to allow this process to occur.

The Ischemic Cell Environment

A number of changes occur within the cell during ischemia which alter its environment and tend to favor the formation of oxygen radicals and lipid peroxidation. Very rapidly after the onset of ischemia, the production of ATP by mitochondria ceases and levels of ATP and phosphocreatine fall sharply as the available pool of high energy phosphates is consumed. Although the actual magnitude of the change in ATP and phosphocreatine may vary in different brain regions with ischemia, reductions around 10-fold for ATP and as much as 60-fold for phosphocreatine are generally observed [17, 18]. Coincident with sharp drops in high energy phosphates are large elevations in cellular lactic acid content [17, 18]. Lactate increases during ischemia for two reasons. First, as the cell experiences a reduction in oxygen delivery, it switches to anaerobic glycolysis converting available glucose to lactate. Second, because of the reduction in blood flow, lactic acid is not removed and tissue lactate concentrations may increase as much as 50-fold to around 30 mmol/kg [19]. Accompanying the increase in tissue lactic acid is the production of tissue acidosis. During ischemia, regional brain pH values have been estimated to fall as low as 6.0 with a range of between 5.9 and 6.4 [17, 20, 21].

The ischemic cell also undergoes changes in its ionic environment. Partially as the result of reductions in ATP, ionic pumps within the membrane that normally function to maintain cellular ion homeostasis fail, and as a result the intracellular concentrations of sodium and calcium rise while concentrations of potassium fall [17, 20, 22]. The rise in intracellular calcium has particularly important consequences on the cellular environment with regards to the generation of oxygen radicals as an elevation of intracellular calcium can lead to the activation of various proteolytic and phospholipase enzymes which may alter the bioavailability and reactivity of substrates for radical reactions. In addition, changes in ionic composition may directly affect lipid peroxidation reactions.

Sources of Oxygen Radicals in Mammalian Systems

Sources of O_2^- and H_2O_2

Changes in cellular metabolism and the ensuing alterations in the cellular environment that can result from ischemia or trauma create an environment that is fertile for the production of oxygen radicals and lipid peroxidation. The enhancement of radical generation and lipid peroxidation under conditions of ischemia occurs at several levels particularly: 1) the generation of O_2^-, and 2) the mobilization of iron (Table 2).

Coincident with the consumption of ATP during ischemia is the accumulation of AMP [17, 19] which is degraded to hypoxanthine [23]. Hypoxanthine is a substrate for the enzyme xanthine dehydrogenase that normally converts hypoxanthine to uric acid while generating NADH [24]. McCord has proposed that during ischemia, xanthine dehydrogenase is converted by limited proteolysis to xanthine oxidase [25]. Xanthine oxidase catalyzes the formation of O_2^- (and consequently H_2O_2) in the presence of hypoxanthine or xanthine [26]. This scheme is hypothesized to occur during reoxygenation resulting in a burst of O_2^- and H_2O_2 production that in turn precipitates structural injury. Evidence that O_2^- production by xanthine oxidase occurs in models of reperfusion ischemia is given by the findings that ischemia-induced damage to organs such as intestine [27], liver [28], skin [29], and heart [30] can be prevented by SOD, catalase or allopurinol, an inhibitor of xanthine oxidase. The use of allopurinol as an inhibitor of xanthine oxidase as evidence for the enzyme's role in reperfusion ischemia is not without its complications. However, the specificity of allopurinol is questionable since large doses are generally required in order to observe protection with the compound [29, 30]. Second, allopurinol and its primary active metabolite oxypurinol, are extremely potent scavengers of OH [31]. Thus, protective effects of allopurinol or oxypurinol in systems alone cannot be taken as conclusive evidence that O_2^- generated by xanthine oxidase is involved.

While the possible role of xanthine oxidase in the generation of O_2^- is fairly convincing in certain non-neuronal tissues, the issue is less clear. On the one hand, Chan et al. have demonstrated that the infusion of xanthine and xanthine oxidase into brain results in histopathological changes which mimic those seen

Table 2. The generation of oxygen radicals associated with ischemia-reperfusion injury

Injury:

- Xanthine dehydrogenase converted to xanthine oxidase which leads to the generation of O_2^-
- NADPH oxidase production of O_2^- associated with neutrophil activation
- Cyclogenase production of O_2^- due to arachidonic acid mobilization
- Catechol autoxidation associated with the release of catecholamines generates O_2^-
- Hemoglobin autoxidation associated with hemorrhage into tissue generates O_2^-
- Mitochondrial leak of O_2^- if electron chain becomes uncoupled
- Iron mobilized from ferritin or transferrin at reduced tissue pH readily catalyzes free radical reactions

following ischemia [32]. Cerchiari et al. have demonstrated that some level of neurological recovery can be achieved in dogs treated with a cocktail containing, among other things, SOD [33]. Badylak et al. have shown that allopurinol will prevent reperfusion injury associated with cardiac arrest followed by resuscitation in the rat [34]. Finally, Kontos et al. demonstrated that O_2^- is indeed generated in brain tissue following fluid percussion injury [35]. Clearly, such studies suggest that O_2^- (perhaps derived from xanthine oxidase) contributes to the pathophysiology of CNS ischemia. On the other hand, a recent study by Kim et al. has raised some doubt concerning the role of xanthine oxidase in the generation of O_2^- in the injured brain [36]. These investigators reported that following experimental subarachnoid hemorrhage, delayed vasospasm of the basilar artery was associated with large elevations in cerebrospinal fluid uric acid levels, suggesting that xanthine oxidase was active. Nevertheless, while allopurinol completely abolished the rise in CSF uric acid, it did not prevent vasospasm. It may be argued that subarachnoid hemorrhage differs considerably from ischemia despite the fact that there is a progressive cerebral ischemia which develops following subarachnoid hemorrhage [37]. It is increasingly clear however, that oxygen radicals and lipid peroxidation play a major role in the pathophysiology of subarachnoid hemorrhage and cerebral vasospasm [38, 39].

While there is evidence that xanthine oxidase generated O_2^- may contribute to ischemic damage associated with ischemia in a variety of tissues including brain, the level of the enzyme's involvement in different experimental models and human disease remains to be determined. Observations that SOD provides some protection against damage in models of cerebral ischemia certainly are consistent with the involvement of O_2^-. The source of O_2^- remains in question. Early studies had suggested that the concentration of xanthine dehydrogenase in brain tissue itself was zero [40]. More recently, however, Beckman et al. have reported that brain does indeed contain low, but measurable concentrations of xanthine dehydrogenase that is converted to xanthine oxidase during reperfusion of ischemic brain [41]. Furthermore, the brain vasculature contains substantial xanthine dehydrogenase [42]. Thus, xanthine dehydrogenase in plasma, brain endothelial cells or brain tissue itself may provide sufficient xanthine oxidase activity to catalyze the formation of O_2^- particularly in the presence of large amounts of hypoxanthine, which is known to accumulate rapidly in the ischemic brain [23, 36]. Xanthine oxidase needs not be the only source of O_2^- within the ischemic brain. Coenzyme Q or ubiquinone, a component of the electron transport chain, normally exists as a semiquinone free radical during active electron transport [43]. Even under normal circumstances, however, some mitochondrial leak of O_2^- and H_2O_2 is known to occur [44, 45]. When O_2^- supplies are reduced, the components of the electron chain may uncouple [46] and mitochondrial leak of O_2^- may increase [45, 47, 48].

Another important source of O_2^- in the injured or ischemic brain is the respiratory burst associated with neutrophil activation in response to tissue injury. Synthesis of O_2^- by the NADH oxidase of neutrophils may result in significant cellular damage by exposing tissues to localized high concentrations of neutrophil-derived oxygen radicals [49]. Several laboratories have provided evidence for the recruitment of phagocytic cells into regions of ischemic or traumatic CNS injury [50–52].

Superoxide may also be generated in the CNS as the result of arachidonic acid metabolism by the cyclooxygenase pathway. As will be discussed later, traumatic or ischemic injury results in the release of large amounts of free arachidonic acid. Kontos and coworkers have hypothesized that the generation of O_2^- in injured brain [35] occurs as released arachidonic acid is converted first to PGG_2 and then to PGH_2 [53]. According to their scheme, prostaglandin synthetase operates as an enzyme free radical during the conversion of PGG to PGH_2 and can oxidize the reduced forms of either NADH or NADPH to their respective radicals (e.g. NAD or NADP). The nucleotide radicals can be readily oxidized by molecular oxygen to generate O_2^-. Although this process probably occurs normally, it may be markedly enhanced during ischemia as high concentrations of arachidonic acid and reduced nucleotides accumulate.

Another source of O_2^- is the autoxidation of catecholamines. The CNS is rich in dopamine, epinephrine and norepinephrine. Any of these can autoxidize and form O_2^-, a process that is enhanced in the presence of metals such as iron [54]. In addition to the autoxidation of catecholamines resulting in the formation of O_2^-, their degradation by the enzyme monoamine oxidase results in the formation of H_2O_2 [12]. The re-uptake of catecholamines from the synaptic cleft by neurons and its repackaging into vesicles are energy requiring processes. With the onset of ischemia, catecholamines released through neurotransmission will accumulate within cells and synapses [55] to react with monamine oxidase. In addition, brain catecholamines may directly affect radical processes within brain tissue as demonstrated by the fact that depletion of brain catecholamines by reserpine markedly reduces the susceptibility of brain tissue to lipid peroxidation [56].

Following trauma, intracerebral or subarachnoid hemorrhage, the CNS is directly exposed to blood derived hemoglobin. In addition to providing a rich source of iron (see below), the slow autoxidation of hemoglobin may give rise to O_2^- [54].

Sources of Iron

The involvement of iron in the generation of oxygen radicals and the process of lipid peroxidation have been discussed. The brain is an extremely rich source of iron and its regional distribution varies in parallel with the sensitivity of various brain regions to *in vitro* lipid peroxidation [57]. Under normal circumstances, low molecular weight forms of redox active iron is maintained, at extremely low or non-existent levels. Extracellularly in plasma, the iron transport protein transferrin tightly binds iron in the Fe^{III} form. Intracellularly, Fe^{III} is sequestered by the iron storage protein ferritin. While both ferritin and transferrin have very high affinity for iron at neutral pH and effectively maintain iron in a noncatalytic state [60], both proteins readily give up their iron at pH values of 6.0 or less. In the case of ferritin, its iron can also be released through reductive mobilization by O_2^- [6, 58]. Once iron is released from ferritin or transferrin it can actively catalyze oxygen radical and lipid peroxidation reactions [6].

A second source of catalytically active iron is hemoglobin. Hemorrhage resulting from mechanical trauma is an obvious source of hemoglobin. Ischemia associated with hemorrhage also provides hemoglobin as will cellular necrosis leading to a disruption of the blood brain barrier. While hemoglobin itself has been reported to stimulate lipid peroxidation [59], it is more likely iron released from hemoglobin which is responsible for hemoglobin mediated lipid peroxidation. Gutteridge however, has shown that hemoglobin can directly stimulate lipid peroxidation through decomposition of preexisting LOOH [60], in agreement with earlier studies by O'Brien [61]. Iron is released from hemoglobin by H_2O_2 or lipid hydroperoxides [60] and this release is further enhanced as the pH falls to 6.5 or below [Braughler, unpublished observations]. In the ischemic cellular environment, therefore, hemoglobin may catalyze oxygen radical formation and lipid peroxidation either directly or through the release of iron by H_2O_2, LOOH and/or acidic pH.

Treatment of Experimental Central Nervous System Trauma and Ischemia: Use of a Novel 21-Aminosteroid

General Comments

There is an urgent need for new therapeutic modalities in the treatment of CNS trauma and ischemia. Physicians often look upon the treatment of CNS trauma and ischemia with reservation because effective therapy in these areas has not significantly advanced over recent years. Moreover, treatment is often delayed in these entities as a consequence of inadequate and inefficient emergency medical care. The therapeutic window is frequently closed as a result. Therapeutic nihilism however is unwarranted. A better understanding of the pathophysiology of these conditions has led to more directed research which doubtless will lead to new and effective therapies. Moreover, recognition of the emergency nature of these conditions has resulted in the formation in many metropolitan areas, of elaborate and effective emergency medical systems. This has allowed many patients to reach medical facilities in time for effective treatment.

A complex series of pathophysiological events follow an initial traumatic or ischemic insult to the CNS [4, 62]. These "secondary" factors include such events as:

1. ion shifts into and out of cells,
2. activation of destructive enzymes,
3. accumulation of harmful neurotransmitters and amino acids,
4. the excess formation of toxic free radicals.

Free radical induced lipid peroxidation is potentially one of the most critical factors leading to secondary CNS injury following trauma or ischemia. The following information will describe a series of experimental studies in CNS trauma and ischemia with a new and novel compound, U-74,006F - a 21-aminosteroid which is a potent inhibitor of free radical induced lipid peroxidation. The 21-aminosteroids were the result of an effort to develop nonglucocorticoids that mimicked the protective effects of high doses of synthetic glucocorticoids (e.g. methylprednisolone) in the injured CNS. It was hypothesized that the beneficial effect of methylprednisolone in the CNS was a nonglucocorticoid action, most likely the ability of the compound to inhibit lipid peroxidation both in vivo and in vitro [63–65]. An effort ensued to synthesize compounds that were potent inhibitors of lipid peroxidation that lacked glucocorticoid activity. Since 1985, several hundred of these compounds have been synthesized, one of which, U-74,006F, was selected for clinical development.

The Basic Mechanism of Action of U-74,006F

The 21-aminosteroids have been shown to be potent inhibitors or iron-catalyzed lipid peroxidation in vitro [66]. In rat brain homogenates or purified brain synaptosomes micromolar concentrations of U-74,006F have been shown to inhibit lipid peroxidation in the presence of iron. While the mechanism by which U-74,006F inhibits lipid peroxidation is not completely clear, it does appear to involve the inhibition of lipid chain reactions through scavenging of both LO· and LOO· [5]. Using in vitro systems involving pure LOO· or LO· inhibition constants for U-74,006F have been determined as 1.4×10^3 and 3.3×10^6 M-1 sec-1, respectively, suggesting that reactivity toward LOO· is considerably greater than for LO·. The ability of U-74,006F to scavenge LOO· or LO· is considerably less than Vitamin-E; nevertheless, U-74,006F is nearly as effective as Vitamin-E at inhibiting lipid peroxidation in intact membranes [66]. In fact, U-74,006F can actually spare Vitamin-E from utilization during lipid peroxidation [67] suggesting that mechanisms in addition to scavenging LOO· or LO· may be involved in its action.

In addition to its ability to scavenge radicals and inhibit lipid peroxidation, U-74,006F has other stabilizing effects of cell membranes. The release of free arachidonic acid from injured cell membranes is blocked by U-74,006F [68]. In other unpublished studies using cultured bovine brain microvessel endothelial cells, the 21-aminosteroids have been shown to localize within the hydrophobic core of cell membranes and cause an increase in lipid ordering (e.g. decrease fluidity) of the phospholipid bilayer [Audus and Braughler, unpublished observations].

In summary, U-74,006F has been shown to inhibit lipid peroxidation and to scavenge radicals. This activity is believed to be responsible for its activity in vivo in experimental models of cerebral ischemia. Evidence for an antioxidant effect of U-74,006F has been obtained from studies demonstrating its ability to preserve tissue and plasma Vitamin-E in experimental animals following experimental stroke or global ischemia associated following cardiac arrest [69, 70].

Effects of U-74,006F in Models of Central Nervous System Trauma

Treatment of Experimental Head Injury with U-74,006F

U-74,006F has been tested in three different experimental head injury models consistently showing a beneficial effect. In an initial study, acute/intravenous administration of the compound to male CF-1 mice was shown to facilitate the early neurological recovery and one week survival after severe concussive head injury [71]. One hour post-traumatic recovery (grip test score) was significantly benefitted over a broad range of doses (0.003-30.0 mg/kg) as a single i.v. bolus within 5 min after injury. A 1 mg/kg dose given within 5 min and again at 1.5 h after severe injury increased 1 week survival by nearly three fold, 27.3% in vehicle treated mice versus 78.6% in the U-74,006F treated. U-74,006F was also effective in improving recovery after more moderate injury.

In a cat severe concussive head injury model, U-74,006F given in a 1 mg/kg i.v. dose at 30 min post-injury and again at 2.5 h has been shown to significantly reduce 4 h cerebral cortical and white matter lactic acid accumulation [72]. In view of the likelihood that the brain tissue lactic acidosis is the result post-traumatic ischemia, its attenuation to near normal levels by U-74,006F suggests a beneficial effect of the compound on cerebral blood flow. While direct blood flow studies have not been carried out in experimental head injury, U-74,006F has been shown to attenuate post-traumatic spinal cord ischemia after either contusion or concussion injury [73, 74].

U-74,006F has further been demonstrated to facilitate 72 h neurological recovery in rats subjected to moderate fluid percussion head injury plus a secondary 45 min period of hypoxia [L. H. Pitts, personal communication].

Treatment of Experimental Spinal Cord Injury with U-74,006F

U-74,006F has been shown to promote recovery from compression injury of the spinal cord in cats [75] and prevent the phenomenon of posttraumatic hypoperfusion of the contused spinal cord also in cats [73]. Anderson et al., in a randomized blinded placebo controlled study, evaluated the dose-response characteristics and capability of U-74,006F to promote functional recovery in cats subjected to compression trauma of the lumber spinal cord [75]. U-74,006F was administered i.v. in doses ranging from 0.048 to 160.0 mg/kg. The animals were evaluated weekly for neurological recovery and animals receiving accumulated doses of U-74,006F ranging from 1.6 to 160.0 mg/kg/48 h exhibited nearly 75% of normal neurological function by 4 weeks after injury. These findings show that over a 100-fold dose range, U-74,006F has a remarkable capacity to promote functional recovery in spinal cord injured cats. Hall studied the effect of U-74,006F on the phenomenon of post-trauma hypoperfusion in the cat spinal cord 30 min after contusion injury of the lumbar area [73]. Blood flow in the spinal cord white matter was measured with the hydrogen clearance technique, and blood flow in the vehicle treated group was reduced by 63.5% compared to pre-injury controls. U-74,006F in contrast, almost completely prevented the development of post-traumatic hypoperfusion at a single dose of 10 mg/kg. In more recent unpublished studies, U-74,006F in doses as low as 1 mg/kg, was found to antagonize the development of post-traumatic ischemia in the spinal cord in a compression injury model [Hall, unpublished observation].

Treatment of Experimental Subarachnoid Hemorrhage with U-74,006F

Delayed cerebral vasospasm following subarachnoid hemorrhage (SAH) is a leading cause of death and long term disability [76]. There is an urgent need for effective treatment of vasospasm following SAH. Studies have been conducted in cats [77], rabbits [78], and monkeys [79] using U-74,006F for the treatment of cerebral vasospasm. Initial studies using a single intravenous bolus of U-74,006F following the introduction of autologous blood into the subarachnoid space of cats, prevented post-SAH induced cerebral hypoperfusion as measured in the caudate nucleus [77]. Vollmer et al. conducted a study to determine if U-74,006F would prevent the development of delayed cerebral vasospasm after experimental SAH in a rabbit model [78]. Autologous blood was introduced into the subarachnoid space of rabbits and U-74,006F (1 mg/kg) or placebo was injected once every 12 h for a total of 6 doses, starting 12 h prior to the SAH. The animals were sacrificed 24 h after SAH and the luminal diameter of the basilar artery was measured. U-74,006F treated animals showed only a 15% reduction in luminal diameter while a 44% reduction occurred in the luminal diameter of placebo animals. Steinke et al. evaluated U-74,006F in the prophylaxis of chronic cerebral vasospasm in a randomized, blinded, placebo-controlled trial in monkeys [79]. Experimental SAH was produced by introducing autologous clot next to the middle cerebral artery following craniectomy. U-74,006F or placebo were administered from day 1 to 6, i.v. every 8 h. Angiography was performed at baseline and at 7 days. CT-scan or MRI were done if there was evidence of delayed ischemic deficit. There was a significant difference in the degree of angiographic vasospasm in the internal carotid and middle cerebral arteries between the placebo and U-74,006F treated animals due to a greater degree of vasospasm in the control group.

Treatment of Experimental Cerebral Ischemia with U-74,006F

Initial focus ischemia studies with U-74,006F in gerbils demonstrated that treatment (10 mg/kg i.p.) 10 min before and immediately after a 3 h period of unilateral carotid occlusion improved 28 and 48 h survival. A histological examination of the brain at 24 h post-ischemia in another group of vehicle treated animals revealed marked neuronal loss in the hippocampus and lateral cerebral cortex. In contrast, the neuronal densities in the ischemic hemisphere of U-74,006F treated gerbils were significantly preserved in both brain regions [78]. More recent physiological studies in the same model have shown that U-74,006F acts to reduce the post-ischemic depletion of brain Vitamin-E at 2 and 24 h after reperfusion together with a facilitated recovery of extracellular calcium

[E. D. Hall and J. M. Braughler unpublished data]. The protection of brain Vitamin-E supports the view that the U-74,006F cereprotective effect is due to inhibition of post-ischemic lipid peroxidation. The enhanced recovery of calcium (i. e. reversal of intracellular accumulation) may be due to the consequent protection of membrane calcium extrusion mechanisms.

U-74,006F has also been shown to reduce post-ischemic brain damage in the cat following a 1 h temporary occlusion of the middle cerebral artery [79]. Beginning 15 min after occlusion release, U-74,006F was administered as a multiple bolus regimen that was continued for 12 h. At one week, using classical histological and quantitative 2-deoxy-glucose autoradiographic techniques, the area of cerebral infarction was significantly reduced compared to that in vehicle treated cats.

The effects of U-74,006F on brain ionic shifts and edema have been examined in a permanent middle cerebral artery occlusion model in rats [80]. In those studies, U-74,006F given as a 3 mg/kg intravenous bolus dose 10 min and 3 h after occlusion significantly reduced 24 h post-ischemic brain Na^+ accumulation, K^+ loss and edema around the infarct site. In other studies, U-74,006F pretreatment has been found to block the formation of vasogenic edema in the brain of rats induced by intracerebral injection of arachidonic acid [78].

U-74,006F has also been demonstrated to improve post-ischemic cerebral blood flow (CBF). In cats, following a 5 min period of near total global cerebral ischemia, CBF was found to decline progressively during the 3 h post-ischemic period in vehicle-treated animals [81]. In comparison, CBF remained significantly greater in animals receiving a single 1 mg/kg intravenous bolus of U-74,006F at 15 min post-ischemia. In addition, U-74,006F treatment significantly enhanced the recovery of somatosensory evoked potentials, reduced post-ischemic arterial acidosis, and improved post-ischemic blood pressure. The improved support of CBF is probably due to both a better maintenance of cerebral perfusion pressure (i. e. arterial blood pressure) and a direct protection of the cerebral microvasculature.

Summary

In summary, U-74,006F has proven to be an effective therapy in the treatment of experimental head trauma, SAH, global cerebral ischemia and stroke. Clinical trials are planned in the near future with this compound in traumatic head injury, SAH and stroke.

References

1. Aust SD, Morehouse LA, Thomas CE (1985) Role of metals in oxygen radical reactions. J Free Rad Biol Med 1:3–25
2. Halliwell B, Gutteridge JMC (1985) Free radicals in biology and medicine. Claredon Press, Oxford
3. Miller JD (1985) Head injury and brain ischemia-implications for therapy. Br J Anaesth 57:120–129

4. Means ED, Anderson DK (1987) Pathophysiology of acute spinal cord injury. In: Davidoff RA (ed) Handbook of the spinal cord, vol 4–5. Dekker, New York, pp 19–61
5. Braughler JM, Hall ED (1989) Central nervous system trauma and stroke: biochemical considerations for oxygen radical formation and lipid peroxidation. J Free Rad Biol Med (in press)
6. Thomas CE, Morehouse LA, Aust SD (1985) Ferritin and superoxide-dependent lipid peroxidation. J Biol Chem 260:3275–3280
7. Fee JA (1982) On the question of superoxide toxicity and the biological function of superoxide dismutases. In: King TE, Mason HS, Morrison M (eds) Oxidases and related redox systems. Pergamon Press, New York, pp 101–149
8. Girotti AW, Thomas JP (1984) Damaging effects of oxygen radicals on resealed erythrocyte ghosts. J Biol Chem 259:1744–1752
9. Braughler JM, Duncan LA, Chase RL (1986) The involvement of iron in lipid peroxidation: importance of ferric to ferrous ratios in irritation. J Biol Chem 261:10282–10289
10. Minotti G, Aust SD (1987) The requirement for ferric in initiation of lipid peroxidation by ferrous hydrogen peroxide. J Biol Chem 262:1098–1104
11. Braughler JM, Chase RL, Pregenzer JF (1987) Oxidation of ferrous iron during peroxidation of lipid substrates. Biochim Biophys Acta 921:457–464
12. Marker HS, Weiss C, Silides DJ, Cohen G (1981) Coupling of dopamine oxidation (monoamine oxidase acitivity) to glutathione oxidation via the generation of hydrogen peroxide in rat brain homogenates. J Neurochem 36:589–593
13. Yamamoto S (1983) Enzymes in the arachidonic acid cascade. In: Pace-Ascieak C, Granstrom E (eds) Prostaglandins and related substances. Elsevier, Amsterdam, pp 171–202
14. Fantone JC, Ward PA (1982) Role of oxygen-derived free radicals and metabolites in leukocyte-dependent inflammatory reactions. Am J Pathol 107:397–418
15. Sevaniar A, Kim E (1985) Phospholipase A_2 dependent release of fatty acids from peroxidized membranes. J Free Rad Biol Med 1:263–271
16. van Kuijk FIGM, Sevanian A, Handelman GJ, Dratz EA (1987) A new role for phospholipase A: protection of membranes from lipid peroxidation damage. TIBS 12:31–34
17. Siesjö BK (1981) Cell damage in the brain: a speculative synthesis. J Cereb Blood Flow Metab 1:155–185
18. Marcy VR, Welsh FA (1984) Correlation between cerebral blood flow and ATP content following tourniquet-induced ischemia in cat brain. J Cereb Blood Flow Metab 4:362–367
19. Welsh FA (1984) Acidosis and energy metabolism. In: Bes A, Braquet P, Paoletti R, Siesjö BK (eds) Elsevier, Amsterdam, pp 177–186
20. Siesjö BK (1984) Brain acid-base metabolism in health and disease. Cereb Blood Flow Metab 1:157–166
21. von Hanwehr R, Smith M, Siesjö BK (1986) Extra- and intra-cellular pH during nearcomplete forebrain ischemia in the rat. J Neurochem 46:331–339
22. Young W, Rappaport ZH, Chalif DJ, Flamm ES (1987) Regional brain sodium, potassium and water changes in the middle cerebral artery occlusion model of ischemia. Stroke 18:751–759
23. Kleihues P, Kobayashi K, Hossmann KA (1974) Purine nucleotide metabolism in the cat brain after one hour of complete ischemia. J Neurochem 23:417–425
24. Batteli MG, Corte ED, Stripe F (1972) Xanthine oxidase type D (dehydrogenase) in the intestine and other organs of the rat. Biochem J 126:747–749
25. McCord JM (1985) Oxygen-derived free radicals in post ischemic tissue injury. N Engl J Med 312:159–163
26. McCord JM, Fridovich I (1968) The reduction of cytochrome c by milk xanthine oxidase. J Biol Chem 243:5753–5760
27. Parks DA, Bulkley GB, Granger DN, Hamilton SR, McCord JM (1982) Ischemic injury in the cat small intestine: role of superoxide radicals. Gastroenterology 82:9–15
28. Adkison D, Hollwarth ME, Benoit IN, Parks DA, McCord JM, Granger DN (1986) Role of free radicals in ischemia-reperfusion injury to the liver. Acta Physiol Scand (suppl) 548:101–107

29. Im MJ, Manson PN, Bulkley GB, Hoopes JE (1985) Effects of superoxide dismutase and allopurinol on the survival of acute island skin flaps. Ann Surg 201:357–359
30. Chambers DE, Parks DA, Patterson G, et al (1985) Xanthine oxidase as a source of free radical damage in myocardial ischemia. J Mol Cell Cardiol 17:145–152
31. Moorhouse PC, Grootveld M, Halliwell B, Quinlan JG, Gutteridge JMC (1987) Allopurinol and oxypurinol are hydroxyl radical scavengers. FEBS Lett 213:23–28
32. Chan PH, Schmidley JW, Fishman RA, Langar SM (1984) Brain injury, edema, and vascular permeability changes induced by oxygen-derived free radicals. Neurology 34:315–320
33. Cerchiari EL, Hoel TM, Safar P, Schlabassi RI (1987) Protective effects of combined superoxide dismutase and desferrioxamine on recovery of cerebral blood flow and function after cardiac arrest in dogs. Stroke 18:869–878
34. Badylak SF, Babbs CF, Kougias C, Blaho K (1986) Effect of allopurinol and dimethylsulfoxide on long-term survival in rats after cardiorespiratory arrest and resuscitation. Am J Emerg Med 4:313–318
35. Kontos HA, Wei EP (1986) Superoxide production in experimental brain injury. J Neurosurg 64:803–807
36. Kim P, Yaksh TL, Romero SD, Sundt TM (1987) Production of uric acid in cerebrospinal fluid after subarachnoid hemorrhage in dog: investigation of the possible role of xanthine oxidase in chronic vasospasm. Neurosurg 21:39–44
37. Ecker A, Reimenschneider PA (1951) Arteriographic demonstration of spasm of the intracranial arteries with special reference to saccular arterial aneurysms. J Neurosurg 8:660–667
38. Sano K, Asano T, Tanishima T, Sasaki T (1980) Lipid peroxidation as a cause of cerebral vasospasm. Neurol Res 2:253–272
39. Travis MA, Hall ED (1987) The effects of chronic two-fold dietary vitamin E supplementation on subarachnoid hemorrhage-induced brain hypoperfusion. Brain Res 408:366–370
40. Stirpe F, Della Corte E (1969) The regulation of rat liver xanthine oxidase. J Biol Chem 244:3855–3863
41. Beckman JS, Liu TH, Hogan EI, Freeman BA, Hsu CY (1987) Oxygen free radicals and xanthine oxidase in cerebral ischemic injury in the rat. Soc Neurosci (Abstr) 13:1498
42. Betz AL (1985) Identification of hypoxanthine transport and xanthine oxidase activity in brain capillaries. J Neurochem 44:574–579
43. Ruzicz FJ, Beinert H, Schilper KL, Dunham WR, Sands RH (1975) Interaction of ubisemiquinone with a paramagnetic component in heart tissue. Proc Natl Acad Sci 72:2886–2891
44. Turrens JF, Alexandre A, Lehninger A (1985) Ubisemiquinone is the electron donor for superoxide formation by complex III of heart mitochondria. Arch Biochem Biophys 237:408–414
45. Patole MS, Swaroop A, Ramasarma T (1986) Generation of H_2O_2 in brain mitochondria. J Neurochem 47:1–8
46. Demopoulos HB (1973) The free radical pathology. Fed Proc 32:1859
47. Boveris A, Cadenas E, Stoppani AOM (1976) Role of ubiquinone in mitochondrial generation of hydrogen peroxide. Biochem J 156:5435–5444
48. Demopoulos HB, Flamm ES, Pietronigro DD, Seligman ML (1980) The free radical pathology and microcirculation in the major central nervous system disorders. Acta Physiol Scand (suppl) 492:91–119
49. McCord JM (1987) Oxygen-derived radicals: a link between reperfusion injury and inflammation. Fed Proc 46:2402–2406
50. Means ED, Anderson DK (1983) Neuronophagia by leukocytes in experimental spinal cord injury. J Neuropath Exp Neurol 42:707–719
51. Hallenbeck JM, Dutka AJ, Tanishima T, et al (1986) Polymorphonuclear leukocyte accumulation in brain regions with low blood flow during the early post ischemic period. Stroke 17:246–253
52. Grome JJ, Gojowczyk G, Hofmann W, Graham DI (1988) Quantitation of photochemically induced focal cerebral ischemia in the rat. J Cerebr Blood Flow Metabol 8:89–95
53. Kukreja RC, Kontos HA, Hess MH, Ellis EF (1986) PGH synthase and lipoxygenase generate superoxide in the presence of NADH or NADPH. Circ Res 59:612–619

54. Misra HP, Fridovich I (1972) The generation of superoxide radical during the autoxidation of hemoglobin. J Biol Chehem 247:6960–6962
55. Lavyne MH, Moskowitz MA, Larin F, Zervas NT, Wurtman RJ (1975) Brain H^3-catecholamine metabolism in experimental cerebral ischemia. Neurology 25:483–485
56. Chakrabarti S, Komar S, Shankar R (1986) Reserpine inhibition of lipid peroxidation and protein phosphorylation in rat brain. Biochem Pharmacol 35:1611–1613
57. Zaleska MM, Floyd RA (1985) Regional lipid peroxidation in rat brain in vitro: possible role of endogenous iron. Neurochem Res 10:397–410
58. Koster JF, Slee RG (1986) Ferritin, a physiological iron donor for microsomal lipid peroxidation. FEBS Lett 199:85–88
59. Sadrzadeh SM, Graf E, Panter SS, Hallaway PE, Eaton JW (1984) Hemoglobin, a biological Fenton reagent. J Biol Chem 259:14354–14356
60. Gutteridge JMC (1986) Antioxidant properties or proteins ceruloplasmin, albumin and transferrin: a study of their activity in serum and synovial fluid from patients with rheumatoid arthritis. Biochim Biophys Acta 869:119–127
61. O'Brien PI (1969) Intracellular mechanisms for the decomposition of a lipid peroxide I. Decomposition of a lipid peroxide by metal ions, nerve compounds and nucleophiles. Can J Biochem 47:485–492
62. Siesjö BK (1988) Mechanisms of ischemic brain damage. Crit Care Med 16:954–963
63. Hall ED, Braughler JM (1981) Acute effects of intravenous glucocorticoid pretreatment on the *in vitro* peroxidation of cat spinal cord tissue. Exp Neurol 73:321–324
64. Anderson DK, Means ED (1983) Lipid peroxidation in spinal cord: $FeCl_2$ induction and protection with antioxidants. Neurochem Path 1:249–264
65. Kurihara M (1985) Role of monamines in experimental spinal cord injury: relationship between $Na^+ + K^+$ ATPase and lipid peroxidation. J Neurosurg 62:743–749
66. Braughler JM, Pregenzer JF, Chase RL, Duncan LA, Jacobsen EI, McCall JM (1987) Novel 21-aminosteroids as potent inhibitors of iron-dependent lipid peroxidation. J Biol Chem 262:10438–10440
67. Braughler JM, Pregenzer JF (1989) The 21-aminosteroid inhibitors of lipid peroxidation: reactions with lipid peroxyl and phenoxy radicals. J Free Rad Biol Med (in press)
68. Braughler JM, Chase RL, Neff GL, et al (1988) A new 21-aminosteroid antioxidant lacking glucorticoid activity stimulates ACTH secretion and blocks arachidonic acid release from mouse pituitary tumor (AtT-20) cells. J Pharmacol Exp Ther 244:423–427
69. Hall ED, Berry KP, Braughler JM (1988) The 21-aminosteroid lipid peroxidation inhibitor U-74,006F protects against cerebral ischemia in gerbils. Stroke 19:997–1002
70. Natale JE, Schott RJ, Hall ED, Braughler JM, D'Alecy LG (1988) The 21-aminosteroid U-74,006F reduces systemic lipid peroxidation, improves neurological function, and reduces mortality after cardiopulmonary arrest in dogs. Stroke 19:1371–1378
71. Hall ED, Yonkers PA, McCall JM, Braughler JM (1988) Effects of the 21-aminosteroid U-74,006F on experimental head injury in mice. J Neurosurg 68:456–461
72. Dimlich RVW, Tornheim PA, Kindel RM, Hall ED, Braughler JM, McCall JM (1989) The effects of a 21-aminosteroid on cerebral metabolites and edema after severe experimental head injury. Adv Neurol (in press)
73. Hall ED (1988) Effect of the 21-aminosteroid U-74,006F on post-traumatic spinal cord ischemia. J Neurosurg 68:462–465
74. Hall ED, Yonkers PA, Braughler JM (1988) Attenuation of post-traumatic ischemia by the lipid peroxidation inhibitor U-74,006F: comparison in a contusion vs compression model. Neurosc Abst 14:1154
75. Anderson DK, Braughler JM, Hall ED, Waters TR McCall JM, Means ED (1988) Dose-response effects of U-74,006F on neurological recovery in an experimental model of spinal cord injury. J Neurosurg 69:562–567
76. Heros RC, Zervas NT, Varsos V (1983) Cerebral vasospasm after subarachnoid hemorrhage: an update. Ann Neurol 14:599–608
77. Hall ED, Travis MA (1989) Effects of the non-glucorticoid 21-aminosteroid U-74,006F on progressive brain hypoperfusion following experimental subarachnoid hemorrhage. Exp Neurol (in press)

78a. Hall ED, Travis MA (1988) Inhibition of arachidonic acid-induced vasogenic brain edema by the non-glucocorticoid 21-aminosteroid U-74,006F. Brain Res 451:350–352
78b. Vollmer DG, Kassell NE, Hongo K, Ogawa H, Tsukahara T (1989) Effect of the non-glucocorticoid 21-aminosteroid U-74,006F in the treatment of experimental cerebral vasospasm. Surg Neurol (in press)
79a. Silvia RC, Piercey MF, Hoffmann WE, Chase RL, Braughler JM, Tang AH (1987) U-74,006F, an inhibitor of lipid peroxidation protects against lesion development following experimental stroke in the cat: Histological and metabolic analysis. Neurosci Abst 13:1499
79b. Steinke DE, Weir BKA, Findlay JM, Tanabe T, Grace M, Krushelnychy BD (1989) A trial of the 21-aminosteroid U-74,006F in a primate model of chronic cerebral vasospasm. Neurosurgery (in press)
80. Young W, Wojak JC, DeCrescito V (1988) Aminosteroid lipid peroxidation inhibitor reduces ionic shifts and edema in the rat middle cerebral artery occlusion model of regional ischemia. Stroke 19:1013–1019
81. Hall ED, Yonkers PA (1988) Attenuation of post-ischemic cerebral hypoperfusion by the 21-aminosteroid U-74,006F. Stroke 19:340–344

Brain Ischemia and Reperfusion Injury

J.R. Kirsch, M.A. Helfaer, R.C. Koehler, and R.J. Traystman

Introduction

During ischemia, brain injury results from an inadequate supply of substrate (oxygen and glucose) to meet metabolic needs. The most common clinical etiology for cerebral hypoxia is cerebral ischemia or the lack of an adequate blood supply to meet the brain's metabolic needs. Cerebral ischemia may occur in a variety of clinical settings including head trauma, postsurgical brain swelling, subarachnoid hemorrhage, stroke, and cardiac arrest. Even though ischemia is a recurring theme in each of these clinical settings it is clear from laboratory work that the pathophysiology of brain injury varies with different types of ischemia and therefore requires different therapeutic interventions. We will begin this review with a discussion of blood flow and metabolic changes during ischemia and the role of ion fluxes, ischemia induced release of excitatory amino acids and production of oxygen-derived free radicals in the pathophysiology of ischemic brain injury. We will conclude with a discussion of potential therapeutic options in protecting the brain from ischemic damage.

Pathophysiology

Cerebral Blood Flow: Ischemic Threshold

Normal values for cerebral blood flow (CBF) vary depending upon the conditions under which they are measured (e.g. anesthetized or awake, adult or newborn). Barbiturates and Etomidate decrease CBF whereas inhalation agents and ketamine increase CBF. In newborns CBF is less than in adults but in older children CBF is greater than found in adults. Although the ischemic threshold has not been studied in children, there is some evidence that newborn animals tolerate ischemia better than adult animals. Likewise there is some recent evidence that the ischemic threshold for damage may be different for different anesthetics. In general when adults have a CBF below 15 ml/min/100 g the brain's electrical activity fails and below 10 ml/min/100 g there is evidence for ionic pump failure which results in cell death. However, Ljunggren et al. observed that even though total ischemia in the rat for 3 min is followed by almost complete energy depletion, additional prolongation to 15 min does not preclude complete restoration of energy supply after recirculation [1]. Likewise, in some animal models, ischemia of up to an hour may be associated with recovery of function. Indeed, neurologic recovery is determined by not only the degree of ischemia but also the duration of ischemia and the metabolic environment during ischemia.

At a blood flow between 10 and 15 ml/min/100 g, although there may be functional impairment, cell structural integrity is maintained and recovery of function is possible. The area of brain which surrounds the core of focal ischemia may have flow in this range and has been called the "ischemic penumbra". Improving blood flow to the penumbra in an attempt to decrease the total amount of tissue damage from focal ischemia has become a major therapeutic goal.

Cerebral Blood Flow: Homeostatic Mechanisms

The brain has several homeostatic mechanisms to prevent a decrease in CBF when cerebral perfusion pressure is reduced. Perfusion pressure to the brain is defined as the difference between mean arterial blood pressure and intracranial pressure (or cerebral venous pressure which ever is larger). In normal adults CBF is maintained constant (autoregulated) between a perfusion pressure of 50–150 mm Hg (Fig. 1). Within the autoregulatory range a decrease in perfusion pressure is compensated for by a reduction in cerebral vascular resistance. Below or above the autoregulatory range blood flow is pressure passive. In patients with chronic hypertension, the autoregulation curve is shifted to the right so that the lower limit is greater than 50 mm Hg (depending on the degree of hypertension). In newborns the autoregulation curve is shifted to the left so that the lower limit is less than 50 (approximately 25–30 mm Hg).

When intracranial pressure is globally increased, homeostatic mechanisms (increased sympathetic outflow) cause systemic arterial blood pressure to increase in an attempt to maintain cerebral perfusion pressure (Cushing Response). An increase in intracranial pressure may have many different etiologies (e.g. head trauma, metabolic disturbances, tumor) but each disease process produces a component of injury via the common pathway of decreasing cerebral perfusion pressure, which with failure of homeostatic mechanisms results in decreased ce-

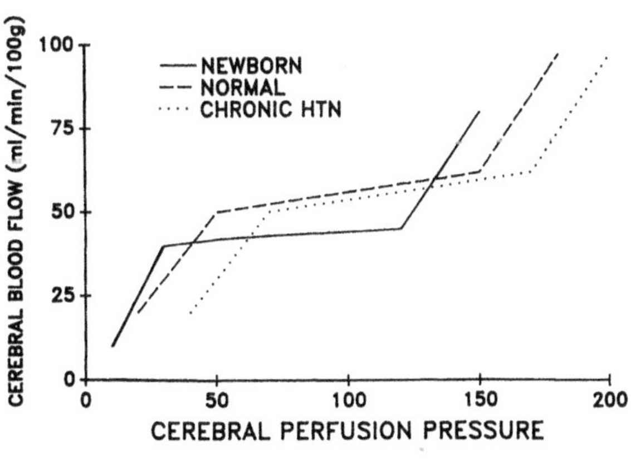

Fig. 1. This graph demonstrates classic cerebral autoregulation for newborn, normal adults and patients with chronic hypertension. The curve is shifted to the left in newborns and to the right in patients with chronic hypertension

rebral blood flow. Increased intracranial pressure may cause either a global or focal blood flow reduction depending on the regionality of the pressure elevation. A global increase in intracranial pressure is more likely to stimulate homeostatic mechanisms to increase arterial blood pressure. A focal increase in intracranial pressure is more likely to cause an immediate reduction in regional blood flow. Clinical diagnosis of regional increases in intracranial pressure may be difficult to make prior to the onset of signs of cerebral ischemia. Direct intracranial monitoring techniques which are currently available (e.g. ventricular drain, subarachnoid bolt) have no regional resolution. Alternatively, CT-scanning and a careful neurologic exam may be helpful for diagnosis and for following a patient's clinical progress.

Normally the brain extracts approximately 40% of the oxygen in arterial blood to drive metabolism (oxygen extraction = (arterial-cerebral venous oxygen content)/arterial oxygen content). When perfusion pressure is below the lower limit of autoregulation oxygen extraction increases to maintain normal oxygen uptake [oxygen uptake = CBF · (arterial-cerebral venous oxygen content)]. Eventually CBF decreases to a level which cannot be compensated for by increasing oxygen extraction and energy failure occurs (Fig. 2).

In the setting of focal ischemia an additional homeostatic mechanism involves dilation of collateral vessels which lead to the tissue at risk of infarction. For example, occlusion of large vessels may be compensated for by a change in flow pattern through the Circle of Willis. Improved blood flow through collateral blood vessels is less likely to prevent ischemia caused by occlusion of small vessels. In any case, therapeutic maneuvers should focus on improving blood flow through whatever collateral blood vessel exists.

Cerebral Blood Flow: Ischemic Penumbra

Focal ischemia (e.g. embolic and thrombotic stroke, transient ischemic attacks, vasospasm) is associated with several attributes which makes its pathophysiology distinct from global ischemia. Whereas in global ischemia flow is reduced throughout the brain, focal ischemia is associated with areas of different gradations of flow reduction. Today, clinical diagnosis of focal ischemia is made ear-

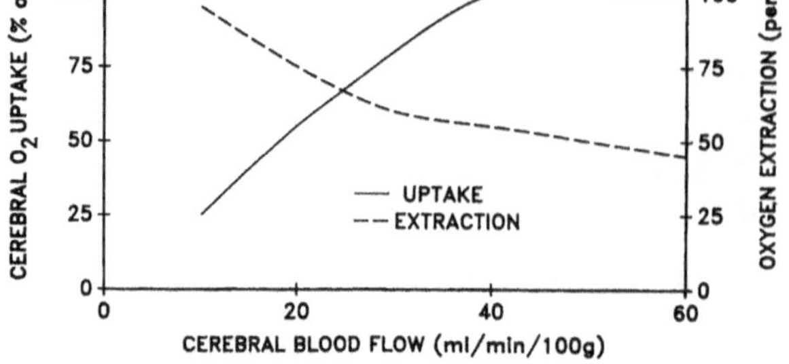

Fig. 2. This graph demonstrates the effect of decreasing cerebral blood flow on cerebral oxygen uptake on the left axis and on oxygen extraction on the right axis. As cerebral blood flow decreases, oxygen extraction increases, but not enough to avoid a decrease in cerebral oxygen uptake

liest with a careful neurologic exam. CBF measurements (133-Xe, N20, PET scanning, cerebral angiography) and CT-scanning are less helpful acutely but may be important parameters to follow over time. Focal ischemia is associated with three different areas of tissue based on it's blood flow and metabolic state (no flow, "trickle flow", or normal flow). In the center of the ischemic focus, blood flow is below the level required to maintain metabolism and the tissue is not viable. Blood vessels in this tissue do not autoregulate or respond normally to changes in carbon dioxide and oxygen. The penumbra area is tissue that surrounds the focus and has been defined by a reduction in blood flow which is associated with a reduction in electroencephalogram amplitude, spreading electrical depression, reduced cerebrovascular reactivity (e.g. reduced autoregulation, carbon dioxide and oxygen reactivity), minimal initial edema formation, and restricted microfoci of reactive glia in the absence of marked changes in ionic fluxes. The mechanism of flow reduction in the penumbra appears to be multifactorial and may involve vascular spasm from intracellular accumulation of calcium and arachidonic acid metabolites, liberation of excitatory amino acids and oxygen-derived free radicals, and swelling of perivascular glial cells [2]. The penumbra may also be an area which has continued damage from metabolism of glucose to lactic acid when oxygen availability is reduced. Based on this, one would expect hyperglycemia to cause increased tissue damage from focal ischemia.

Cerebral Blood Flow: Reperfusion

After transient complete global cerebral ischemia, reperfusion is initiated with a period of hyperperfusion followed by a prolonged period of hypoperfusion (Fig. 3). Whereas the duration of hyperperfusion may be brief (10–20 min), hypoperfusion may be prolonged (several hours). There appears to be a great deal of heterogeneity of blood flow reduction during the hypoperfusion period with near normal flows in some areas and flows near zero in other areas. During hyperperfusion, metabolic substrates are supplied to the brain in excess of its

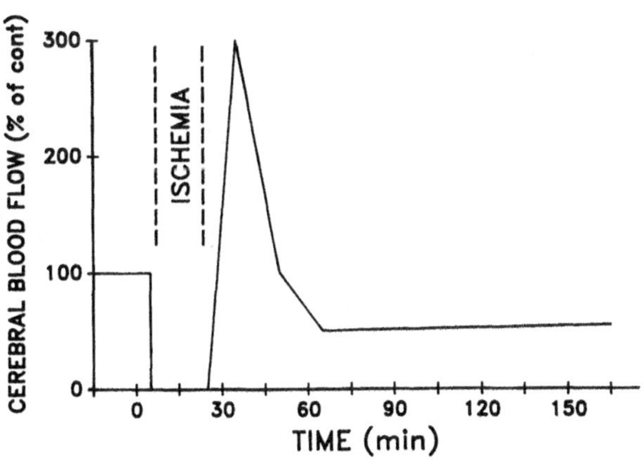

Fig. 3. This graph demonstrates the effect of transient ischemia on cerebral blood flow. In this figure, hyperemia is followed by a period of delayed hypoperfusion

needs and substrate extraction is actually decreased. However, during hypoperfusion there is a concomitant reduction in cerebral metabolism.

The blood flow changes following transient focal ischemia are somewhat different. With short durations of ischemia (5-10 min) hyperperfusion usually occurs without subsequent hypoperfusion. After longer durations of ischemia hypoperfusion usually occurs without preceding hyperperfusion. In experimental models of transient focal ischemia, the exact pattern of blood flow response during reperfusion is dependent on the anesthetic techniques employed during the protocol.

With both transient global and focal cerebral ischemia there is a significant delay in time until blood vessels return to normal physiological responsiveness (e.g. autoregulation, CO_2 and O_2 reactivity). The mechanism for blood flow changes during reperfusion are probably multifactorial involving abnormalities which are initiated during ischemia and brought to fruition with the return of blood flow and substrates. Mechanisms which will be discussed below involve alterations in calcium homeostasis, production of toxic oxygen metabolites, and end products of the cyclooxygenase and lipoxygenase pathways.

Cerebral Metabolism: Insufficient Energy Production

The brain has a high metabolic rate relative to CBF and substrate delivery. It also has a poor ability to store substrates (glucose and oxygen). As a result, even under normal circumstances, the brain in comparison to other organs extracts a large fraction of the substrates supplied by the blood. In the presence of oxygen the brain normally metabolizes glucose via the Krebs Cycle but it may also metabolize other substrates (e.g. ketones, lactic acid) when they are present in high enough quantities. When oxygen supply is limited the brain is only able to metabolize glucose. With severe ischemia substrate supply is limited and after the small amount of stored glucose is used, the brain is unable to meet its metabolic needs. Ischemia causes damage to mitochondria which is exacerbated in the presence of acidosis. Damage to mitochondria further limits aerobic metabolism. Initially during ischemia the small store of glycogen in the brain is converted to glucose which is then metabolized anaerobically (glycolysis) to lactic acid. Anaerobic metabolism of glucose produces much less energy than aerobic metabolism (Krebs Cycle) and is unable to supply sufficient energy for normal brain function. In addition, lactic acid, the byproduct of glycolysis, accumulates during ischemia and directly causes tissue damage [3]. The amount of lactic acid which is produced during ischemia is directly related to the stores of glucose and glycogen in the brain. Parenchymal acidosis in the presence of energy failure is especially damaging to brain. As discussed above, ischemia induced mitochondrial dysfunction is made worse by acidosis. Accumulation of lactic acid and subsequent tissue damage is accelerated during ischemia in the presence of hyperglycemia.

Ion Fluxes

As a result of insufficient energy supply and build up of toxic metabolites, ischemia is associated with failure of adenosine triphosphate (ATP)-dependent ionic pumps (Table 1). During the first minutes after onset of significant ischemia, potassium slowly leaks out of the cell. During this period the brain is able to produce enough ATP to maintain relative ionic homeostasis. This period is prolonged when energy need is reduced (e.g. hypothermia, barbiturate coma) and decreased when energy needs are increased (e.g. seizures). During the next period, which corresponds to the time when ATP and PCr levels are near zero, there is a rapid loss of cellular potassium and influx of sodium, chloride, and calcium [4]. The rapid rate at which these ion fluxes occur, however, make it unlikely that they are caused only by failure of ionic pumps. Rather, a mass opening of ion gates is felt to occur which is unrelated to ionic pump failure. In addition, excitatory amino acids, which are released during ischemia, also increase influx of sodium, calcium, and chloride.

Regardless of source, an increase in cellular calcium leads to increased sequestration of calcium into mitochondria. The increase in mitochondrial calcium leads to a decrease in electrochemical gradient across the mitochondrial membrane, and subsequently uncoupling of oxidative phosphorylation. This uncoupling results in inability to produce amounts of ATP sufficient to maintain cellular viability.

The influx of calcium during ischemia has also been hypothesized to cause accumulation of free fatty acids by stimulating phospholipases which breakdown lipid membranes. Phospholipase activity is greatest when there is a long duration of ischemia [5] and tissue levels of ATP are low. Free fatty acids themselves may cause tissue damage directly during the period of ischemia. In addition, they probably play a key role indirectly in tissue damage which occurs during reperfusion. Even in the event of successful ischemic resuscitation, brain damage will continue to evolve during the initial phases of reperfusion. One potential explanation for evolution of post-ischemic brain injury is tissue damage related to the production of the byproducts of fatty acid metabolism in the presence of oxygen. For example, during reperfusion the lipoxygenase and cyclooxygenase pathways are stimulated by the large accumulation of the free fatty acid arachidonic acid which occurred during ischemia. Specifically, these pathways cause the production of thromboxanes, leukotrienes, endoperoxides and free oxygen radicals. Prostaglandins may be responsible for vascular sludging and altered vascular reactivity [6]. Oxygen-derived free radicals may cause direct

Table 1. Sequela of insufficient oxygen supply

1. Increased lactic acid production
2. Failure of ATP dependent processes
3. Calcium/sodium/chloride fluxes
4. Intracellular accumulation of free fatty acids
5. Extracellular accumulation of excitatory amino acids

brain injury by initiating free radical chain reactions with cellular lipids and cause vascular paralysis by an unknown mechanism [7]. Cellular influx of calcium is also important in conversion of xanthine dehydrogenase to xanthine oxidase which facilitates production of oxygen-derived free radicals during reperfusion via post ischemic oxidation of adenosine metabolites.

Another mechanism of calcium mediated injury occurs in vascular smooth muscle cells. Here the influx of calcium during ischemia may cause vascular spasm and be responsible for delayed hypoperfusion. If the entry of calcium is blocked, vasoconstriction and, therefore, postischemic hypoperfusion may be ameliorated.

Excitatory amino acids: When the brain is exposed to ischemia, certain areas are more prone to suffer damage than others. In particular, the hippocampus is selectively vulnerable to damage not only from ischemia but also from seizures. Ischemia in rats produces large increases in the concentration of excitatory amino acids (e.g. glutamate and aspartate) in the hippocampus [8]. Under normal circumstances the hippocampus has a high density of receptors for the excitatory amino acid glutamate as well as a high capacity for glutamate uptake [9]. Depolarization of excitatory amino acid containing neurons causes release of excitatory neurotransmitters. After release from a nerve terminal, glutamate increases sodium and calcium permeability in postsynaptic neurons (mostly of dendritic origin) causing rapid neuronal depolarization [10]. Three types of excitatory amino acid receptors have been identified based on activation by kainate, quisqualate, or N-methyl-D-aspartate (NMDA). Specifically, glutamate acts on kainate and quisqualate receptors to increase sodium and chloride influx into the cell. In the setting of depolarization glutamate also stimulates NMDA receptors to increase calcium influx. The rapid accumulation of cellular electrolytes causes osmotically induced swelling and eventual lysis. Neurons not killed by this pathway may be damaged directly from the slower influx of calcium [11]. The potential mechanisms for neuronal damage related to calcium were described above. Influx of calcium caused by stimulation of the NMDA receptor may be inhibited by magnesium in a voltage-dependent manner.

Since microscopically neuronal damage which occurs as a result of excitotoxic lesions resembles that which is a result of ischemia, it is reasonable to hypothesize that damage during ischemia may involve an excitatory amino acid pathway. Further support for this hypothesis has come from the finding that cells in culture are protected from anoxia with excitatory amino acid antagonists. In ischemia, release of excitatory amino acids is stimulated and reuptake mechanisms are impaired [12] which causes a large extracellular accumulation of these toxins. Interstitial concentrations of excitatory amino acids in fetal brain also increase dramatically when exposed to asphyxia. During reperfusion from ischemia the interstitial concentration of excitatory amino acids fall rapidly. As a result, glutamate and other excitatory amino acids become prime candidates as important mediators of brain injury during cerebral ischemia but not during reperfusion. It is interesting to note that in concert with newborn animals tolerating cerebral ischemia better than adults; when exposed to ischemia newborn animals have a 2–6 fold decreased binding to excitatory amino acid receptors as compared to adults. The potential therapeutic role of excitatory amino acid receptor antagonists will be discussed below.

Oxygen-Derived Free Radicals

Oxygen-derived free radicals are likely important mediators of brain injury during reperfusion from ischemia and within the penumbra in focal ischemia. In ischemia and reperfusion there is a period of energy failure followed by reoxygenation. In the penumbra there are areas of brain with inadequate energy supply with some continued oxygen availability and there are probably small areas which are exposed to alternating periods of ischemia and reperfusion.

Multiple pathways exist for production of oxygen-derived free radicals in brain but under normal circumstances free radicals are rapidly detoxified by endogenous antioxidants (e.g. ascorbic acid, alpha-tocopherol) or free radical scavengers (e.g. superoxide dismutase, catalase, peroxidases). In pathologic states production of free radicals overwhelms the cell's ability to quickly detoxify and tissue damage results from chain reactions occurring with free radicals and lipid membranes. The potential pathways for free radical production in brain include: mitochondrial respiration, arachidonic acid metabolism via cyclooxygenase and lipoxygenase, xanthine oxidase metabolism, and autoxidation of compounds like catecholamines. The arachidonic acid and xanthine oxidase pathways appear to be predominant pathways for production of oxygen-derived free radicals in response to ischemia and reperfusion.

As discussed above, with the onset of ischemia several pathways exist leading to an increase in intracellular calcium concentration. In an ATP deficient environment increased intracellular calcium leads to stimulation of phospholipases, breakdown of lipid membranes and accumulation of high concentrations of free fatty acids. During reperfusion and with reintroduction of oxygen to tissue, the free fatty acid, arachidonic acid is metabolized via the cyclooxygenase and lipoxygenase pathways which leads to the production of superoxide anion.

Oxygen-derived free radicals may also be produced during reperfusion through a mechanism which requires the degradation of ATP to yield adenosine and hypoxanthine. With the onset of ischemia brain adenine nucleotides are metabolized to nucleosides and purine bases, and there is a rapid rise in interstitial concentration of adenosine [13]. Adenosine is metabolized to hypoxanthine which then acts as a substrate for xanthine oxidase during reperfusion and superoxide anion is produced as a byproduct. In order for the adenosine pathway to be considered as an important source of oxygen derived free radicals during reperfusion, the brain must have adequate amounts of xanthine oxidase. Under normal circumstances whole brain has low xanthine oxidase activity [14]. However, xanthine oxidase activity in brain microvessels is approximately four-fold that of the cerebral cortex [15]. Thus it is likely that endothelial cells are important in the production of toxic oxygen metabolites during reperfusion. Furthermore, during cerebral ischemia, another enzyme xanthine dehydrogenase is rapidly converted to xanthine oxidase increasing the brain's potential for production of oxygen derived free radicals during reperfusion [16]. This conversion is increased during ischemia because of the increase in intracellular calcium.

In general free radicals are very reactive molecules because they have one or more unpaired electrons. As such they react avidly with molecules containing polyunsaturated double bonds in order to regain the thermodynamically lowest energy state. Superoxide anion in and of itself is not a particularly reactive species and is therefore thought to cause most of its tissue damage through other intermediates. For example superoxide anion may protonate to HO_2 which can directly attack and damage polyunsaturated fatty acids. However, superoxide anion is believed to produce most of its damage through the increased production of hydroxyl radicals. Superoxide anion acts to reduce iron in ferritin which allows iron to escape into free solution. Superoxide anion also dismutes to form hydrogen peroxide and in so doing converts iron to the ferrous state (Fe^{2+}). Ferrous ions and hydrogen peroxide then react via the Fenton Reaction to yield hydroxyl radicals which are very reactive and able to damage most biologic molecules.

Opiates: It has been hypothesized that opiates are released in cerebral ischemia and may be responsible for brain damage related to stimulation of central opiate receptors. In support of this, morphine (μ-receptor agonist) administration has been reported to worsen ischemic neurologic deficits and administration of an enkephalin analogue (delta-receptor agonist) has been shown to worsen blood flow to ischemic brain [17, 18]. On the other hand, several kappa receptor agonists have been shown to decrease the amount of neuronal damage following transient focal ischemia [19]. In fact, the degree of protection is increased with agents having more potent kappa receptor agonist activity and is abolished in structurally similar agents with no kappa receptor agonist activity [19]. Therefore, if an opiate pathway was important in the pathophysiology of brain damage from ischemia it would appear that the mechanism would involve stimulation of mu or delta receptors but not kappa receptors.

Medical Management

Introduction

Options for the treatment of ischemia stem from an understanding of the pathophysiology described above. Treatments have been stratified into the following areas: flow promotion; decreasing the brain's metabolic needs (barbiturates, etomidate); decreasing production of toxic metabolites during ischemia (calcium antagonists, excitatory amino acid inhibitors, opiate receptor antagonists); decreasing toxicity of metabolites during reflow (corticosteroids, prostaglandin inhibitors, free radical scavengers) (Table 2).

Table 2. Medical management of cerebral ischemia

Treatment	Proposed mechanism
1. CPR Hypertension Decrease ICP	1. Blood flow promotion
2. Barbiturate	2. Decrease $CMRO_2$ Reduce free radical mechanisms
3. Calcium antagonists	3. Blood flow promotion Prevent cellular calcium influx
4. Corticosteroids	4. Prevent vasogenic edema
5. Free radical scavengers	5. Decrease reperfusion injury
6. Excitatory amino acid inhibitors	6. Block agonist operated calcium channels
7. Opitate receptor antagonists	7. Block effect of endogenous opiate release
8. Etomidate	8. Decrease $CMRO_2$

Blood Flow Promotion

When global ischemia is produced by cardiac arrest the first treatment for cerebral ischemia should be effective cardiopulmonary resuscitation (CPR). Although much work has been done to optimize cardiac resuscitation, little is known about the efficacy of cerebral resuscitation with conventional CPR. For example in a study of 459 patients resuscitated in the field and admitted to a community hospital only about half had significant neurologic recovery. Of these survivors, one third had persistent neurologic deficits [20]. As compared to conventional CPR, simultaneous compression and ventilation CPR causes an increase in carotid blood flow which is associated with an increase in CBF but not necessarily in an improved neurologic recovery [21]. Epinephrine administered during either conventional or simultaneous compression and ventilation CPR increases CBF presumably by constricting extracerebral vessels to effectively shunt blood flow to the brain [22]. Epinephrine administration also increases electroencephalographic activity and allows for greater success initiating spontaneous circulation. Open-chest CPR as compared to conventional CPR is associated with greater CBF [23] brain electrical activity and brain recovery [19]. The practical clinical implications of these preliminary studies continue to be investigated.

Global ischemia may also be caused by increases in intracranial pressure. An increase in volume of any of the constituents (either normally occurring or pathologic) of the intracranial vault may cause an increase in intracranial pressure. Regardless of the cause of increased intracranial pressure, in the acute setting, the treatment begins with obtaining control of the patient's airway. Airway control protects against aspiration when level of consciousness is decreased, allows for early institution of therapeutic hyperventilation and assures adequate oxygenation. Hyperventilation decreases the blood volume component of the intracranial vault. Normal brain blood vessels respond to the decrease in arterial carbon dioxide tension by constriction. Hyperventilation decreases intracranial pressure by decreasing blood flow to normal brain but by decreasing downstream pressure (intracranial pressure) it increases blood flow to abnormal tissue. Hypoxia causes cerebral vessels to dilate which could increase cerebral blood volume and increase in intracranial pressure and therefore must be avoided. If increased intracranial pressure is accompanied by diffuse tissue swelling, diuretics may be of therapeutic value. Osmotic diuretics (e.g. mannitol) rapidly cause fluid loss from brain tissue but acutely may increase intracranial pressure by increasing intravascular volume. This effect can be avoided by pretreatment with a loop diuretic (e.g. furosemide), initiating hyperventilation prior to administration of the osmotic diuretic, or use of the loop diuretic in the absence of osmotic diuretics.

Barbiturate therapy: Barbiturates (e. g. pentobarbital, thiopental) have been tested for efficacy in the setting of pure cerebral hypoxia, global cerebral ischemia, focal cerebral ischemia, and increases in intracranial pressure. Theoretically, barbiturates may be of therapeutic value because they could decrease the brain's metabolic needs in the setting of decreased energy supply, decrease the production of free fatty acids during ischemia, have an effect on free radical mechanisms, attenuate cerebral edema, and improve the microcirculation [24]. The decrease in metabolic needs of the brain produced by barbiturate administration actually does prolong the time to when massive changes in cellular electrolytes occur during ischemia (normally at approximately 2 min of ischemia). However, it must be realized that even a doubling of time overall could reflect only a small improvement in ischemic tolerance.

Barbiturates may have therapeutic efficacy in decreasing brain injury from oxygen-derived free radicals via one of three mechanisms: limiting free radical production, free radical scavenging, or blocking the initiation of free radical chain reactions. If production of oxygen-derived free radicals results from metabolism of free fatty acids during reperfusion, then decreasing production of free fatty acids during ischemia by barbiturate administration may decrease the production of oxygen-derived free radicals. However, for efficacy the barbiturate would have to be administered prior to ischemia which in most clinical cases is impossible. In experimental models our understanding of the efficacy of barbiturates to decrease production of oxygen-derived free radicals is incomplete because free radicals have been difficult to measure directly. However, the lack of efficacy for barbiturate pretreatment to decrease accumulation of other cyclooxygenase and lipoxygenase byproducts (eicosanoids) during reperfusion [25] makes this hypothesis unlikely. The ability of barbiturates to scavenge free radicals has been evaluated more completely. Although thiopental is a relatively potent free radical scavenger, other barbiturates (e.g. phenobarbital, pentobarbital) which appear to have equivalent efficacy treating cerebral ischemia have no ability to scavenge oxygen-derived free radicals [26]. In evaluating the free radical scavenging properties of barbiturates an interesting finding has been that barbiturates appear to stabilize heme-coordinated iron complexes [27]. Theoretically, if iron is not available to facilitate conversion of superoxide anion to hydroxyl radical less free radical tissue damage would occur. This specific role of barbiturates has not yet been tested in animal models.

Although initially there was much enthusiasm over their potential ability to ameliorate tissue damage from ischemia, barbiturates have been found to have very limited clinical use. In global ischemia (cardiac arrest and resuscitation) initial animal studies suggested that barbiturates were effective in ameliorating brain damage when administered either prior to or following the insult [28]. These initial studies, however, were plagued with methodological problems and subsequently other laboratories have been unable to demonstrate a therapeutic role for barbiturates in global ischemia [29]. Despite these consistent negative results in animals, human studies were initiated. In humans, barbiturates were found not to be therapeutic when given after isolated cerebral ischemia or near-drowning or during resuscitation from cardiac arrest [30].

In the laboratory, barbiturates have been found to be of therapeutic benefit in focal ischemia [31]. However, in order to be effective they must be given within one hour of arterial occlusion. Furthermore, the dose required to obtain protection in most studies is much larger than what would be safe to administer to patients. At high doses, barbiturates cause alteration in level of consciousness and profound hypotension with myocardial depression. Although barbiturates may be used intraoperatively to protect the brain during intracranial revascularization [32] and to decrease postoperative neuropsychiatric complications in patients undergoing open ventricle operations requiring cardiopulmonary bypass the profound myocardial depression they cause makes their utility limited.

Barbiturates decrease intracranial pressure by decreasing cerebral metabolism and cerebral blood flow. However, there is yet little evidence that this effect of barbiturates favorably alters the outcome of any disease entity. In isolated cases barbiturates may control intracranial pressure when other agents are not effective. We frequently use short acting barbiturates (e.g. thiopental) to blunt increases in intracranial pressure seen during endotracheal intubation or suctioning particularly in patients at risk for herniation. The clinician must always remember that barbiturates should be used with caution because they decrease the level of consciousness and may cause profound depression of cardiovascular function.

Calcium antagonists: As discussed above, alterations in calcium homeostasis may occur both during ischemia and reperfusion. Calcium influx into neurons facilitates the liberation of free fatty acids and into blood vessels causes vasoconstriction. Several calcium antagonists have been found to be relatively specific for brain (nimodipine, lidoflazine, flunarizine, nicardipine) although all of these agents currently are used only for investigational purposes in the United States. The more common calcium antagonists (e.g. nifedipine, verapamil, diltiazem) appear to have little or no efficacy for the brain.

In animal models of focal ischemia nimodipine administration was associated with improved blood flow, improved electrical activity, improved metabolism and decreased infarct size [33]. Preliminary observations in patients suggest that nimodipine may improve cerebral blood flow during acute ischemia. In subarachnoid hemorrhage approximately 60% of patients suffer from angiographically documented cerebral vasospasm [34]. The exact cause for this vasospasm has not been delineated, however, calcium antagonists have been shown to decrease the amount of vasculature constriction in vitro and in animal models [35]. More importantly they improve the neurologic outcome of patients suffering from subarachnoid hemorrhage [36].

The efficacy of calcium antagonists for global ischemia and reperfusion is in question. In animal models of global ischemia and reperfusion, nimodipine pretreatment appears to improve survival and cerebral blood flow during resuscitation [37]. However, when given during recirculation nimodipine administration caused an improved post-ischemic blood flow in both dogs and monkeys but only improved neurologic function in monkeys [38]. Likewise, in animal models flunarizine administration at the time of resuscitation appears to improve blood flow [39] but does not improve postischemic neurologic function [40]. Lidoflazine, on the other hand improves postischemic neurologic function without necessarily improving blood flow. Because the results have not been consistent in animal models, we agree with Shapiro [41] that a human study at this time seems premature.

Corticosteroids: Steroids are efficacious for treating vasogenic edema around brain tumors [42] and in doing so may prevent local ischemia. However, steroids do not treat edema caused by other types of ischemia [43], steroids are also not efficacious for the treatment of brain injury which results from focal ischemia in patients. The use of steroids in the clinical setting is not without risks. For example, steroids increase risks of infection, cause derangement in patients' nutritional status, and decrease wound healing. Currently we do not recommend steroids as treatment for cerebral ischemia.

Prostaglandins: As described above, during ischemia there is an accumulation of free fatty acids in brain. During reperfusion these fatty acids allow for a large production of prostaglandins [44]. When animals are treated with the prostaglandin inhibitor indomethacin prior to ischemia there is a decrease in the degree of perfusion abnormalities [45] and improved neurologic recovery [44]. When indomethacin is given only during reperfusion no therapeutic effect is found [46]. Indomethacin has also been found not to be of therapeutic value in the setting of focal ischemia [47] yet prostacyclin afforded neurologic improvement to patients with focal cerebral ischemia [48]. Much more work needs to be done in this area before these agents should be used clinically to prevent tissue damage from cerebral ischemia.

Free Radical Scavengers

There are several strategies available for interrupting oxygen-derived free radical processes. The drugs that are currently used experimentally include alpha-tocopherol, allopurinol, superoxide dismutase, catalase, deferoxamine, dimethyl sulfoxide, and mannitol. Since there has not been any human trials to evaluate the efficacy of exogenously administered free radical scavengers on neurologic outcome following cerebral ischemia, the following discussion will be entirely based on animal studies. Taken in total these studies suggest that there may be therapeutic potential for free radical scavengers in decreasing tissue damage resulting from cerebral ischemia.

Alpha-tocopherol is an endogenous antioxidant. Animals deficient in alpha-tocopherol are more prone to tissue damage from oxygen-derived free radicals. Animals administered excess alpha-tocopherol are less prone to tissue damage from oxygen-derived radicals in vitro, and have reduced brain injury and improved neurologic outcome when exposed to ischemia and reperfusion in vivo.

Allopurinol blocks xanthine oxidase and therefore blocks the production of superoxide anions which are generated via the oxidative metabolism of adenosine byproducts. It has no effect on the production of oxygen-derived free radicals by other mechanisms. When allopurinol is given prior to global ischemia, so that it has time to cross the blood brain barrier, it improves survival, neurologic outcome, and biochemical evidence of damage during reperfusion [49]. In the setting of focal ischemia it decreases infarct size [50].

Both superoxide dismutase and catalase are endogenous free radical scavengers. Superoxide dismutase catalyzes the conversion of superoxide anion to hydrogen peroxide. There appears to be two intracellular superoxide dismutase isoenzymes (CuZn SOD, MW 32,000 Dalton; Mn SOD, MW 90,000 Dalton) and one extracellular isoenzyme (EC-SOD, MW 135,000). Because of its large molecular weight superoxide dismutase does not cross the blood brain barrier easily when given systemically. In addition, superoxide dismutase is rapidly cleared from the circulation after it is administered parenterally. Therefore, experimentally it must be infused in high concentration. In this setting superoxide dismutase caused a dose related improved neurologic recovery in animals exposed to transient spinal cord ischemia [51]. Likewise when given during permanent focal ischemia superoxide dismutase causes stabilization of brain pH and cortical blood flow [32]. In an attempt to decrease clearance from the circulation and to increase transit across the blood brain barrier other investigators have either linked superoxide dismutase to polyethylene glycol or have entrapped it in liposomes. As would be expected, when polyethylene glycol linked superoxide dismutase was administered at the time of reperfusion in gerbils exposed to transient forebrain ischemia, overall survival was improved.

Catalase catalyzes the conversion of hydrogen peroxide to water. Catalase has four tetrahedrally arranged subunits (MW 240,000 Dalton). Catalase has not been tested by itself for global ischemia but we have not found it to be efficacious in the setting of transient focal ischemia. When given as a small single dose in combination with a small single dose of superoxide no improvement in neurologic recovery was found in dogs subjected to transient global ischemia. On the contrary, when catalase linked with polyethylene glycol is given with superoxide dismutase linked with polyethylene glycol, infarct size is decreased in rats exposed to focal ischemia [52].

Deferoxamine inhibits the conversion of hydrogen peroxide to hydroxyl radical by removing iron from the reaction. Deferoxamine reduces brain injury and although it improves overall survival rate following global ischemia, by itself, it does not improve neurologic outcome of the survivors [53]. However, when deferoxamine is administered during reperfusion from global ischemia in combination with superoxide dismutase there is an improvement in both CBF and functional recovery (somatosensory evoked potentials).

Dimethyl sulfoxide and mannitol are both hydroxyl radical scavengers. Dimethyl sulfoxide decreases intracranial pressure by an unknown mechanism and improves neurologic outcome and microscopic evidence of damage when administered to animals prior to reperfusion from spinal cord ischemia [54]. Dimethyl sulfoxide improves neurologic outcome and brain histology in the setting of transient focal cerebral ischemia but not after more prolonged periods of focal ischemia [55]. Mannitol has been shown to attenuate ischemic neuronal damage with prolonged focal ischemia [56] and to stabilize cortical blood flow and intracellular brain pH in the ischemic penumbra but not the ischemic core [32].

Excitatory amino acid inhibitors: Several different inhibitors of excitatory amino acid receptors exist but until recently evaluation of potential therapeutic efficacy has been limited by the need to obtain high concentrations in the brain for compounds which have poor penetration of the blood brain barrier. 2-amino-7-phosphonoheptanoic acid (2-APH) is a specific competitive antagonist of the NMDA receptors which is usually administered by focal injection or microdialysis. This drug has been used experimentally to determine which areas of the brain may benefit from blockade of NMDA receptors during ischemia. (+)-5-methyl-10, 11-dihydro-5H-dibenzo(a,d)cyclohepten-5,10-imine maleate (MK 801) is a noncompetitive use-dependent blocker of NMDA receptors which crosses the blood brain barrier readily. This drug has been used experimentally to determine whether blocking NMDA receptors during ischemia may have any clinical relevance. As described above since the concentration of excitatory amino acids peaks during ischemia and then rapidly returns to control during reperfusion one would predict that administering blockers prior to ischemia would be most effective. During focal ischemia (but not during complete global ischemia) it may also be possible to administer a blocker that would have access to the penumbra and decrease the overall volume of brain at risk for damage. In fact as predicted, when NMDA receptor antagonists are administered prior to the onset of ischemia, brain damage is ameliorated [57]. In the setting of prolonged focal ischemia MK 801 also reduced infarct size when given 2 h after middle cerebral artery occlusion. Although one laboratory [58] has shown less histologic damage to animals administered inhibitors of excitatory amino acids at the end of ischemia, other laboratories do concur on the efficacy of these agents when given at reperfusion. Much more work is needed in this new and exciting area to determine clinical efficacy of NMDA antagonists.

Opiates receptor agonists and antagonists: Naloxone is an opiate receptor antagonist which has no effect on cerebral blood flow in awake normal animals. However, because of the finding that brain levels of opiates increase in response to ischemia, naloxone has been tested for therapeutic efficacy. The results have been mixed. At least in animal studies, naloxone administration is associated with improved neurologic recovery from spinal cord trauma or ischemia presumably by blocking either kappa or μ-receptors. Although early studies demonstrated some therapeutic benefit for opiate antagonists in treatment for cerebral ischemia more recent studies have been less encouraging. One potential explanation for these mixed findings is that when naloxone is given in large quantities it will block all opiate receptors. Since agonists acting on kappa receptors may actually protect the brain from ischemic damage and agonists acting on other receptors (e.g. μ-receptors) may exacerbate ischemic damage, blocking all receptors will have overall no effect. The use of more specific opiate receptor antagonists in future studies may help clarify the role of opiates in the pathophysiology of ischemic brain damage.

Etomidate

Etomidate is an anesthetic which decreases cerebral oxygen consumption. Theoretically etomidate could have similar therapeutic potential compared with barbiturates. However, as explained for barbiturates, the ability to decrease metabolic needs of the brain at the onset of ischemia has not improved neurologic recovery from clinically relevant durations of ischemia. Etomidate has been shown to shorten the time needed for resuscitation in a cardiac arrest model of cerebral ischemia [59] and may provide protection in patients being maintained on extracorporeal circulation for cardiac surgery [60]. Etomidate has not been enthusiastically investigated because it is also known to cause adrenal suppression even after single dose.

Summary

In this review the authors have discussed the pathophysiology and several therapeutic strategies for cerebral ischemia. It seems likely that there will never be simple therapeutic answers to the complex pathophysiology of cerebral ischemia as we now understand it. Ultimate therapies will probably involve combinations of interventions designed to block several ongoing pathophysiologic processes in neuronal death. Progress in this field will likely be slow and difficult.

References

1. Ljunggren B, Ratcheson RA, Siesjö BK (1974) Cerebral metabolic state following complete compression ischemia. Brain Res 73:291–307
2. Little JR, Kerr FWL, Sundt TM Jr (1975) Microcirculatory obstruction in focal cerebral ischemia: relationship to neuronal alterations. Mayo Clin Proc 50:264–270
3. Kalimo H, Rehncrona S, Sonderfedt B, Olsson Y, Siesjö BK (1981) Brain lactic acidosis and ischemic cell damage: II. Histopathology . J Cereb Blood Flow Metab 1:313–327
4. Siesjö BK (1984) Cerebral circulation and metabolism. J Neurosurg 60:883–908
5. Bazan NG Jr, DeBazan HEP, Kennedy WG, et al (1971) Regional distribution and rate of production of free fatty acids in rat brain. J Neurochem 18:1387–1393
6. Kontos HA, Wei EP, Povlishock JT, Christman CW (1984) Oxygen radicals mediate the cerebral arteriolar dilation form arachidonate and bradykinin in cats. Circ Res 55:295–303

7. Wei EP, Christman CW, Kontos HA, et al (1985) Effects of oxygen radicals on cerebral arterioles. Am J Physiol 248:H157–H162
8. Benveniste H, Drejer J, Schousboe A, Diemer NH (1984) Elevation of the extracellular concentrations of glutamate and aspartate in rat hippocampus during transient cerebral ischemia monitored by intracerebral microdialysis. J Neurochem 43:1369–1374
9. Greenamyre JT, Young AB, Penney JB (1984) Quantitative autoradiographic distribution of L-[3H]glutamate binding sites in rat central nervous system. J Neurosci 4:2133–2144
10. Curtis DR, Phillis JW, Watkins JC (1959) Chemical excitation of spinal neurones. Nature 183:611–612
11. Farber JL, Chien KR, Mittnachts (1981) The pathogenesis of irreversible cell injury in ischemia. Am J Physiol 102:271–281
12. Drejer J, Benveniste H, Diemer MH, Schousboe A (1985) Cellular origin of ischemia-induced glutamate release from brain tissue in vivo and in vitro. J Neurochem 45:145–151
13. Van Wylen DGL, Park TS, Rubio R, Berne RM (1986) Increases in cerebral interstitial fluid adenosine concentration during hypoxia, local potassium infusion, and ischemia. J Cereb Blood Flow Metab 6:522–528
14. Al-Khalidi UAS, Chaglassian TH (1965) The specific distribution of xanthine oxidase. Biochem J 97:318–320
15. Betz AL (1985) Identification of hypoxanthine transport and xanthine oxidase activity in brain capillaries. J Neurochem 44:574–579
16. Beckman JS, Campbell GA, Freeman BA (1986) Conversion of brain xanthine dehydrogenase to oxidase contributes to cerebral ischemic injury in the gerbil. Free radicals in biology and medicine: Ischemia/Reperfusion injury. Presented at the Grand Hotel Point Clear, Alabama, March 17–19
17. Hosobuchi Y, Basins DS, Woo SK (1982) Reversal of induced ischemic neurologic deficit in gerbils by the opiate antagonist naloxone. Science 215:69–71
18. Sandor P, Gotoh F, Tomita M, Tanahashi M, Gogolak I (1986) Effects of a stable enkephalin analogue, (D-Met2, Pro5)-enkephalinamide, and naloxone on cortical blood flow and cerebral blood volume in experimental brain ischemia in anesthetized cats. Cereb Blood Flow Metab 6:553–558
19. Hall ED, Pazara KE (1988) Quantitative analysis of effects of k-opioid agonists on postischemic hippocampal CAl neuronal necrosis in gerbils. Stroke 19:1008–1012
20. Longstreth WT, Invi TS, Cobb LA, Copass MK (1983) Neurologic recovery after out-of-hospital cardiac arrest. Ann Intern Med 98:588–592
21. Bircher N, Safar P (1985) Cerebral preservation during cardiopulmonary resuscitation. Crit Care Med 13:185–190
22. Michael R, Guerci AD, Koehler RC, et al (1984) Mechanisms by which epinephrine augments cerebral and myocardial perfusion during cardiopulmonary resuscitation in dogs. Circulation 69:822–835
23. Arai T, Dote K, Tsuahara I, Nitta K, Nagaro T (1984) Cerebral blood flow during conventional, new and open-chest cardiopulmonary resuscitation in dogs. Resuscitation 12:147–154
24. Shiu GK, Nemoto EM (1981) Barbiturate attenuation of brain free fatty acid liberation during global ischemia. Neurochem 37:1448–1456
25. Dorman RV (1988) Effects of cerebral ischemia and reperfusion on prostanoid accumulation in unanesthetized and pentobarbital-anesthetized gerbils. J Cereb Blood Flow Metab 8:609–612
26. Smith DS, Rehncrona S, Siesjö BK (1980) Barbiturates as protective agents in brain ischemia and as free radical scavengers in vitro. Acta Physiol Scand 42:129–134
27. Godin DV, Mitchell J, Saunders BA (1982) Studies on the interaction of barbiturates with reactive oxygen radicals: implications regarding barbiturate protection against cerebral ischemia. Can Anaesth Soc J 29:203–210
28. Goldstein A Jr, Wells BA, Keats AS (1966) Increased tolerance to cerebral anoxia by pentobarbital. Arch Int Pharmacodyn Ther 161:138–143

29. Todd MM, Chadwick HS, Shapiro HM, Dunlop BS, Marshall LF, Dueck R (1982) The neurologic effects of thiopental therapy following experimental cardiac arrest in cats. Anesthesiology 57:76–86
30. Abramson NS, Safar P, Detre KM, et al (1986) Randomized clinical study of thiopental loading in comatose survivors of cardiac arrest. N Engl J Med 314:397–403
31. Smith AL, Hoff T, Nielsen SL, et al (1974) Barbiturate protection in acute focal cerebral ischemia. Stroke 5:1–7
32. Meyer FB, Sundt TM, Yanagihara, Anderson RE (1987) Focal cerebral ischemia: Pathophysiologic mechanism and rationale for future avenues of treatment. Mayo Clin Proc 62:35–55
33. Meyer FB, Anderson RE, Yaksh TL, et al (1986) Effect of nimodipine on intracellular NV brain pH, cortical blood flow, and EEG in experimental focal cerebral ischemia. J Neurosurg 64:617–626
34. Weir B, Grace M, Hansen J, et al (1978) Time course of vasospasm in man. J Neurosurg 48:173–178
35. Leblanc R, Feindel W, Yamamoto L, Milton JG, Frojmovic MM (1984) Reversal of acute experimental cerebral vasospasm by calcium antagonism with verapamil. Can J Neurol Sci 11:42–47
36. Guggiari M, Taquoi G, Philippon J, et al (1987) Curative treatment with intravenous nimodipine for cerebral vasospasm after subarachnoid haemorrhage due to aneurysm rupture. Anesthesiology (abstr) 67:A584
37. Steen PA, Newberg LA, Milde H, et al (1983) Nimodipine improves cerebral blood flow and neurologic recovery after complete cerebral ischemia in the dog. Cereb Blood Flow Metab 3:38–43
38. Steen PA, Newberg LA, Milde H, et al (1984) Cerebral blood flow and neurologic outcome when nimodipine is given after complete cerebral ischemia in the dog. J Cereb Blood Flow Metab 4:82–87
39. White BC, Gadzinski DS, Hoehner P, et al (1982) Effect of flunarizine on canine cerebral cortical blood flow and vascular resistance post cardiac arrest. Ann Emerg Med 111:119–126
40. Newberg LA, Steen PA, Milde JH, et al (1984) Failure of flunarizine to improve cerebral blood flow or neurologic recovery in a canine model of complete cerebral ischemia. Stroke 15:666–671
41. Shapiro HM (1985) Postcardiac arrest therapy. Calcium entry blockade and brain resuscitation. Anesthesiology 62:384–387
42. French LA, Galicich JH (1964) The use of steroids for control of cerebral edema. Clin Neurosurg 10:212
43. Siegel BA, Studer RK, Potchen E (1972) Sterioid therapy of brain edema: ineffectiveness in experimental cerebral microembolism. Arch Neurol 27:209–212
44. Gaudet RJ, Levine L (1979) Transient cerebral ischemia and brain prostaglandins. Biochem Biophys Res Commun 86:893–901
45. Furlow TW, Hallenbeck JM (1978) Indomethacin prevents impaired perfusion of the dog's brain after global ischemia. Stroke 9:591–594
46. Hallenbeck JM, Furlow TW (1979) Prostaglandin I2 and indomethacin prevent impairment of post-ischemic brain reperfusion in the dog. Stroke 10:629–637
47. Boulu RG, Plotine M, Gueniau C, Sofeir M, Wiernspeger N (1982) Effect of indomethacin in experimental cerebral ischemia. Pathol Biol 30:278–281
48. Gryglewski RJ, Nowak S, Kostka-Trabka E, et al (1983) Treatment of ischemic stroke with prostacyclin. Stroke 14:197–202
49. Itoh T, Kawakami M, Yamauchi Y, et al (1986) Effect of allopurinol on ischemia and reperfusion-induced cerebral injury in spontaneously hypertensive rats. Stroke 17:1284–1287
50. Martz D, Rayos G, Schielke GP, et al (1988) Allopurinol limits infarct size in partial ischemia. The seventh international symposium on intracranial pressure and brain injury, June 19–23, Ann Arbor, Michigan USA, p 33
51. Lim KH, Connolly M, Rose D, et al (1986) Prevention of reperfusion injury of the ischemic spinal cord: use of recombinant superoxide dismutase. Ann Thorac Surg 42:282–286

52. Linsay SL, Beckman JS, Liu TH, et al (1988) The effect of superoxide dismutase and catalase on focal cerebral ischemia. Anesthesiology A215
53. Fleischer JE, Lanier WL, Milde JH, et al (1987) Failure of deferoxamine, an iron chelator, to improve neurologic outcome following complete cerebral ischemia in dogs. Stroke 18:124-127
54. Coles JC, Ahmed SN, Mehta HU, et al (1986) Role of free radical scavenger in protection of spinal cord during ischemia. Ann Thorac Surg 41:551-556
55. McGraw CP (1983) Treatment of cerebral infarction with dimethyl sulfoxide in the Mongolian gerbil. Ann NY Acad Sci 411:278-285
56. Little JR (1979) Treatment of acute focal cerebral ischemia with intermittent, low dose mannitol. Neurosurgery 5:687-691
57. Simon RP, Swan JH, Griffiths T, Meldrum BS (1984) Blockade of N-methyl-D-aspartate receptors may protect against ischemic damage in the brain. Science 226:850-852
58. Izumiyama K, Kogure K (1988) Prevention of delayed neuronal death in gerbil hippocampus by ion channel blockers. Stroke 19:1003-1007
59. Mullie A, Hermans C, Vandevelde K, et al (1981) Resuscitability of the heart with brain protective drugs during cardiopulmonary resuscitation in dogs. Crit Care Med 9:183
60. Hempelmann G, Dieter K, Volker L, et al (1982) Cerebral protection in neurosurgery, cardiac surgery, and following cardiac arrest. J Cereb Blood Flow Metab 2:S66-S71

Anaerobic Metabolism Within the Brain: Its Relationship to Brain Failure in Head-Injured Patients

C. S. Robertson

Introduction

Anaerobic glycolysis is a characteristic feature of central nervous system ischemic metabolism. With complete cerebral ischemia, such as occurs with cardiac arrest, oxygen supplies are depleted within 30 s. Oxidative phosphorylation ceases, but endogenous stores of glucose maintain anaerobic glycolysis for a few moments. The amount of lactic acid accumulation is primarily dependent upon the preischemia tissue glucose stores, which are proportional to the blood glucose concentration. After 2–3 min, ATP stores become depleted, and the adenylate energy charge reaches minimal values after approximately 5 min.

With incomplete ischemia, the metabolic consequences are dependent upon the residual blood flow. If the reduction in blood flow is severe enough to limit oxidative phosphorylation, a deterioration of tissue energy metabolism occurs similar to complete ischemia. The continued supply of glucose, however, may permit development of a more severe lactic acidosis.

Causes of Ischemia/Infarction After Severe Head Injury

Increased Intracranial Pressure (ICP)

Increases in intracranial pressure can cause global ischemia, or local ischemia due to compression of intracranial vessels. Global ischemia usually results from severe intracranial hypertension where cerebral perfusion pressure is reduced to <50 mmHg (Fig. 1). Refractory intracranial hypertension of this severity occurs in approximately 10–15% of all comatose head-injured patients, and is associated with a mortality of $>90\%$ [1]. With less severe intracranial hypertension, circulation may be compromised in certain susceptible areas. Compression of the posterior cerebral arteries against the tentorium causes ischemia of the occipital lobes, resulting in the classical pathological finding of intracranial hypertension, called "medial occipital necrosis". This type of infarction has been found at autopsy in 33% of patients who die of head injury [2]. The CT-scan appearance is that of lucent areas in the occipital lobes, which can be unilateral or bilateral (Fig. 2).

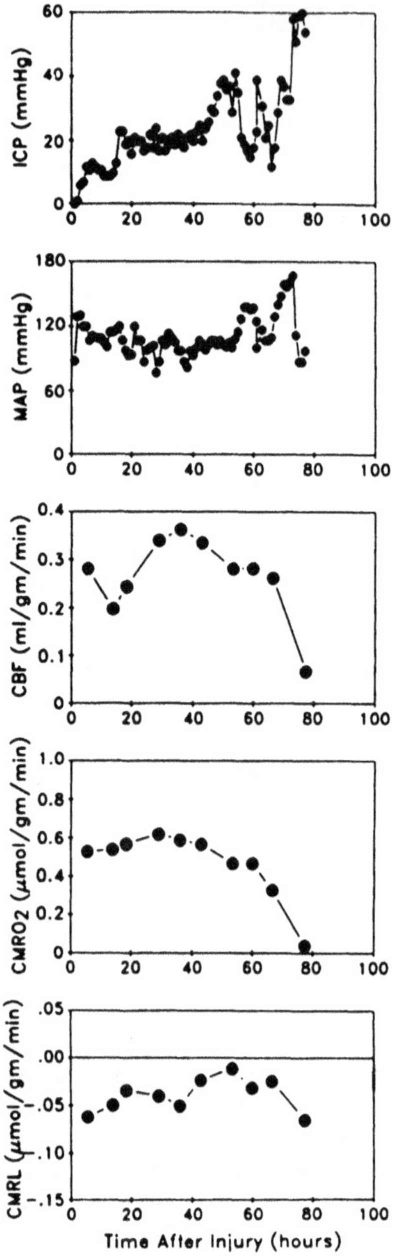

Fig. 1. Cerebral blood flow and metabolism variables in a patient who developed uncontrollable intracranial hypertension 3 days postevacuation of a subdural hematoma. Despite treatment, when cerebral perfusion pressure dropped to 30 mmHg, CBF and $CMRO_2$ decreased to very low values, and CMRL increased

Hypotension

Normally the brain regulates cerebral blood flow in a normal range despite variations in mean arterial pressure from 50 to 130 mmHg. The ability of the brain to autoregulate cerebral blood flow is commonly impaired following severe head

Table 1. List of abbreviations used in text

ICP	= intracranial pressure
CPP	= cerebral perfusion pressure
CBF	= cerebral blood flow
$PjvO_2$	= jugular venous pO_2
$SjvO_2$	= jugular venous oxygen saturation
$AVDO_2$	= cerebral arteriovenous oxygen difference
AVDL	= cerebral arteriovenous lactate difference
$CMRO_2$	= cerebral metabolic rate of oxygen
CMRL	= cerebral metabolic rate of lactate

injury [3, 4]. Hypotension of a degree which would normally be compensated for without neurological consequences, can reduce cerebral blood flow to critical levels (Fig. 3) and result in ischemic injury following head trauma. In clinical studies, the presence of a systolic blood pressure <90 mmHg on admission to the hospital, has been found to double mortality rate for head injured patients, from 34% to 65% [5, 6]. Experimental studies have shown a greater reduction in high energy phosphates and in pH when an impact injury is coupled with hypotension [7]. The watershed areas of the brain, typically between the anterior and middle cerebral artery distributions, are the most susceptible to ischemia due to hypotension. This type of boundary zone infarction has been found at autopsy in 22% of patients who die of their head injury [2].

Vasospasm or Injury of Intracranial Vessels

Infarctions in the distribution of arterial territories (other than posterior cerebral artery) occur in 9% of patients who die of head injury [2]. The most likely causes of these infarctions include arterial vasospasm, compression of vessels by mass lesions, and injury of major intracranial vessels (Figs. 4 and 5).

Angiographic evidence of vasospasm has been reported to occur in 19% of patients with moderate to severe head injury [8–10]. The incidence of ischemic injury due to vasospasm is more difficult to estimate because the neurological signs of ischemia are superimposed upon the neurological deficits of the traumatic injury. In a group of patients with fatal head injuries, selected because they had both angiographic and neuropathological examinations, the incidence of arterial spasm on the preoperative angiogram was 41%. The factors most strongly correlating with the subsequent development of arterial territory infarctions were the presence of intracranial hematomas and vasospasm. These studies suggested that mechanical factors generated by distortion and displacement of an intracranial hematoma can reduce regional cerebral blood flow to critical levels, especially when vasospasm is present [11].

Injuries of the major intracranial arteries range from intimal dissection with thrombosis to complete transection. The incidence of this type of ischemic injury is not known, but is probably less common than the other causes of arterial distribution infarctions. A review of 31 cases of intracranial carotid artery injury

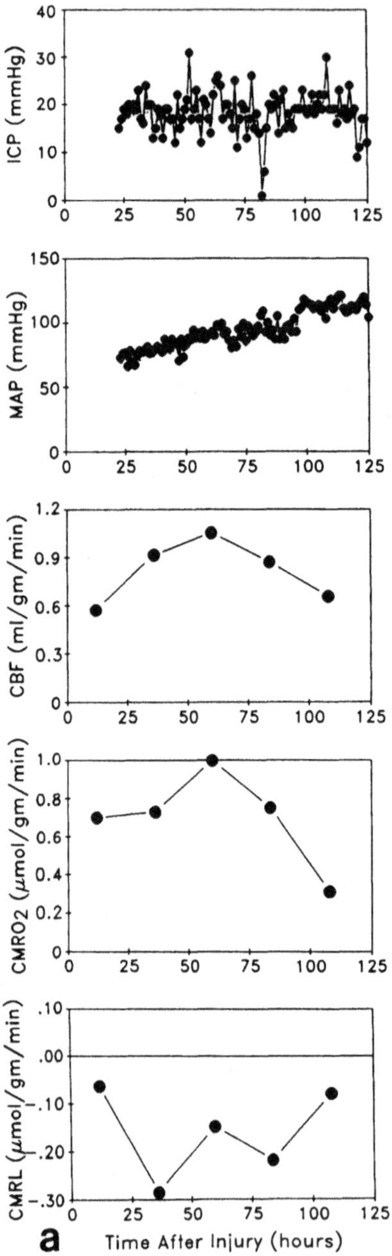

Fig. 2. a Cerebral blood flow and metabolism variables in a patient who developed a posterior cerebral artery infarction. The patients was admitted with a GCS 4 and a CT-scan demonstrating a basilar skull fracture and diffuse swelling (**b**). Two days later, a CT-scan showed a wedge-shaped low density area in the left occipital lobe (**c**). The characteristic metabolic pattern of an evolving infarction included an elevated CMRL, and a $CMRO_2$ that tended to decrease over time

reported in the literature through 1987 demonstrated generally a poor outcome with 16/31 (51%) dying and 7/31 (23%) surviving with a major neurological deficit [12].

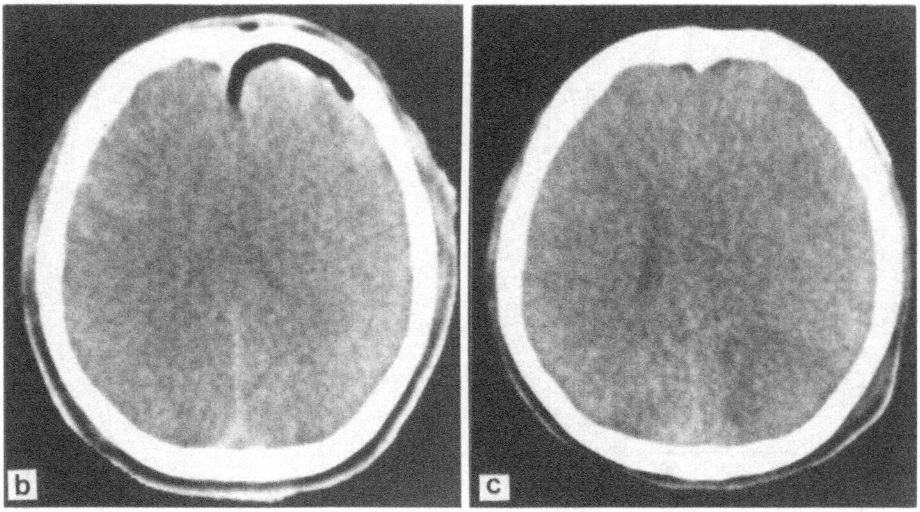

Fig. 2b, c

Consequences of Anaerobic Metabolism

Consequences of Anaerobic Metabolism on Energy Metabolism

The energy generated by the anaerobic metabolism of glucose is 1/19 that obtained from aerobic metabolism, i.e., 2 mol ATP/mol glucose compared to 38 mol ATP/mol glucose. Anaerobic metabolism of even large stores of glucose is not able to delay membrane depolarization more than 2–3 min during global ischemia [13]. The additional energy gained with anaerobic metabolism is at the expense of developing a more severe lactic acidosis. The late neurological sequalae of temporary ischemia are consistently worse when the blood glucose level is elevated during ischemia, suggesting that lactic acidosis or other metabolic consequences of glucose metabolism damages nervous tissue [13–18].

Consequences of Anaerobic Metabolism on Neurological Outcome from Head Trauma

Numerous studies have reported a correlation between the CSF concentration of the end-product of anaerobic metabolism, lactic acid, and neurological outcome following head injury [19–25]. CSF lactate was commonly elevated immediately postinjury. In patients who recovered neurological function, CSF lactate rapidly returned to normal. Persistence of CSF lactic acidosis was associated with a poor neurological outcome or death [25].

Mortality rate after head injury is increased from 25 to 56%, and neurological recovery is usually poor in survivors when cerebral ischemia is a complicating factor [26]. In one large autopsy study, 91% of all patients who died of their head injury had histological evidence of ischemic injury [2].

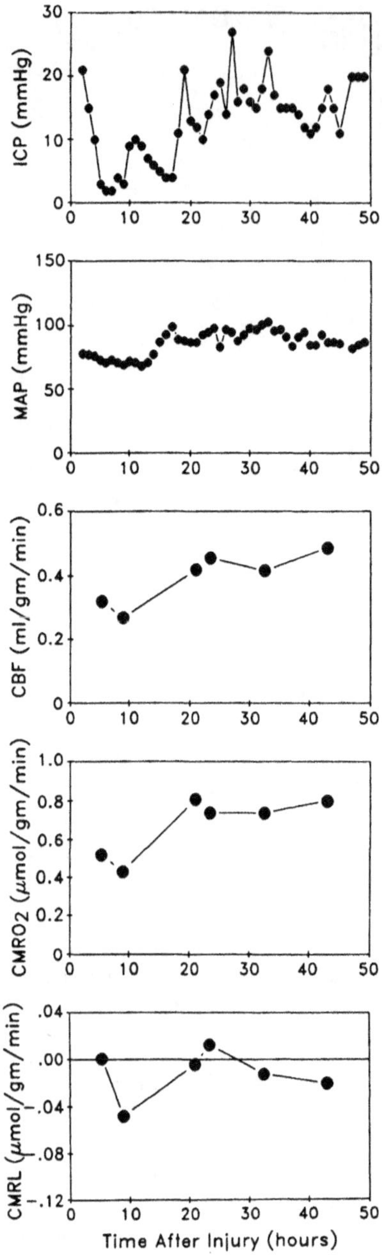

Fig. 3. Cerebral blood flow and metabolism variables in a patient with a diffuse brain injury who developed cerebral ischemia when he became hypovolemic. As the mean arterial pressure decreased, CBF and $CMRO_2$ decreased, and CMRL increased. He was treated with infusions of blood and crystalloid, and as his blood pressure increased, the cerebral blood flow increased, and cerebral metabolism variables returned to values more typical of a comatose patient

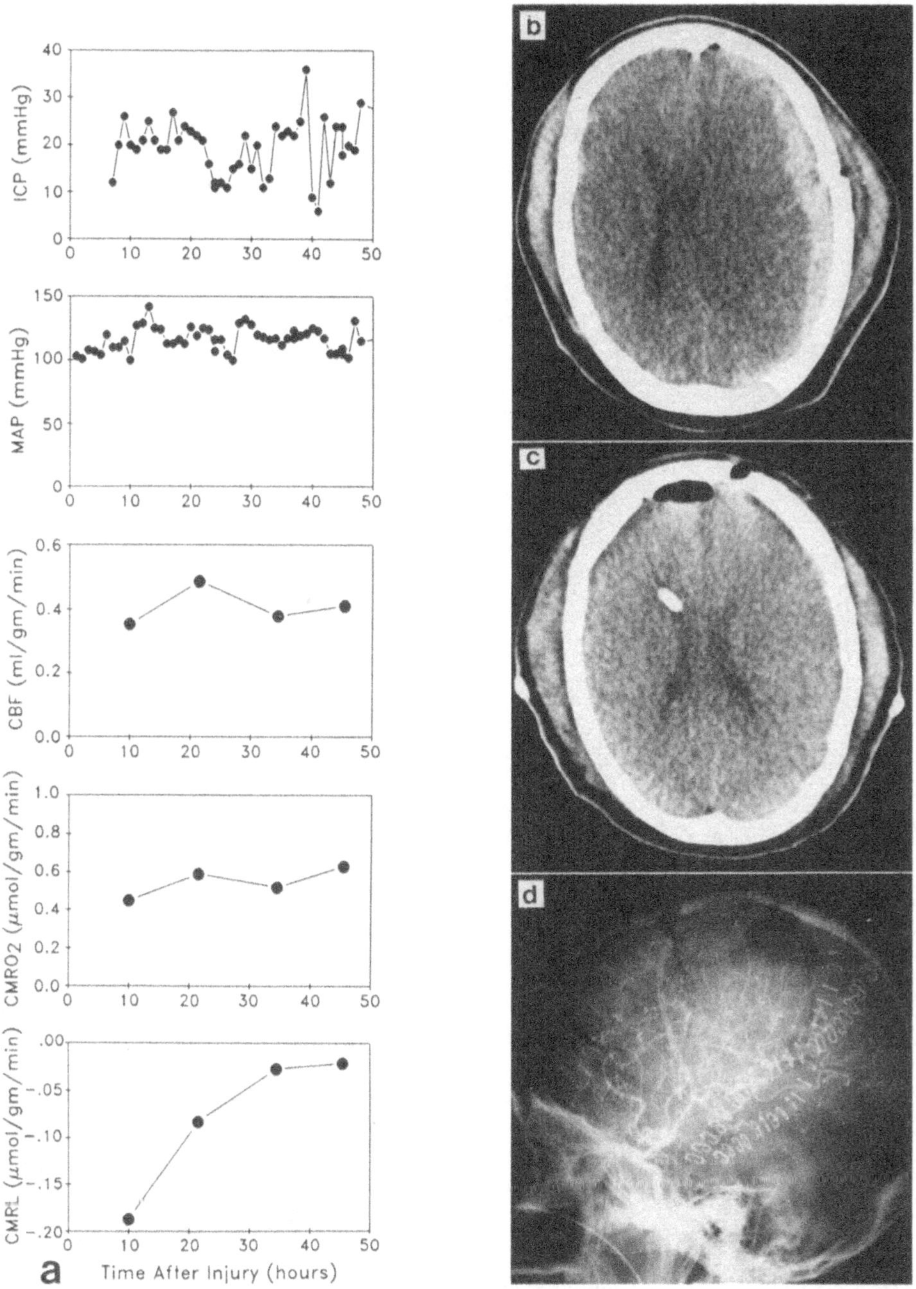

Fig. 4. a Cerebral blood flow and metabolism variables in a patient who developed a middle cerebral artery infarction following evacuation of a large intracerebral hematoma. The CT-scans show the intracerebral hematoma at admission (**b**), successful evacuation of the hematoma on day 1 postinjury (**c**), and the appearance of a large middle cerebral artery distribution infarction on day 4 postinjury (**d**). The characteristic cerebral metabolic patterns of an evolving infarction included a CMRL, and a low $CMRO_2$

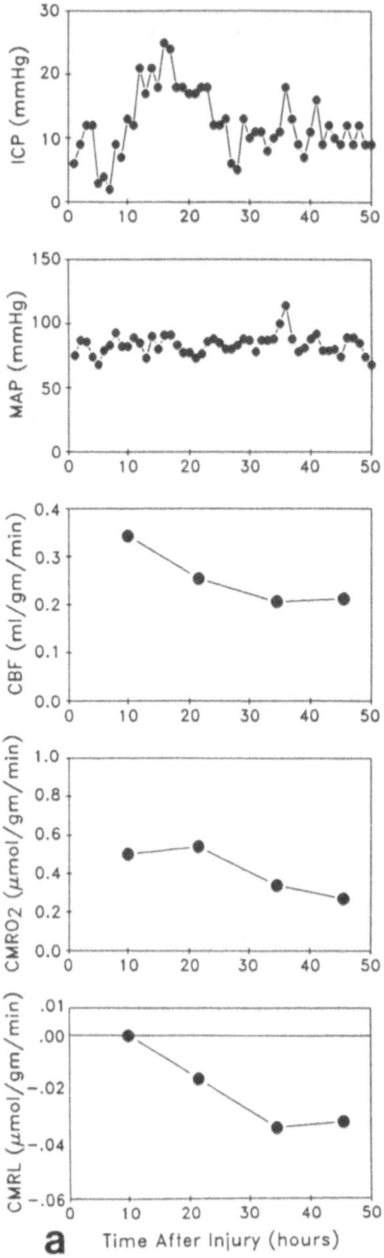

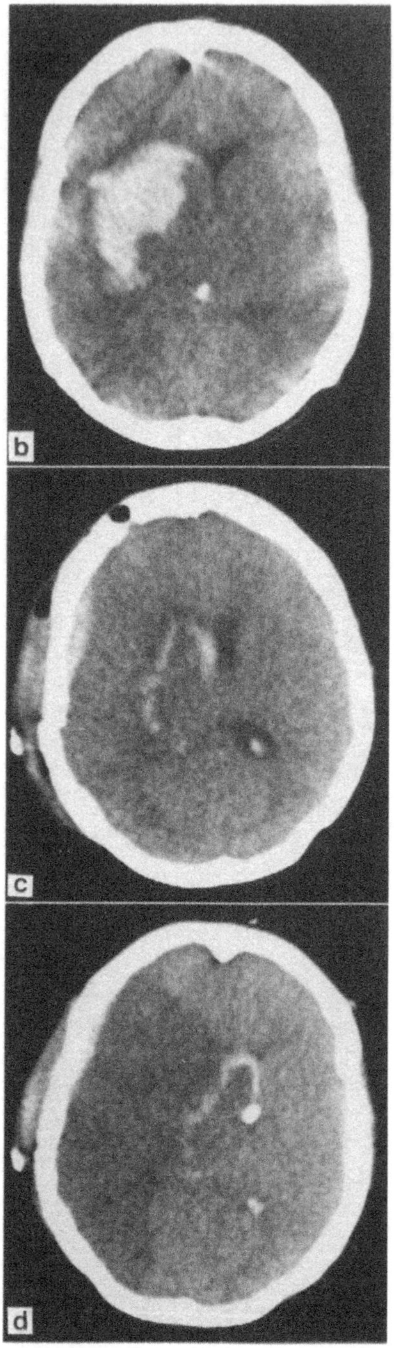

Fig. 5. a Cerebral blood flow and metabolism variables in a patient who developed cerebral vasospasm following a gunshot wound. The CT-scans show the subdural hematoma caused by the gunshot wound which was present at admission (**b**), and the successful evacuation of the hematoma on postinjury day 1 (**c**). The patient's cerebral blood flow was initially near normal values. However, over the subsequent 48 h, the cerebral blood flow decreased, eventually compromising cerebral oxygen consumption and resulting in increased cerebral lactate production. An arteriogram (**d**) demonstrated a markedly slow circulation time and diffuse vasospasm. He was treated with hypervolemic hemodilution, and eventually recovered with a severe disability

Determining Adequate Cerebral Perfusion in the Comatose Patient

Normal CBF Values

Although the consequences of cerebral ischemia on neurological recovery are well-known, assessing the adequacy of cerebral perfusion in comatose patients remains one of the most difficult clinical problems. Cerebral blood flow in patients has been compared to levels measured in normal adults. However, because the cerebral metabolic rate of patients who are comatose due to an injury are in general reduced, it has been argued that a reduced cerebral blood flow may, in fact, be appropriate. Evidence supporting this argument is that the incidence of intracranial hypertension is lower, and mortality rate, in some studies, is better in patients with a reduced cerebral blood flow [27].

Neurophysiological Ischemic Thresholds

Information regarding the adequacy of cerebral blood flow is available from experimental models of cerebral ischemia. While a cerebral blood flow of 0.4–0.6 ml/gm/min is normal, consciousness is altered and the EEG is suppressed when cerebral blood flow drops below 0.25 ml/gm/min [28, 29]. The EEG becomes isoelectric at cerebral blood flows of 0.18–0.20 ml/gm/min [28–31]. The sodium-potassium pump fails and evoked potentials are lost at cerebral blood flow of 0.12–0.16 ml/gm/min [32, 33]. Ion pump failure occurs at cerebral blood flow values of 0.10–0.15 ml/gm/min, and calcium channels open at values <0.10 ml/gm/min [30, 33]. The degree of reduction of cerebral blood flow and the length of time that cerebral blood flow remains reduced are the two crucial factors in determining the survival of neuronal tissue. Irreversible ischemic injury may not occur for several hours when cerebral blood flow is reduced to 0.18 ml/gm/min, while infarction results in minutes when cerebral blood flow is <0.10 ml/gm/min [34, 35].

From this experimental information, a cerebral blood flow in a comatose patient of <0.18 ml/gm/min can be reasonably interpreted as inadequate to support basal metabolic functions. However, the consequences of a cerebral blood flow between 0.18 and 0.25 ml/gm/min is uncertain. The reduced cerebral blood flow may be limiting neuronal function or may be adequate for the reduced cerebral metabolic requirements caused by the injury. A single measurement of cerebral blood flow may not identify all patients with inadequate cerebral perfusion. Observations of cerebral blood flow and cerebral metabolism over time and in response to elevation of the reduced cerebral blood flow may be more informative.

Cerebral Perfusion Variables in Patients with Cerebral Ischemia

Physiological variables which might be of value in assessing the adequacy of cerebral perfusion have been evaluated in a large group of head-injury patients with an initial GCS $\leq$ 8. In the first study, cerebral ischemia was identified by

Table 2. Demographic characteristics of patients studied

	Correlation with CT-scan	Response to treatment of CBF
Total number	41	58
Type of injury:		
diffuse brain injury	11	13
epidural hematoma	2	5
subdural hematoma	9	17
intracerebral hematoma	13	16
gunshot wound	6	7
Sex: male	34	39
female	7	19
Glasgow Coma Score: 3–5	9	15
6–8	32	43
Glasgow Outcome Scale:		
good recovery/moderate disability	20	18
severe disability/vegetative	13	26
dead	8	14

the subsequent development of an infarction on CT-scan. In the second study, cerebral ischemia was defined by an increase in $CMRO_2$ following treatment of the reduced CBF. The demographic characteristics of these patients are summarized in Table 2.

The clinical management is described in detail in previous publications [26, 36]. All patients were treated by a standard protocol that emphasized early surgical evacuation of intracranial hematomas, controlled ventilation, and monitoring of intracranial pressure. Routine medications included phenytoin, morphine for sedation, and antibiotics. Intracranial pressures greater than 20 mmHg were treated with hyperventilation (pCO_2 25 to 30 mmHg), cerebrospinal fluid drainage, sedation and paralysis, mannitol, and (if necessary) barbiturates.

Cerebral blood flow was measured by the Kety-Schmidt technique, using N_2O as the indicator [37–39]. An 18 gauge catheter was inserted percutaneously into the internal jugular vein and positioned so that the tip was in the jugular bulb. The catheter was placed on the side of the most severe injury, or on the right side if the injury was diffuse. The correct position of the catheter tip was confirmed by and x-ray study. A 20 gauge catheter was placed in the radial artery. Ten percent N_2O was introduced into the patient's inspired gases in a stepwise fashion, and 10 timed samples of arterial and jugular venous blood were anaerobically collected during the first 15 min of N_2O saturation. The N_2O concentration was measured in the blood samples on an infrared analyzer using an extraction system modified from that described by Swedlow and Lewis [39]. the CBF was calculated from curves fit to the measured N_2O concentrations and integrated to 15 min [40].

Arterial and jugular venous blood samples were obtained simultaneously with measurement of CBF for determination of blood gases, oxygen saturation, hemoglobin, and lactate concentration. The $CMRO_2$ and CMRL values were calculated by multiplying the CBF by the $AVDO_2$ and AVDL, respectively. CPP was calculated by subtracting the ICP from the mean arterial pressure.

Correlation of cerebral perfusion variables with CT-scan findings: Forty-one patients had sequential daily measurements of CBF during days 1–5 postinjury. All of the CBF values were in the range generally accepted as being adequate to prevent infarction (i.e., ≥ 0.18 ml/gm/min). Nonenhanced cranial CT-scans were obtained as clinically indicated. Generally, CT was performed on admission, postoperatively, and several times during the first 3–6 weeks after injury. Based on the CT-scans, the patients were divided into three groups (cerebral infarction, possible cerebral ischemia, and no cerebral ischemia). Physiological variables, including CPP, CBF, $PjvO_2$, $SjvO_2$, $AVDO_2$, $CMRO_2$, CMRL, and (-AVDL)/$AVDO_2$ were examined to determine which variables were associated with the CT-scan development of cerebral infarction.

Six patients developed areas of low density on serial CT-scans which were characteristic of cerebral infarction. The criteria for distinguishing an infarction from edema were the restriction of a hypodense area to the distribution of an arterial territory with distinct margins, and persistence of the hypodense area after the acute phase of injury. The distribution of the infarctions were: posterior cerebral artery (2 patients), middle cerebral artery (2 patients), anterior cerebral artery (1 patient), and cerebral hemisphere (1 patient). Examples of typical infarctions are shown in Figs. 2 and 4.

Eight of the patients had no low density areas on serial CT-scans. It was assumed that the patients in this group were the least likely to have had significant ischemic injury, and could therefore serve as comatose, but nonischemic controls.

The remaining 27 patients showed low density areas in the regions of previous intracerebral hematomas or contusions. This was a heterogeneous group with the low density areas resulting from edema and/or infarction, but the difference could not be distinguished with certainty on the basis of the CT-scan. The area of tissue involvement was, in general, smaller than in the patients with cerebral infarction.

Of the physiological variables examined, the two measures of anaerobic metabolism, CMRL and (-AVDL)/$AVDO_2$, provided the clearest identification of the patients with cerebral infarction (Fig. 6).

In the patients without cerebral ischemia, CMRL and (-AVDL)/$AVDO_2$ were consistently near zero, indicating low cerebral lactate production. Patients who developed a cerebral infarction had a markedly negative CMRL and an elevated ratio (-AVDL)/$AVDO_2$, indicating an elevated cerebral production of lactate, on days 1–2 after injury. The cerebral lactate production tended to return toward normal by days 3–5 postinjury (Figs. 2 and 4).

$CMRO_2$ in the patients without ischemic injury was consistently greater than the $CMRO_2$ of the patients who developed a cerebral infarction. These differences in $CMRO_2$ were most prominent on day 1 postinjury, and did not appear to be due to differences in degree of coma, since the distribution of the GCS scores was similar in the 2 groups.

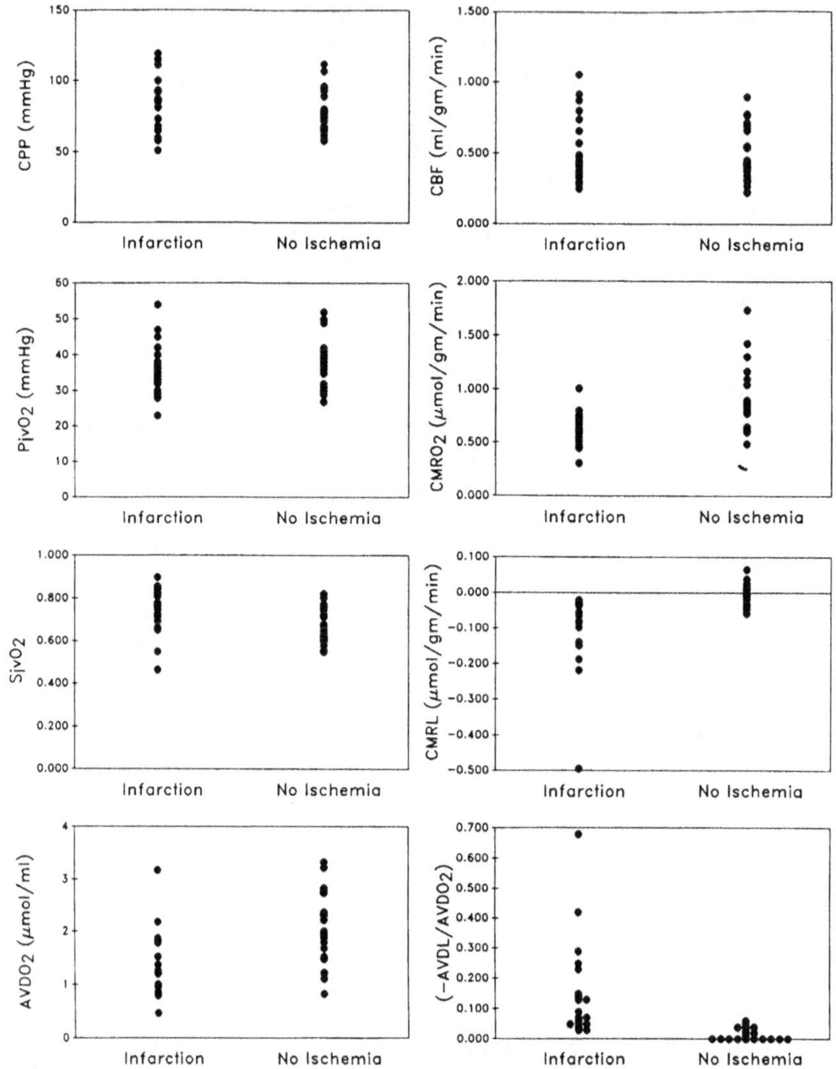

Fig. 6. Cerebral perfusion variables comparing patients who developed cerebral infarction on CT-scan, and patients without evidence of cerebral ischemia. The major differences were the higher anaerobic metabolism measured by CMRL and the ratio (-AVDL)/$AVDO_2$ and the lower $CMRO_2$ in the group who developed infarctions

None of the other physiological variables, including $PjvO_2$, $SjvO_2$, $AVDO_2$, CPP, were different in the 2 groups of patients. The tendency was, in fact, for these variables to suggest a relative hyperemia in the patients who developed a cerebral infarction.

Correlation of cerebral perfusion variables with response to treatment of the reduced CBF: Fifty-eight patients had sequential q8h measurements of CBF,

$CMRO_2$, and CMRL for 5–10 days post-injury. When a CBF $\leq$0.25 ml/gm/min accompanied by an increased oxygen extraction ($AVDO_2 \geq 3.0$ µmol/ml) or increased anaerobic metabolism ($-AVDL/AVDO_2 \geq 0.08$) was identified, attempts were made to increase CBF. Treatments varied from patient to patient, but included allowing pCO_2 to increase to 35 mmHg, hypervolemic hemodilution, and/or dopamine-induced hypertension. CBF, $CMRO_2$, and CMRL were repeated after treatment.

A total of 26 (45%) patients had CBF values $\leq$ 0.25 ml/gm/min at some time during the CBF monitoring period. The reduced CBF was acompanied by increased oxygen extraction ($AVDO_2 \geq 3.0$ µmol/ml) in 10 patients, and by increased anaerobic metabolism ($-AVDL/AVDO_2 \geq 0.08$) in 10 patients. The response to treatment of the reduced CBF was determined most clearly by the presence or absence of increased cerebral lactate production.

In the 10 patients identified with increased oxygen extraction, pretreatment CBF averaged 0.221 ± 0.038 ml/gm/min. Two of the patients, with intracranial hypertension being treated with mechanical hyperventilation, were treated by permitting the pCO_2 to increase to 35 mmHg. The remainder of the patients were treated with hypervolemic hemodilution, and one patient was treated, in addition, with dopamine-induced hypertension. All of the patients had an increase in CBF with treatment, to a mean value of 0.336 ± 0.050 ml/gm/min (Fig. 7). In all of the patients, $AVDO_2$ decreased into the normal range as CBF was increased by the therapy, from 3.92 ± 0.84 to 2.61 ± 0.39 µmol/ml. $CMRO_2$ was unchanged by the treatment.

In the 10 patients with increased anaerobic metabolism, the pretreatment CBF averaged 0.163 ± 0.038 ml/gm/min. In 2 patients, where the cerebral ischemia was due to intractable intracranial hypertension, it was not possible fo follow treatment of the ischemia with CBF measurements, since they died despite aggressive treatment. In the remaining 8 patients, the effects of treatment of the reduced CBF on cerebral metabolism was documented by CBF, $CMRO_2$, and CMRL measurements before and after treatment. The treatments that were examined included: increasing pCO_2 to 35 mmHg (3 patients), hypervolemic hemodilution (4 patients), and dopamine-induced hypertension (1 patient). CBF increased with treatment in all 8 cases to 0.303 ± 0.107 ml/gm/min (Fig. 8). In 7 of the patients, an increase in $CMRO_2$ accompanied the increase in CBF, from a mean value of 0.26 ± 0.17 to 0.68 ± 0.14 µmol/gm/min. In one patient, $CMRO_2$ remained unchanged, although CBF was increased by the therapy. The change in $AVDO_2$ was quite variable and it was not possible to determine whether $CMRO_2$ was improved or not from the changes in $AVDO_2$. However, the ratio $(-AVDL)/AVDO_2$ decreased in the 7 patients where treatment resulted in an increase in $CMRO_2$, and, in contrast, increased in the patient in whom $CMRO_2$ remained unchanged.

Categories of CBF adequacy: From these studies, it was concluded that the presence of increased anaerobic metabolism following a severe head injury indicated either an evolving infarction or hypoperfusion of a sufficient degree to impair cerebral metabolism. The CBF patterns defined in Table 3 have been proposed as a clinically practical method for categorizing CBF adequacy in comatose pa-

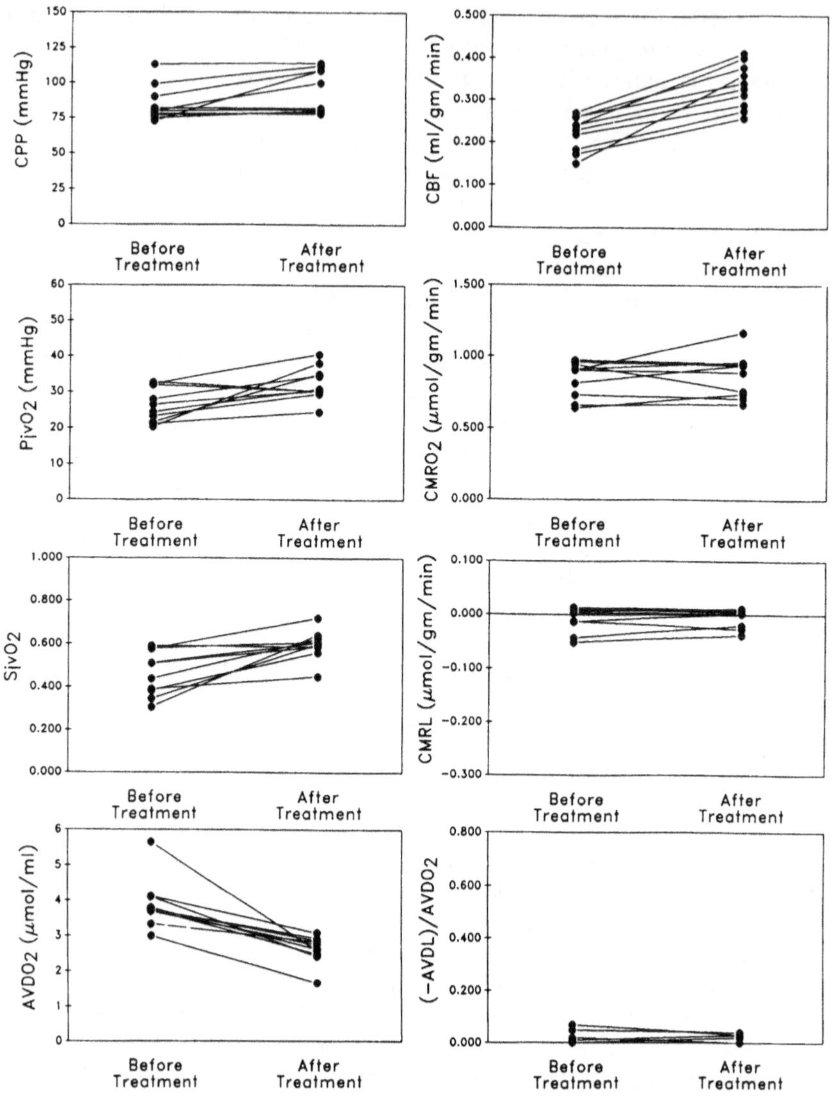

Fig. 7. Cerebral perfusion variables before and after treatment of a reduced cerebral blood flow in patients with increased cerebral oxygen extraction. CBF increased and $AVDO_2$ decreased in all patients. $CMRO_2$ and CMRL were unchanged by treatment

tients, and identifying patients that are likely to benefit from therapy to increase CBF.

The pattern of increased cerebral oxygen extraction, called compensated hypoperfusion, may be the most important to recognize clinically. The increased $AVDO_2$ sugests that the brain is compensating for the decreased blood flow by extracting oxygen more completely, but because anaerobic metabolism is not increased and because $CMRO_2$ does not change as CBF is increased, the low

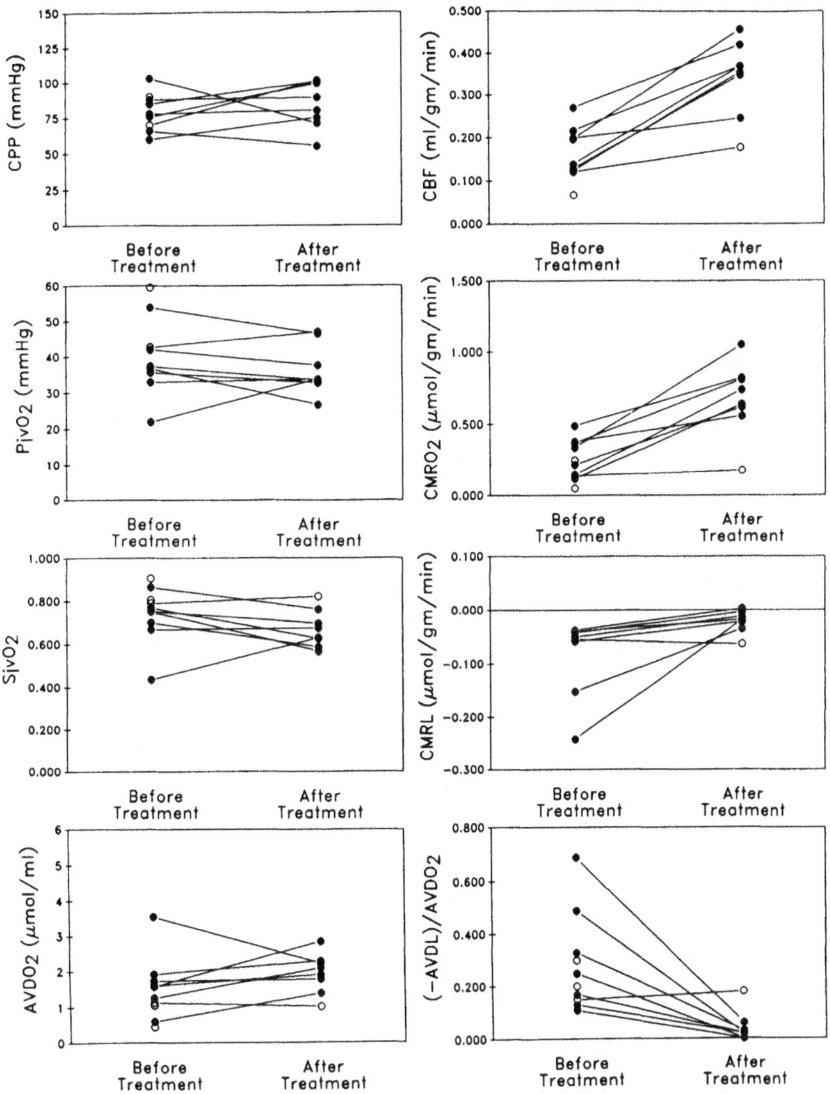

Fig. 8. Cerebral perfusion variables before and after treatment of a reduced cerebral blood flow in patients with increased anaerobic metabolism. The open circles identify the 2 patients in whom posttreatment data were not obtained, and the one patient in whom increasing CBF did not improve cerebral metabolism. In the remaining patients, $CMRO_2$ increased, and CMRL decreased as the CBF was increased by treatment

blood flow does not appear to have altered overall cerebral energy metabolism. Although the patients are not truly ischemic at the moment of the CBF measurement, they have exhausted the brain's compensatory mechanism for maintaining cerebral metabolism in the presence of decreased oxygen availability. In such

Table 3. Categories of CBF adequacy

	$AVDO_2$ (μmol/ml)	$-(AVDL)/AVDO_2$
Nonischemic CBF patterns:		<0.08
hyperemia	<1.3	
normal CBF	1.3–3.0	
compensated hypoperfusion	>3.0	
Ischemia/infarction	Variable	≥0.08

cases, small decreases in either CBF or arterial oxygen content could produce significant cerebral ischemia.

The pattern of increased anaerobic metabolism, indicating ischemia or evolving infarction, was also important to identify, because sometimes this ischemia pattern was reversible. Because $ABDO_2$ is often normal or low, this pattern may be assumed to indicate that brain tissue is irreversibly injured and that the CBF is adequate for the markedly reduced metabolic requirements. Although this is sometimes the case, the presence of reversible ischemic changes is best dermined by a trial of increasing CBF. The reason for the low $AVDO_2$ in patients with reversible ischemia is not entirely clear. It may be that the blood flow is not homogenous and that areas of very low flow and markedly increased oxygen extraction are mixed with areas of normal oxygen extraction. Alternatively, it may be that with very low CBF, venous blood in the jugular bulb is contaminated with more extracerebral blood than when blood flow is normal. Studies conducted in normal adults have shown that extracerebral contamination is only 2–3% [41]. However, no studies have documented that this remains the case when blood flow to the brain is markedly reduced.

References

1. Bowers SA, Marshall LF (1980) Outcome in 200 consecutive cases of severe head injury treated in San Diego County: a prospective analysis. Neurosurgery 6:237–242
2. Graham DI, Adam JH, Doyle D (1978) Ischaemic brain damage in fatal non-missile brain injuries. J Neurol Sci 39:213–234
3. Lewelt W, Jenkins LW, Miller JD (1980) Autoregulation of cerebral blood flow after experimental fluid percussion injury. J Neurosurgery 53:500–511
4. Wei EP, Dietrich WD, Povlishock JT, Navari RM, Kontos HA (1980) Functional, morphological, and metabolic abnormalities of the cerebral microcirculation after concussive brain injury in cats. Circ Res 46:37–47
5. Miller JD (1985) Head injury and brain ischaemia-implications for therapy. Br J Anaesth 57:120–129
6. Neufield P, Pitts L, Kaktis JV (1980) The influence of shock on mortality after head trauma. Crit Care Med 8:254
7. Ishige N, Pitts LH, Berry I, Nishimura MC, James TL (1988) The effects of hypovolemic hypotension on high-energy phosphate metabolism in traumatized brain in rats. J Neurosurg 68:129–136
8. Friedenfelt H, Sunstrom R (1963) Local and general spasm in the internal carotid system following trauma. Acta Radiol (Diagn)1:278–283

9. Suwanweh C, Suwanweh N (1972) Intracranial arterial narrowing and spasm in acute head injury. J Neurosurg 26:314–323
10. Wilkins RH, Odom GL (1970) Intracranial arterial spasm associated with craniocerebral trauma. J Neurosurg 32:626–633
11. MacPherson P, Graham DI (1978) Correlation between angiographic findings and the ischemia of head injury. J Neurol Neurosurg Psychiat 41:122–127
12. Morgan MK, Besser M, Johnston I, Chaseling R (1987) Intracranial carotid artery injury in closed head trauma. J Neurosurg 66:192–197
13. Hansen AJ (1978) The extracellular potassium concentration in brain cortex following ischemia in hypo- and hyperglycemic rats. Acta Physiol Scand 102:324–329
14. Ginsberg MD, Welsh FA, Budd WW (1980) Deleterious effect of glucose pretreatment on recovery from diffuse cerebral ischemia in the cat. I. Local cerebral blood flow and glucose utilization. Stroke 11:347–354
15. Myers RE, Yamaguchi M (1976) Effects of serum glucose concentration on brain response to circulatory arrest. J Neuropathol Exp Neurol 35:301
16. Rehncrona S, Roser I, Siesjö BK: Brain lactic acidosis and ischemic cell damage. 1. Biochemistry and neurophysiology. J Cereb Blood Flow Metab 1:297–311
17. Siemkowicz E, Hansen AJ (1978) Clinical restitution following cerebral ischemia in hypo-, normo-, and hyperglycemic rats. Acta Neurol Scand 58:1–8
18. Robertson CS, Grossman RG (1987) Protection against spinal cord ischemia with insulin-induced hypoglycemia. J Neurosurg 67:739–744
19. Cold G, Enevoldsen E, Malmros R (1975) Ventricular fluid lactate, pyruvate, bicarbonate, and pH in unconscious brain-injured patients subjected to controlled ventilation. Acta Neurol Scand 52:187–195
20. Crockard HA, Taylor AR (1972) Serial CSF lactate/pyruvate values as a guide to prognosis in head injury coma. Eur Neurol 8:151–157
21. Enevoldsen EM, Cold G, Jensen FT, Malmros R (1976) Dynamic changes in regional CBF, intraventricular pressure, CSF pH, and lactate levels during the acute phase of head injury. J Neurosurg 44:191–214
22. King LR, McLaurin RL, Knowles HC Jr (1974) Acid-base balance and arterial and CSF lactate levels following human head injury. J Neurosurg 40:617–625
23. Metzel E, Zimmerman WE (1971) Changes of oxygen pressure, acid-base balance, metabolites, and electrolytes in cerebrospinal fluid and blood after cerebral injury. Acta Neurochir 25:177–188
24. Seitz HD, Ocker K (1977) The prognostic and therapeutic importance of changes in the CSF during the acute stage of brain injury. Acta Neurochir 38:211–231
25. DeSalles AAF, Kontos HA, Becker DP, et al (1986) Prognostic significance of ventricular CSF lactic acidosis in severe head injury. J Neurosurg 65:615–624
26. Robertson CS, Grossman RG, Goodman JC, Narayan RK (1987) The predictive value of cerebral anaerobic metabolism with cerebral infarction after head injury. J Neurosurg 67:361–368
27. Obrist WD, Langfitt TW, Jaggi JL, Cruz J, Gennarelli TA (1984) Cerebral blood flow and metabolism in comatose patients with acute head injury. Relationship to intracranial hypertension. J Neurosurg 61:241–253
28. Gregory PC, McGeorge AP, Fitch W, Graham DI, MacKenzie ET, Harper AM (1979) Effects of hemorrhagic hypotension on the cerebral circulation. II. Electrocortical function. Stroke 10:719–723
29. Williams LF Jr (1968) Hemorrhagic shock as a source of unconsciousness. Surg Clin N Am 48:236–272
30. Symon L (1985) Flow thresholds in brain ischaemia and the effects of drugs. Br J Anaesth 57:34–43
31. Trojaborg W, Boysen G (1973) Relation between EEG, regional cerebral blood flow and internal carotid artery pressure during carotid endarterectomy. Electroencephalogr Clin Neurophysiol 34:61–60
32. Branston NM, Symon L, Crockard HA, Pasztor E (1974) Relationship between the cortical evoked potential and focal cortical blood flow following acute middle cerebral artery occlusion in the baboon. Exp Neurol 45:195–208

33. Astrup J, Symon L, Branston NM, Lassen NA (1977) Cortical evoked potentials and extracellular K^+ and H^+ at critical levels of brain ischemia. Stroke 8:51–57
34. Hossman KA, Schuier FJ (1980) Experimental brain infarcts in cats. 1. Pathophysiological observations. Stroke 11:583–592
35. Jones TH, Morawetz RB, Crowell RM, et al (1981) Thresholds of focal cerebral ischemia in awake monkeys. J Neurosurg 54:773–782
36. Robertson CS, Narayan RK, Gokaslan ZL, et al (1989) Cerebral arteriovenous oxygen difference as an estimate of cerebral blood flow in comatose patients. J Neurosurg (in press)
37. Kety SS, Schmidt CF (1945) The determination of cerebral blood flow in man by the use of nitrous oxide in low concentrations. Am J Physiol 143:53–66
38. Kety SS, Schmidt CF (1948) The nitrous oxide method for the quantitative determination of cerebral blood flow in man: theory, procedure, and normal values. J Clin Invest 27:476–483
39. Swedlow DB, Lewis LE (1980) Measurement of cerebral blood flow in children. Anesthesiology 53(Suppl):S160
40. Kety SS (1951) The theory and applications of the exchange of inert gas at the lungs and tissues. Pharmacol Rev 3:1–41
41. Shenkin HA, Harmel MH, Kety SS (1948) Dynamic anatomy of the cerebral circulation. Arch Neurol Psychiatry 60:242–252

Pathophysiology of the Encephalopathies Associated with Uremia and Hyponatremia

C. L. Fraser and A. I. Arieff

Introduction

Among patients with renal failure, nervous system dysfunction remains a major cause of disability. Depite the widespread use of dialysis therapy, such patients continue to manifest a variety of neurologic disorders [1]. Patients with chronic renal failure who have not yet received dialytic therapy may develop symptoms ranging from mild sensorial clouding to delirium and coma [2]. Even after the institution of adequate maintenance dialysis therapy, patients may continue to manifest more subtle nervous system dysfunction such as impaired mentation, generalized weakness, sexual dysfunction and peripheral neuropathy [3, 4].

Uremic Encephalopathy

Uremic encephalopathy may occur in patients with either acute or chronic renal failure when glomerular filtration rate falls below approximately 10% of normal [2]. In common with other organic brain syndromes these patients display variable disorders of consciousness that can affect psychomotor behavior, thinking, memory, speech, perception and emotion [2, 5]. In patients with acute renal failure, uremic symptoms are generally more severe and progress more rapidly than in patients with number and severity of symptoms may vary cyclically, with intervals of well-being in an otherwise progressive downhill course. The symptoms are usually improved by dialysis and are almost entirely relieved by successful renal transplantation [2].

Differential Diagnosis of Uremic Encephalopathy

Uremic encephalopathy should be suspected in patients with renal failure if there are clinical signs and symptoms consistent with central nervous system deterioration. However, the presenting symptoms of uremic encephalopathy may be similar to those of other metabolic encephalopathies [6] so that there is some risk of misdiagnosis and mistreatment. The problem of differential diagnosis is increased by the fact that patients with renal failure may develop other intercurrent illnesses capable of inducing encephalopathy. If a patient with renal insufficiency is taking a drug with potential central nervous system toxicity that is normally excreted or metabolized by the kidney, the ensuing central nervous system symptoms may be due either to which has reached toxic levels of the drug at ordinary dose rates or to uremia [2]. In patients with both advanced liver and renal diseases, it is often difficult to determine whether the encephalopathy is due to either hepatic or renal causes or both [7]. In such patients the blood urea nitrogen and serum creatinine do not always adequately reflect the degree of functional renal impairment [8].

Central Nervous System Consequences of Acute and Chronic Renal Failure

Electroencephalograms (EEGs) in patients with acute renal failure are generally grossly abnormal when the diagnosis of acute renal failure is first made [9]. In most instances, the percentage of electroencephalogram power less than either 5 Hz or 7 Hz is 20 times greater than the normal value. The abnormal percentages of electroencephalogram frequencies both above 9 Hz and below 5 Hz are not usually improved by dialysis within the first eight weeks of treatment, although they may return to normal with recovery of renal function. If renal failure continues, the electroencephalogram may transiently worsen both during and after hemodialysis and this pattern may continue for up to six months after the initiation of dialytic therapy [9–11].

Electroencephalogram abnormalities in patients with chronic renal failure are usually not as severe as those reported in patients with acute renal failure. In general there is a good correlation between both the percentage of electroencephalogram frequencies and power below 7 Hz and the decline of renal function as estimated by serum creatinine [11, 12]. After the initiation of dialysis there may be an initial period of clinical stabilization during which time the electroencephalogram continues to deteriorate. However, after approximately six months of dialysis treatment the EEG tends to normalize. Normal values may not be reached however, unless the patient receives a kidney transplant [10]. In patients with chronic renal failure, certain cognitive functions are also impaired. These include attention span, speed of decision making, short-term memory and mental manipulation of symbols [5, 13].

Subcellular Studies on Uremic Brain

Because of the difficulty of establishing a causal relationship between brain content of electrolytes, neurotransmittors, parathyroid hormone (PTH) and the symptoms of uremic encephalopathy, investigators have more recently evaluated effects of uremia on the brain by studying brain subcellular fractions. This subcellular analysis has been undertaken primarily with synaptosomes [3, 14–16] which are vesicles derived from the presynaptic nerve terminal in brain [3, 17]. The reasons for studying synaptosomal function in uremia were based on their anatomical location and *in vivo* physiological role in the process of information transfer.

When a neuron in the central nervous system (CNS) is stimulated, an action potential is generated which travels the length of the neuron to the nerve terminal where it results in an increase in the membrane permeability of the plasma membrane to calcium. This change results in calcium influx from the extracellular space into the cytosol of the nerve terminal [1, 18]. The mechanisms by which calcium enters cells include sodium channels, calcium channels and the Na-Ca exchanger [15, 19]. As opposed to non-excitable cells, in excitable cells such as neurons and myocardium, the exchanger participates in both influx and efflux of calcium [20, 21]. In order to maintain calcium balance, the calcium which enters the cell from the extracellular space has to be pumped out after its effect has been achieved. In nerve terminals, the outward movement of calcium is accomplished primarily by both the Na-Ca exchanger and the Ca-ATPase pump [22]. Regardless of which transporter is utilized, the overall effect is to maintain a calcium gradient of 10000:1 (outside:inside cells). In a steady state, the net calcium flux across the plasma membrane is zero. In cellular regulation of calcium, the Ca-ATPase pump modulates subtle changes in cytosolic calcium, while the Na-Ca exchanger is important in regulating major changes in calcium flux [15].

Utilizing synaptosomes, Fraser and associates have demonstrated that in the brains of uremic rats, several defects in synaptosomal function exist [3, 14–16]. Both the Na- Ca exchanger and the Ca-ATPase pumps were shown to be abnormal [14]. The presence of uremia resulted in an enhancement of calcium transport by both transport mechanisms. These defects were shown to be primarily dependent on PTH, and in addition, PTH administered to nonuremic rats could reproduce the transport abnormalities found in uremia [15]. Further studies by this group have demonstrated that the action of PTH on calcium transport in uremic synaptosomes was independent of cAMP [16]. Although PTH stimulates calcium transport in brain synaptosomes, it was unable to stimulate cAMP production in the same synaptosomes [16].

In other studies on synaptosomes, it was also shown that in addition to the effects of uremia on Ca transport, the Na-K ATPase pump function was affected by uremia as well [3]. The ouabain sensitive component of both sodium and potassium transport was significantly decreased in the brains of uremic rats. In crude brain preparation, Na-K ATPase enzyme activity was found to be normal to decreased [1]. Contrary to the detrimental effects of uremia on brain ion transport, water and urea transport were not affected by uremia [23].

There is substantial evidence that neurotransmitter substance regulation may be altered in acute uremia [12, 24–27]. Since the mid sixties, it has been shown that neurotransmitter substances such as norepinephrine, 5-hydroxytryptamine, acetylcholine and dopamine are transported in the brain by sodium dependent mechanisms. It has also been shown that the Na-K ATPase and potassium participate directly in the transport of the biogenic amines [28–31]. Quabain, an inhibitor of the Na-K ATPase pump, is not only capable of inhibiting the pump but it also inhibits neurotransmitter transport [28, 32]. Inhibition of the pump results in inhibition of the neurotransmitter. In uremic rats, norepinephrine uptake, tyrosine hydroxlase activity and catecholamines, such as dopamine, norepinephrine and epinephrine concentrations were found to be substantially decreased [33, 34]. Autopsy material from brains of hemodialysis patients who died with renal failure showed a 40% decrease in gamma aminobutyric acid (GABA) content and a 25–35% decrease in acetylcholine transferase activity [35]. This decrease in transferase activity could result in decrease synthesis of acetylcholine. The findings in brain synaptosomes, which have demonstrated both decreased function of the Na-K ATPase pump and decreased transport of both sodium and potassium in acutely uremic rat brain is consistent with these observations [3].

Hyponatremia

Hyponatremia is the most common electrolyte abnormality seen in a general hospital population, with a prevalence of about 2.5% [7]. It is commonly seen in association with many different systemic disease states and is almost always the result of dilution of extracellular fluid solute. It may be either acute or chronic, and total body water may be either high, low, normal or "uncertain" [36].

Pathophysiology of Hyponatremic Encephalopathy

In recent years, there has been an increased awareness that acute symptomatic hyponatremia in women of child bearing age can lead to death and/or permanent brain damage [8, 36]. The reasons for the apparent protection of men from the complications of acute hyponatremia is unclear. However, it appears that the female brain may be less able to defend itself against hyponatremia than that of the male. In response to acute hyponatremia, the brain is able to lower its intracellular osmolality to match that of plasma by the extrusion of osmotically active cations (sodium and potassium). The cation loss serves to lessen the development of an osmolar gradient between brain and plasma, and consequently moderate the development of cerebral edema [38]. This compensatory mechanism of the brain occurs quite rapidly after the onset of hyponatremia, beginning within thirty minutes of the initial insult. The loss of brain electrolytes occurs both directly across the blood brain barrier into the plasma and indirectly into the cerebrospinal fluid for ultimate removal [39]. If this compensation is adequately achieved, brain water content will not be significantly increased above normal and cerebral edema will not develop. However, if there is interference with the extrusion of one or both of the cations, then the resulting osmotic disequilibrium between the brain and plasma will result in inward movement of water into the brain. Persistence of the hyponatremia may lead to cerebral edema, cerebral herniation and ultimately, death or permanent brain damage. The increased death rate in females from acute hyponatremia is not restricted only to human subjects [40–42]. In fact, in both rabbit and rat models of acute hyponatremia, the female animals are much more likely to die than do the males. The mortality among female rabbits is greater than 85% for sodium <110 mEq/l, and $<25\%$ among the males [43, 44].

The extrusion of sodium from the brain occurs primarily by the Na-K ATPase pump [3], and recent evidence has suggested that sex hormones can directly affect the function of this pump [17, 45, 46]. Moreover, it has been shown that female sex hormones (estrogen and progesterone) can inhibit Na-K ATPase enzyme activity in many tissues, while the male sex hormone (testosterone) may stimulate enzyme activity [45].

Recent data from our laboratory indicates that Na-K ATPase pump function in female rat brain synaptosomes in markedly less than it is in males [45]. The reason for this reduced pump activity in females appears to be due to increased affinity of the pump in females to bind to circulating ouabain-like substances which irreversibly alters its function. This observation has substantial clinical implications, since there is now overwhelming evidence to indicate that the female sex hormones, such as estrogen and progesterone have ouabain-like actions on the Na-K ATPase in the heart, ilium, liver and certain regions of the brain [46–48]. In isolated heart muscle, it was shown that progesterone and its derivatives bind to ouabain binding sites of the Na-K ATPase pump in dog, cat, rat and guinea pig. The binding of these compounds to the Na-K ATPase were shown to displace ouabain from its binding site in a dose dependent manner which is similar to that observed with the cardiac glycosides [46]. It was also observed that the male sex hormone, testosterone, did not displace ouabain from its binding sites even at very high concentrations. In another study, the estrous cycle in female rats was found to influence the Na-K ATPase enzyme activity in both the mediobasal hypothalamus and the preoptic suprachiasmatic areas within the brain [49]. It was shown that enzyme activity varies substantially with the various phases of the cycle. Activity was highest prior to the estrogen surge before ovulation, and lowest during the estrus phase (estrogen and progesterone surge). Norephinephrine content of both the preoptic suprachiasmatic and mediobasal hypothalamus regions also vary during the cycle as well [17].

The inhibitory effect of the female sex hormones on the Na-K ATPase has also been demonstrated in other tissues [26, 48, 50, 51]. In the intestine, estrogen exerts an inhibitory effect on specific activity of the Na-K ATPase in the ileal basolateral membranes [48]. In the liver, reduction in membrane fluidity by estrogen results in inhibition of both hepatocellular bile excretion and liver plasma membranes Na-K ATPase activity [26, 50]. Based on these studies, it appears that both estrogen and progesterone exert inhibitory effects on the Na-K ATPase pump in many biological membranes. A number of other hormones have also been shown to influence electrolyte status. These include atrial natriuretic peptide, aldosterone, adrenocorticotropic hormone, prolactin, angiotensin, vasopressin as well as progesteronc, estrogen and testosterone [36].

As opposed to the inhibitory effects of the female sex hormones on the Na-K ATPase activity, there is evidence suggesting that the male sex hormone testosterone, stimulates Na-K ATPase activity [47]. Testosterone was shown to significantly increase enzyme activity in the preoptic suprachiasmatic region of the brain in castrated male rats, while orchiectomy (testosterone absence) resulted in a significant decrease in enzyme activity in the mediobasal hypothalamus [47]. These results directly contrast the inhibitory action of estrogen in these regions of the brain. The data from these studies are consistent with the observation that receptors for the principal ovarian and testicular gonadal hormones are found in many regions of the brain.

Symptoms of Acute Hyponatremia

The symptoms of acute hyponatremia are dependent on several factors, which include the age and sex of the patient as well as the etiology, magnitude and acuteness of the condition [6, 52]. Neurological manifestations of acute to subacute hyponatremia may be observed when the plasma sodium is below 130 mM. These include headache, nausea and emesis in most cases, as well as several possible additional symptoms [36, 37]. More severe symptoms such as grand mal seizures, respiratory arrest and coma occur in a substantial number of patients. When the degree of brain swelling exceeds about 5 to 8% of brain volume, herniation may occur, leading to a symptom complex which may include sudden apnea, bradycardia, unequal pupils, dilated pupils (unilateral or bilateral), hypoventilation, cardiovascular instability, impaired temperature regulation (hyperthermia or hypothermia), urinary and/or fecal incontinance and respiratory arrest [6, 36, 37, 53]. In general, symptoms are more severe and occur at a higher level of serum sodium in younger women (age 16–45 years) than in either men or older women. Acute symptomatic hyponatremia with plasma sodium below 120 mM has a mortality above 35% with a substantial morbidity, which is usually permanent brain damage. However, when plasma sodium is more slowly (several days to several weeks) lowered to 120 mM or less patients usually are less symptomatic. In male or elderly female patients (above 60 years) whose plasma sodium is above 120 mM and are not symptomatic, both morbidity and mortality are minimal.

In experimental animals with acute water intoxication, coma and seizures may be seen when serum sodium is acutely lowered to levels below 128 mM over a period of 4 h or less, but when serum sodium is reduced below 120 mM over several days, many animals are asymptomatic; more profound hyponatremia (serum sodium less than 110 mM) usually results in varying degrees of paralysis, lethargy, coma and seizures but this depends on the age, sex and hormonal status of the animals. For example, adult male rats with chronic serum sodium of about 110 mM are relatively asymptomatic [54]. Thus, both in patients and experimental animals, the neurological manifestations seem to correlate only grossly with both the degree of hyponatremia and with the rapidity of the fall in serum sodium. More recent observations indicate that the age and sex of the individual may be at least as important as the aforementioned factors [36, 37, 43, 44].

When the brain swells such that the swelling exceeds about 5 to 8% of brain volume, herniation may occur, leading to a symptom complex which may include unequal pupils, dilated pupils, hypoventilation, cardiovascular instability, impaired temperature regulation, urinary and/or fecal incontinance and respiratory arrest [37, 40, 42, 55]. Hypoxic brain damage will usually develop [37] and there may also be delayed postanoxic encephalopathy [40]. Increased intracranial pressure may lead to damage to other brain structures such as the pituitary gland, hypothalamus or cranial nerves. Other changes which have been reported include necrosis of the cerebellum, medulla, hypothalamus, pituitary, pons and basal ganglia. Permanent brain damage in such patients in virtually always associated with hypoxic brain damage, which is largely secondary to increased intracranial pressure, leading to decreased tissue oxygenation [37].

Symptoms of Chronic Hyponatremia

Patients with chronic hyponatremia generally have less severe symptoms and a lower morbidity and mortality. However, since chronic hyponatremia is more common in both men and elderly women, this may be due not so much to the degree or duration of the hyponatremia as to the age, sex and hormonal status of the patient. Young women are not prone to many of the disorders which may be associated with chronic hyponatremia. Chronic hyponatremia is commonly observed in patients with any of several edematous states, such as congestive heart failure [36], nephrotic syndrome, liver failure [8] or renal insufficiency. In all of the aforementioned conditions, both total body water and sodium tend to be increased [36]. It is also frequently seen in patients with the syndrome of inappropriate secretion of antidiuretic hormone (SIADH), which may be caused by various tumors (which secrete ADH or similar acting polypeptides), as well as a large variety of diseases of either the central nervous system or lungs [6]. Among hospitalized patients, an inappropriate ADH-like syndrome is commonly seen with the administration of various drugs, including oral hypoglycemics, tricyclic antidepressant agents, certain anticancer agents, diuretics, clofibrate, and morphine like analgesics. Chronic hyponatremia may also be seen in patients with salt losing states, such as salt-losing renal disease, idiosycratic reaction to diuretics, excessive sweating, Addison's disease, AIDS or gastrointestinal electrolyte loss. It has also been reported in patients ingesting massive quantities of beer [36].

Consequences of Hyponatremic Encephalopathy

Hyponatremia may affect brain function and lead to permanent damage by any of several ways. Initially, the symptoms of acute hyponatremia are probably due to brain swelling, with a secondary increase of intracranial pressure. With more prolonged hyponatremia, the brain becomes depleted of both sodium and potassium, thereby somewhat limiting the increase in brain cell volume [38, 39]. The loss of brain sodium and potassium may result in both inhibition in brain energy metabolism and interference with neurotransmitter amino acid release at the synaptic level. These changes may affect brain function and may in part be responsible for the encephalopathy of hyponatremia. With swelling which exceeds about 5 to 8% of brain volume, herniation may occur. Hypoxic brain damage will usually develop and there may also be delayed postanoxic encephalopathy. Increased intracranial pressure may lead to damage to other brain structures such as the pituitary gland or cranial nerves. Thus, survival in acute hyponatremia depends on the ability of the brain to lower its intracellular osmolality by extruding electrolytes, rather than gaining water, the latter of which can lead to brain swelling and herniation [52]. In patients with protracted hyponatremia then, it can be assumed that the cell content of sodium, potassium and chloride is low and brain water is modestly elevated [38, 39, 52]. The possible effects of any therapy must be evaluated against such a background.

Differential Diagnosis of Hyponatremic Encephalopathy

Hyponatremic encephalopathy often occurs in apparently healthy patients who have been hospitalized for routine elective problems. Because such patients appear to be generally healthy, the diagnosis of hyponatremic encephalopathy may not be suspected. Moreover, when similar patients develops a symptom complex which can include unexpected findings such as opisthotonus, respiratory depression, impaired response to verbal and/or painful stimuli, bizarre behavior, incontinance of urine or feces, visual and/or auditory hallucinations, lethargy, decorticate and decerebrate posturing and seizure activity, there is an extensive differential diagnosis. Additionally, within 24 h after respiratory arrest, patients can develop fixed dilated pupils and hypothermia [1]. The respiratory arrest is usually diagnosed as being somehow related to the administration of morphine or meperidine (Demerol). There is no response to the intravenous administration of naloxone HCI (Narcan). The decorticate and decerebrate posturing is frequently diagnosed as a reaction to phenothiazine drugs (promazine [Sparine], promethazine HCI [Phenergan] or prochlorperazine [Compazine]), which have been administered for the nausea. These have been treated by discontinuing the agent and administrating diphenhydramine HCI (Benadryl) or benztropine mesylate (Cogentin), again without any response. The sudden obtundation has occasionally been diagnosed as acute viral encephalitis, but this can generally be ruled out by examination of the cerebrospinal fluid. The fixed dilated pupils are often thought to be indicative of brain death, and largely for this reason, many patients have received no therapy for their low serum sodium. The fixed dilated pupils are most likely caused by cerebral herniation, with pressure of the temporal lobe on the third (oculomotor) nerve or occlusion of the posterior cerebral artery near the third nerve. Many patients develop some combination of unilateral and then bilateral dilated pupils, absent pain response, apnea and positive Babinski. These signs and symptoms are frequently interpreted as being consistent with various drug reactions (see above) or acute intracranial events, such as subarachnoid bleeding episodes. Acute intracranial episodes can and should be ruled out by computed axial tomography (CAT-scan) or magnetic resonance imaging (MRI) of the head. All of the above events are consistent with acute (less than 24 h) progressive brain herniation, and this can generally be diagnosed by modern imaging techniques (CT-scan and/or MRI).

Treatment of Hyponatremia

Criteria for Treatment of Hyponatremia

Previously, it was often thought that therapy for hyponatremia was not warranted unless the serum sodium was below some arbitrary value, usually taken to be 120 mM. However, recent evidence suggests that the absolute level of serum sodium is not nearly as important as the associated symptomatology, as well as the age and sex (36, 43–45]. Permanent brain damage may occur in patients whose serum sodium is as high as 130 mM if central nervous system manifestations of hyponatremia are present. Thus, in any patient with hyponatremia, a therapeutic decision must be made [6]. In a patient who has symptomatic hyponatremia, therapy with hypertonic NaCl should be considered, but one must bear in mind that hyponatremia per se is not in and of itself a reason to treat with hypertonic NaCl. Male patients with serum sodium of 120 to 130 mM who are asymptomatic may do well when treated with water restriction or intravenous 154 mM NaCl. However, patients who are symptomatic with serum sodium below 130 mM should probably be treated with hypertonic NaCl, particularly if they fall into one of the very high risk patient catagories, such as young women or small children [36].

Cerebral Demyelinating Lesions and Hyponatremia

Cerebral demyelinating lesions and central pontine myelinolysis: It has been suggested in the past that treatment of symptomatic hyponatremia with hypertonic NaCl may lead to central pontine myelinolysis (CPM), a rare neurological disorder of uncertain etiology which was initially described in alcoholic malnourished subjects [6, 56–59]. The lesion described in patients with CPM involved the center of the base of the pons and often extended from mid-brain to nerves of the lower pons. Most medullary sheaths were destroyed within the area of the lesion. The destruction of myelin involved all tracts, but in contrast to the complete destruction of myelin, axis cylinders, nerve cells, and blood vessels were relatively well preserved [56, 57].

More recently, it has been suggested that extrapontine lesions are sometimes also present in patients who have pontine demyelination [58, 60]. These lesions differ from those which are confined to the pons in that they are usually anoxic in nature. The clinical characteristics among patients with documented CPM are variable but the disorder has a very high mortality and improvement is rare. In the original description, patients had flaccid quadriplegia, facial weakness, inability to speak and swallow and impaired response to painful stimuli. Facial and tongue weakness were thought to be a pseudobulbar phenomena.

There is some apparent confusion in the literature over the use of the diagnostic term "central pontine myelinolysis" (CPM). Although originally described as a distinct pathological entity where cerebral demyelinating lesions were confined to the pons the term has been recently been assigned to patients or laboratory animals who had demyelination of the brain which was either:

a) pontine;
b) extrapontine;
c) both pontine and extrapontine;
d) clinical manifestations similar to those of patients with CPM but without autopsy or radiological confirmation of cerebral demyelination.

The term "cerebral demyelinating lesions" should be used to mean any cerebral demyelination which is confirmed by autopsy, MR imaging or CAT-scanning, regardless of the location of the lesions in the brain [53]. Such a description includes both pontine and extrapontine myelinolysis. Patients who have functional neurologic impairment without demyelinating lesions should not be referred to as having either CPM or cerebral demyelinating lesions.

Delayed post-anoxic encephalopathy associated with hyponatremia: An association between hyponatremia and CPM has been suggested by some investigators, but more recent studies have demonstrated that the brain lesions associated with hyponatremia (hyponatremic encephalopathy) are largely due to a combination of hypoxia, herniation and pressure necrosis [36]. Demyelination is usually secondary to anoxia/hypoxia and/or increased intracranial pressure. Patients who are treated for their hyponatremia after an hypoxic episode will often recover consciousness after the hyponatremia has been corrected. In such patients, the clinical manifestations of hypoxia are sometimes delayed, giving a false appearance of some relationship to therapy [12]. Although only recently recognized as being associated with hyponatremia, hypoxic brain damage appears to be an important factor in the neurological disability observed in some hyponatremic subjects [40]. The syndrome of delayed post-anoxic encephalopathy has been known at least since 1925 [37, 61]. The disorder can follow anoxia-hypoxia from any cause but most cases are related to either carbon monoxide intoxication, attempted strangulation, cardio-pulmonary arrest or various miscellaneous intoxications. The vast majority of reported cases are related to either carbon monoxide intoxication or cardio-pulmonary arrest with resuscitation. Whatever the cause, patients are initially deeply comatose, often requiring artificial ventilation. Characteristically, they begin to regain consciousness within one to three days. Initial improvement may be rapid enough that patients are discharged from the hospital within a week of the initial intoxication. As early as two days, or as late as several weeks, patients begin to relapse. The onset may be abrupt and heralded by disorientation, confusion, restlessness, apathy and irritability, often with agitation, mania or other inappropriate behavior. There may be cortical dysfunction which is multifocal in character, with dysphasias, agnosias and apraxias. Motor control is impaired, with resultant rigidity or spasticity.

There are no obvious features during the initial anoxic insult which serve to distinguish those patients destined to relapse from those who have uncomplicated recoveries. Many such patients are initially misdiagnosed and are felt to have primary cerebral pathology, such as subdural hematoma. In the hyponatremic patients the diagnosis must be made on clinical grounds, but appears to be the most likely cause of the recurrent seizures and coma, with either death or a persistent vegetative state as the usual outcome. An unfortunate clinical misinterpretation appears to have occurred in the clinical literature. Patients with symptomatic hyponatremia have been treated (usually with hypertonic NaCl) and appeared to improve [58–60]. Then, after several days, they deteriorated neurologically and often did not survive. At autopsy, these patients often had demyelinating lesions of the brain, often including the pons. Because of an occasional superficial anatomical similarity to central pontine myelinolysis, such patients were said to have such a lesion [58, 60], even though the distribution of lesions invariably involved many other parts of the brain in addition to the pons. The situation was further compounded by the fact that CPM is most common in subjects with cirrhosis, and such patients also have a high incidence of hyponatremia [8]. Thus, in patients with the combination of cirrhosis, hyponatremia and neurological deterioration, the cerebral demyelinating lesions found at autopsy was often mistakenly diagnosed as related to the "therapy" of hyponatremia [58, 59], even though many such patients had received no therapy at all [36, 40]. In fact, the deterioration several days after therapy was virtually always associated with respiratory arrest which occured *before* treatment [37, 40, 60] and the clinical picture and neuropathology were that of hypoxic encephalopathy, often delayed postanoxic encephalopathy [37]. It is now clear that such a sequence frequently occurs in the *absence* of therapy [36, 43]. Similar pontine lesions are found in patients who have had wasting disorders unrelated to hyponatremia, such as burns [62] thus rendering any association with treatment of hyponatremia most unlikely [36]. The actual diagnosis of CPM has in the past been made only by post-mortem exam. Recently, several cases have been diagnosed by CT-scan of the pons and magnetic resonance imaging may be a still more valuable tool in the future.

Effects of Treatment

In general, many physicians do not employ hypertonic NaCl to treat symptomatic hyponatremia because of the presumed hazards of circulatory overload. It should be pointed out that this may be more of a theoretical hazard than a real one; few if any cases of circulatory overload complicating the treatment of hyponatremia have ever been reported. A major argument for "slow" correction of symptomatic hyponatremia is the possible development of cerebral demyelinating lesions (see above). At the present time, there are at least six prospective studies involving over 100 patients who were treated with hypertonic NaCl where serum sodium was corrected at rates of 0.8 to 5 mmol/hr. There was no neurological deterioration or evidence of cerebral demyelinating lesions if respiratory depression or arrest did not occur prior to therapy, or if certain other conditions [53] were not present [23, 41, 63–66].

References

1. Fraser CL, Arieff AI (1988) Neurological complications of uremia. In: Schrier RW, Gottschalk CW (eds) Strauss and Welt: diseases of the kidney, 4th edn. Little & Brown, Boston, pp 3063–3092
2. Teschan PE, Arieff AI (1985) Uremic and dialysis encephalopathies. In: McCandless DW (ed) Cerebral energy metabolism and metabolic encephalopathy. Plenum Publishing, New York, pp 263–286
3. Fraser CL, Sarnacki P, Arieff AI (1985) Abnormal sodium transport in synaptosomes from brain of uremic rats. J Clin Invest 75:2014–2023
4. Said G, Boudier L, Selva J, Zingraff J, Drueke T (1983) Different patterns of uremic polyneuropathy: A clinicopathologic study. Neurology 33:567–574
5. Teschan PE, Ginn HE, Bourne JR, et al (1979) Quantitative indices of clinical uremia. Kidney Int 15:676–697
6. Arieff AI (1985)Effects of water, electrolyte and acid base disorders on the central nervous system. In: Arieff AI, DeFronzo RA (eds) Fluid, electrolyte and acid base disorders. Churchill Livingstone, New York, pp 969–1040
7. Chung HM, Kluge R, Schrier RW, Anderson RJ (1986) Postoperative hyponatremia: A prospective study. Arch Intern Med 146:333–336
8. Papadakis MA, Arieff AI (1988) Hyponatremia and hypernatremia in patients with liver disease. In: Epstein M (ed) The kidney in liver disease, 3rd edn. Williams & Wilkins, Baltimore, pp 73–88
9. Cooper JD, Lazarowitz VC, Arieff AI (1978) Neurodiagnostic abnormalities in patients with acute renal failure: Evidence for neurotoxicity of parathyroid hormone. J Clin Invest 61:1448–1455
10. Hughes JR (1980) Correlation between EEG and chemical changes in uremia. Electroenceph Clin Neurophysiol 48:583–594
11. Kiley JE, Woodruff MW, Pratt KL (1976) Evaluation of encephalopathy by EEG frequency analysis in chronic dialysis patients. Clin Neph 5:245–250
12. Ginsberg MD (1979) Delayed neurolgical deterioration following hypoxia. Adv Neurol 26:21–44
13. Souheaver GT, Ryan JJ, DeWolfe AS (1982) Neuropsychological patterns in uremia. J Clin Psychol 38:490–496
14. Fraser CL, Sarnacki P, Arieff AI (1985) Calcium transport abnormality in uremic rat brain synaptosomes. J Clin Invest 76:1789–1795
15. Fraser CL, Sarnacki P (1988) Parathyroid hormone mediates changes in calcium transport in uremic rat brain synaptosomes. Am J Physiol 254:F837–F844
16. Fraser CL, Sarnacki P, Budayr A (1988) Evidence that parathyroid hormone mediated calcium transport in rat brain synaptosomes is independent of cAMP. J Clin Invest 81:982–988
17. Kucharczyk J, Fraser CL, Arieff AI (1989) Hyponatremia and the central nervous system. In: Griffs RC, Arieff AI (eds) Neurologic manifestations of systemic disorders. Little, Brown & Co., Boston (in press)
18. Katz B, Miledi R (1971) The release of acetylcholine from nerve endings by graded electric pulses. Proc R Soc Lomd B Biol Sci 167:23–38
19. Barritt GJ (1982) Calcium movement across cell membrane. In: The role of calcium in biological systems. Boca Raton, Fl CRC
20. Blaustein MP, Oborn CJ (1975) The influence of sodium and calcium fluxes in pinched-off nerve terminals in vitro. J Physiol (London) 247:657–686

21. Reuter H, Mullins LJ (1979) The dependence of calcium efflux from cardiac muscle on temperature and external ion composition. Q Rev Biphys 12:371-460
22. Phillipson KD, Nishimoto AY (1982) Stimulation of Na-Ca exchange in cardiac sarcolema vesicles by proteinase pretreatment. Am J Physiol 243:C191-C195
23. Verkman AS, Fraser CL (1986) Water and non-electrolyte permeability in brain synaptosomes isolated from normal and uremic rats. Am J Physiol (Regulatory, Integrative and Comparitive Physiology) 250(2):R306-R312
24. Bogdanski TP, Blaszkowski TP, Tissari AH (1970) Mechanisms of biogenic amine transport and storage IV. Relationship between K+ and Na+ requirement for transport and storage of 5-hydroxy tryptamine and norephinephrine in synaptosomes. Biochim Biphys Acta 211:521-532
25. Bogdanski DF, Brodie BB (1966) Role of sodium and potassium ions in storage of norepinephrine by synaptic nerve endings. Life Sci 5:1563-1569
26. Davis RA, Kern F, Showalter R, Sutherland E, Sinesky M, Simon FR (1978) Alterations of hepatic Na-K ATPase and bile flow by estrogen: effects on liver surface membrane lipid structure and function. Proc Natl Acad Sci 75:4130-4134
27. Iversen LL, Kravitz EA (1966) Sodium dependence of transmitter uptake at adrenergic nerve terminals. Mol Pharmacol 2:360-362
28. Bogdanski DF, Tissari AH, Brodie BB (1968) Role of sodium potassium, ouabain and reserpine in uptake, storage and metabolism of biogenic amines in synaptosomes. Life Sci 7:419-428
29. Bogdanski DF, Brodie BB (1969) The effects of inorganic ions on the storage and uptake 3H norepinephrine by rat heart slices. J Pharm Exp Ther 165:181-189
30. Kometiani ZP, Tsakadze LG, Jariashvili (1984) Functional significance of the effects of neurotransmitters on the Na-K ATPase system. J Neurochem 42:1246-1250
31. Paton DM (1968) Cations and metabolic requirements for retention of metaraminol by rat uterine horns. Br J Pharmacol Chemother 33:277-286
32. Tissari AH, Schonhoffer PS, Bogdanski DF, Brodie BB (1969) Mechanism of biogenic transport. II. Relationship between sodium and the mechanism of ouabain blockade of the accumulation of serotonin and norepinephrine by synaptosomes. Mol Pharm 5:593-604
33. Ali F, Tayeb O, Attallah A (1985) Plasma and brain cathecholamines in experimental uremia: Acute and chronic studies. Life Sci 37:1757-1764
34. Hennemann H, Hevendehl G, Horler E, Heidland A (1973) Toxic sympathicopathy in uraemia. Proc Eur Dialysis Transpl Assoc 10:166-170
35. Perry TL, Yon VW, Kish SJ, Ito M, Foulks JG, Godolphin WJ, Sweeney VP (1985) Neurochemical abnormalities in brain of renal failure patients treated by repeated hemodialysis. J Neurochem 45:1043-1048
36. Fraser CL, Arieff AI (1989) Water metabolism and its disorders. In: Cohen RD, Alberti KGMM, Lewis B, Denman AM (eds) The molecular and metabolic basis of acquired disease. Bailliere Tindall, London
37. Arieff AI (1987) Hyponatremia associated with permanent brain damage. Adv Intern Med 32:325-344
38. Arieff AI, Llach F, Massry SG (1976) Neurological manifestations and morbidity of hyponatremia: Correlation with brain water and electrolytes. Medicine 55:121-129
39. Melton JE, Patlak CS, Pettigrew KD, Cserr HF (1987) Volume regulatory loss of NA, Cl, and K from rat brain during acute hyponatremia. Am J Physiol 252:F661-F669
40. Arieff AI (1986) Hyponatremia, convulsions, respiratory arrest, and permanent brain damage after elective surgery in healthy women. N Engl J Med 314:1529-1535
41. Ashouri OS (1986) Severe diuretic-induced hyponatremia in the elderly: A series of eight patients. Arch Intern Med 146:1355-1357
42. Ashraf N, Locksley R, Arieff AI (1981) Thiazide-induced hyponatremia associated with death or neurologic damage in outpatients. Am J Med 70:1163-1168

43. Ayus JC, Krothapalli RK, Arieff AI (1988) Sexual difference in survival with severe symptomatic hyponatremia. Kidney Int 33:180
44. Fraser CL, Kucharczyk J, Arieff AI, Rollin C, Sarnacki P, Norman D (1989) Sex differences result in increased morbidity from hyponatremia in female rats. Am J Physiol: Regul, Integ & Compar Physiol 256:R880–R885
45. Fraser CL, Sarnacki P (1989) Na-K ATPase pump function in rat brain synaptosomes is different in males and females. Am J Physiol: Endocrinology and Metabolism 257 (Aug)
46. Labella FS, Bihle I, Kim RS (1984) Progesterone derivatives that bind to the digitalis receptor: Effects on ^{86}Rb uptake and contractility in the isolated guinea pig heart. Can J Physiol Pharm 62:1057–1064
47. Guerra M, Rodriques del Castillo A, Battaner E, Mas M (1987) Androgens stimulate preoptic area Na+, K+-ATPase activity in male rats. Neurosci Lett 78:97–100
48. Schwarz SM, Bostwick HE, Medow MS (1988) Estrogen modulates ileal basolateral membrane lipid dynamics and Na^+-K^+- ATPase activity. Am J Physiol 254:G687–G694
49. Rodriquez del Castello A, Battaner E, Guerra M, Alonso T, Mas M (1987) Regional changes of brain Na+, K+-transporting adenosine triphosphate related to ovarian function. Brain Res 416:113–118
50. Feefe EB, Scharschmidt BF, Blankenship NM, Ockner RK (1979) Studies of relationships among bile flow, liver plasma membrane Na-K ATPase, and membrane microviscosity in the rat. J Clin Invest 64:1590–1598
51. Lijnen P, Groeseneken D, Lommelen L, M'Buyamba-Kabangu JR, Amery A (1985) In vitro inhibition of renal sodium-potassium ATPase activity by progesterone. Meth Find Exptl Clin Pharmacol 7:347–349
52. Arieff AI, Guisado R (1976) Effects on the central nervous system of hypernatremic and hyponatremic states. Kidney Int 10:41–53
53. Ayus JC, Krothapalli RK, Arieff AI (1987) Treatment of severe symptomatic hyponatremia: A prospective study. N Engl J Med 317:1190–1195
54. Verbalis JG, Drutarosky MD (1988) Adaptation to chronic hypoosmolality in rats. Kidney Int 34:351–360
55. Fraser CL (1989) Neurologic manifestations of uremia and disorders of calcium metabolism. In: Griggs RC, Arieff AI (eds) Neurologic manifestations of systemic disorders. Little, Brown & Co, Boston (in press)
56. Burcar PJ, Norenberg MD, Yarnell PR (1977) Hyponatremia and central pontine myelinolysis. Neurology 27:223–226
57. Messert B, Orrison W, Hawkins M, Quaglieri C (1979) Central pontine myelinolysis. Neurology 29:147–160
58. Norenberg MD, Leslie KO, Robertson AS (1982) Association between rise in serum sodium and central pontine myelinolysis. Ann Neurol 11:128–135
59. Tomlinson BE, Pierides AM, Bradley WG (1976) Central pontine myelinolysis: Two cases with associated electrolyte disturbance. Quart J Med 179:373–386
60. Sterns RH, Riggs JE, Schochet SS (1986) Osmotic demyelination syndrome following correction of hyponatremia. N Engl J Med 314:1535–1542
61. Gillis CN, Paton DM (1967) Cation dependence of sympathetic transmitter retention by slices of rat ventricle. Br J Pharmacol Chemother 29:309–318
62. McKee A, Winkelman M, Banker B (1988) Central pontine myelinolysis in severely burned patients: Relationship to serum hyperosmolality. Neurol 38:1211–1217
63. Ayus JC, Olivero JJ, Frommer JP (1982) Rapid correction of severe hyponatremia with intravenous hypertonic saline. Am J Med 72:43–48
64. Cheng JC, Zikos D, Skopicki HA, Peterson DR, Fisher KA (1988) Correction of symptomatic hyponatremia. Kidney Int 33:186

65. Decaux G, Unger J, Brimioulle S, Mockel J (1982) Hyponatremia in the syndrome of inappropriate secretion of antidiuretic hormone. JAMA 247:471–474
66. Hantman D, Rossier B, Zohlman R, Schrier R (1973) Rapid correction of hyponatremia in the syndrome of inappropriate secretion of antidiuretic hormone: An alternative treatment to hypertonic saline. Ann Intern Med 78:870–875

Encephalopathy Associated with Liver Disease

J. Wendon and R. Williams

Introduction

Hepatic encephalopathy (HE) is a reversible clinical syndrome of which the manifestations range from a slight alteration in mental status to deep coma with a lack of response to painful stimuli. The degree to which symptoms of encephalopathy are seen within an individual patient appears to be directly related to the speed of development of the hepatic failure; thus a paracetamol overdose may proceed from mild disorientation to grade IV coma over the course of several hours.

The cause of hepatic encephalopathy whether arising from fulminant hepatic failure (FHF) or decompensation of chronic liver disease (CLD) has been attributed to the accumulation of toxic substances in the circulation that may act by impairing neuronal function and possibly by causing damage to the blood brain barrier.

There are many potentially toxic substances to be considered; ammonia, mercaptans, fatty acids and phenols; these compounds have been shown not only to induce coma but also to act synergistically inducing coma in normal individuals [1, 2]. These substances arise predominantly from the gut and reduction of their absorption results in some amelioration of encephalopathy in patients with cirrhosis. In addition there has been much interest recently in the role of the inhibitory neurotransmitter gamma amino-butyric acid (GABA) in the disturbance of neurotransmission. In considering the pathogenesis of hepatic encephalopathy it is important always to remember the potentially contributory effects of sepsis, renal failure and pancreatitis which frequently occur in liver failure and are all separately capable of causing coma.

Possible Pathogenetic Mechanisms in the Development of Hepatic Encephalopathy

Blood Brain Barrier Permeability

The blood brain barrier (BBB) plays an essential role in excluding unwanted toxic substances from the brain and maintaining neurotransmitter substances within the brain. This is achieved by the endothelial cells of the cerebral capillaries which, unlike capillary systems elsewhere, are uniquely devoid of fenestrations and have only few pinocytotic vesicles. This barrier is further enhanced by the endothelial basement membrane and astrocyte processes that completely envelope the capillaries.

Several animal studies have demonstrated increases in BBB permeability [3, 4], and the compounds ammonia, methyl-octanoate, mercaptans and phenols have been shown to increase permeability in normal rats [5]. There is some controversy however, relating to increased permeability of the BBB in hepatic encephalopathy, with some studies failing to show evidence of increased permeability. This discrepancy of findings may possibly be explained by the different sensitivity of methods used to measure BBB permeability. Several studies showing both no change and increased permeability have used the Oldendorf technique. This technique involves a single bolus injection of a radio-labelled compound into the carotid artery, and brain uptake is assessed relative to water. Criticisms of this technique relate to the corrections needed for intravascular water content and knowledge of, and changes in cerebral blood flow. Utilization of the permeability surface area product, probably provides a more accurate estimation of BBB permeability for poorly diffusable compounds, and is also independent of changes in cerebral blood flow. Application of this technique in galactosamine treated rats [6, 7] demonstrated no increase in BBB permeability. On the other hand, Zaki et al. [5] have demonstrated increases in BBB by 3–4 fold (Oldendorf technique) in galactosamine-induced FHF. The animals studied were in deep coma and more severely affected than the animal studied by the permeability surface area product studies [6, 7], which may account for the differences in permeability noted. Horowitz et al. [8] have used autoradiographic techniques to identify regional changes in isotope concentration using labelled aminoisobutyric acid, and demonstrated increases in the transfer constant in the medial geniculate body, superior collicullus, central grey substance, area retrosplenius and lateral thalamic nuclei. Transfer constant was not increased in the cortical regions or in the white matter. The difference between this finding and that of the permeability surface area studies may potentially relate to sensitivity of the methods to defect local areas of increased permeability. It would seem that localised changes in BBB permeability may occur, and further work is needed to fully clarify the state of the BBB in hepatic encephalopathy.

Na/K ATPase

Ammonia, phenols, mercaptans, short chain fatty acids and endotoxin (Fig. 1) have been shown to increase BBB permeability [5] and to have a synergistic effect in producing coma in normal animals. In some animal studies of experimentally induced FHF, increases in BBB permeability can be demonstrated [4], and many of the above substances have also been shown to inhibit the activity of Na/K ATPase in vitro [9–11].

Reduced activity of this enzyme is associated with an increase in intracellular sodium and impaired neurotransmission, as well as being a characteristic feature in the cytotoxic form of cerebral edema. Indeed inhibition of Na/K ATPase in endothelial cells of the cerebral capillaries may result in impaired function of the

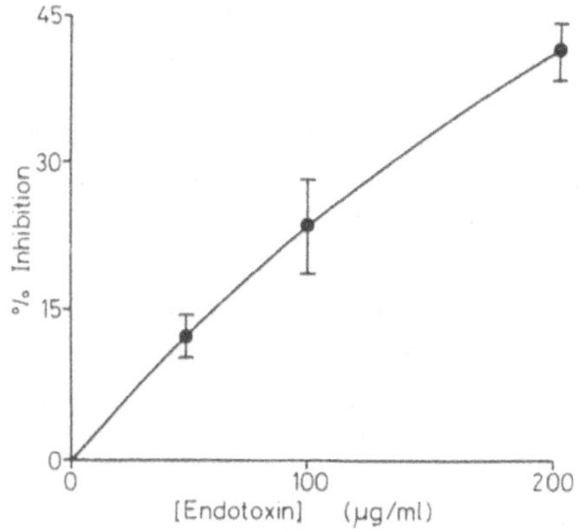

Fig. 1. Inhibition of rat brain Na-K ATPase by endotoxin in vitro. (Reproduced with kind permission from [11])

BBB [12]. Sera from patients with FHF have demonstrated an inhibition in activity of partially purified rat brain Na/K ATPase preparation in vitro [13, 14] (Figs. 2–4). In vivo animal work has also demonstrated significant reductions of Na/K ATPase activity in animals with HE [15] (Fig. 5). Although there was an increase in brain water noted, there was no clear correlation between reduction in Na/K ATPase activity and the development of cerebral edema. The reduction in Na/K ATPase seen in HE is probably due to a toxic substance circulating in the plasma of these patients but this factor remains unidentified!

Hyperammonia

Ammonia is produced in the gastro-intestinal tract as a result of ingestion of protein. The action of colonic bacteria and mucosal enzymes on these and other nitrogenous substances generates ammonia. The ammonia is then transported

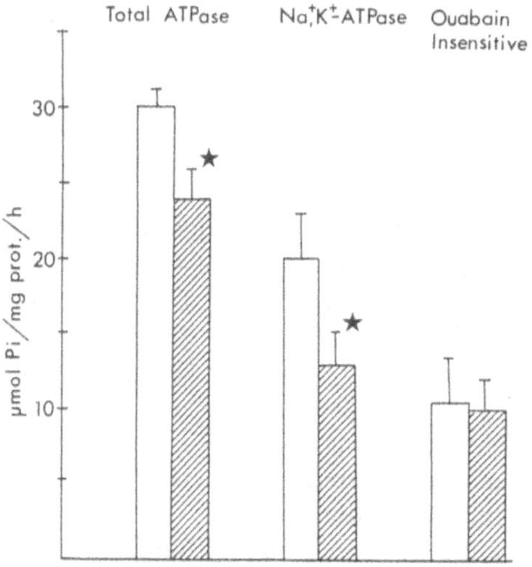

Fig. 2. The effect of fulminant hepatic failure serum on rat brain Na-K ATPase activity in vitro. The unshaded bars represent control serum (n = 11) and the shaded bars represent FHF serum (n = 13), mean ± SD (*p < 0.001 compared with normal serum). (Reproduced with kind permission from [13])

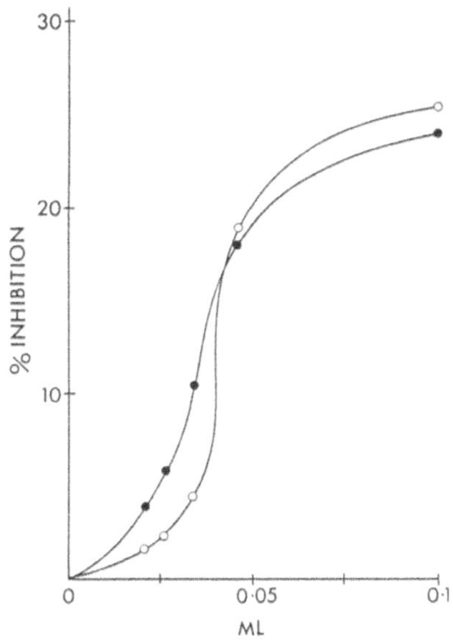

Fig. 3. The inhibition of Na-K ATPase activity with increasing concentration of FHF serum. Volume made up to 0.1 ml with buffer (•) or normal serum (o). (Reproduced with kind permission from [13])

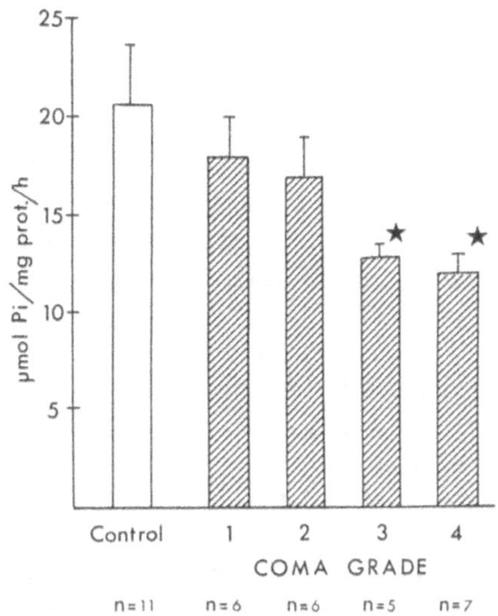

Fig. 4. The effect of FHF serum from patients in different grades of coma on Na-K ATPase activity in vitro. Mean ± SD; *$p < 0.001$ compared to grade 1 coma. (Reproduced with kind permission from [13])

via the portal circulation to the liver where under normal circumstances it would be converted to urea. In liver failure this does not occur and ammonia enters the systemic circulation with a rise in blood ammonia and increased uptake to brain and muscle [16].

The elevation of blood ammonia results in glucagon secretion, which may lead to increased hepatic gluconeogenesis from amino acids, further augmenting ammonia production. Insulin is secreted to maintain normoglycemia, leading to the uptake and metabolism of branched chain amino acids, thus causing a decrease in valine, leucine and isoleucine and elevation of the aromatic amino acids [17, 18].

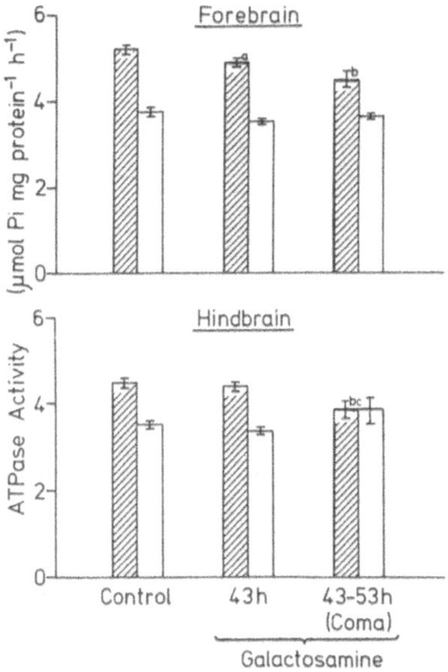

Fig. 5. Na-K ATPase (shaded columns) and ouabain insensitive ATPase (open columns) activities of homogenates of snap frozen brains from control ($n=28$) and galactosamine (2.5 mg/kg) treated rats at 43 h ($n=39$) and in deep coma ($n=7$). Bars represent SEM. ($^{a}p<0.001$ vs. control; $^{b}p<0.005$ vs. control; $^{c}p<0.01$ vs. 43 h treated rats). (Reproduced with kind permission from [15])

Ammonia also combines with glutamate to form glutamine. Correlation between blood ammonia level and encephalopathy in liver failure, although present is poor. However there is a close correlation between CSF glutamine and severity of HE in clinical studies and in animal studies [17]. Glutamine levels in the central nervous system (CNS) will reach a new steady state with the efflux rate being determined by the reaction constant for both glutamine and all other neutral amino acids. This may lead to abnormal plasma and brain amino acid profiles [17].

Although chronic increases in blood ammonia results in characteristic histological and EEG changes similar to those seen in HE [17], the visual evoked responses (VEP) do not resemble those in HE [18]. Also the receptor changes seen following hyperammonemia in rabbits are fundamentally different from those that occur in HE [19]. It is of note however that in congenital urea cycle abnormalities, characterized by hyperammonemia, encephalopathy occurs in association with high blood ammonia levels [17]; and that removal or decrease in ammonia production (e.g.) by emptying the bowel with enema) often results in improvement in early encephalopathy.

Amino Acids

In liver dysfunction there is a reduced capacity for hepatic amino acid oxidation, and the molar ratio of aromatic amino acids to branched chain amino acids is increased [17]. Free plasma levels of tryptophan, tyrosine, tyramine and phenols are also increased in HE and have been shown to correlate with the level of encephalopathy [20]. Of all the amino acids found in the brain or CSF glutamine predominates [17]. Increased brain uptake of free tryptophan, phenylalanine and tyrosine are seen, due to plasma neutral and branched chain amino acid imbalance, which is componded by glutamine efflux from the brain [21]. The result is an excess of serotonin and depletion of dopamine and norepinephrine in the brain. In animal studies however, brain dopamine and norepinephrine can be reduced by 90% without altering conscious level [17]. The arousal response to L-Dopa observed in some patients is more likely to be due to increased renal excretion of ammonia than to cerebral repletion of dopamine. The patients who do respond to L-Dopa do not have associated renal failure [22].

Infusion of branched chain amino acids leads to a reduction in the incremental increases of aromatic amino acids and glutamine seen in hepatic encephalopathy [17]. The toxicity of infused amino acids, resulting in coma or lethargy in animal studies, has been shown to be ameliorated by the addition of 1% arginine or ornithine [23]. In dogs, infusion of phenylalanine plus tryptophan has been reported to cause coma that could be prevented by the addition of branched chain amino acids [24]. However these observations have not been confirmed in other studies [17], and the utilization of branched chain amino acids in the routine treatment of HE cannot be justified at present.

False Neurotransmitters

Several neurotransmitters have been studied in relation to HE, aspartate, glutamate, dopamine, norepinephrine, serotonin, glycine and GABA. Increased CSF levels of neurotransmitters and their metabolites are seen in patients with HE [25], and increased brain aromatic amino acids leads to increased production of brain serotonin and false neurotransmitters, such as octopamine, increased levels of which are found in HE [17]. Plasma norepinephrine is increased, as are its related false neurotransmitters, octopamine and phenylethanolamine, with a positive corelation between octopamine and degree of encephalopathy [17]. However, in experimental animals there is no consistent flux of neurotransmitters in and out of the brain, and in rats, octopamine levels can be increased with a subsequent reduction in dopamine and norepinephrine, without induction of behavior change or coma [17]. Thus the etiological role of such agents in HE in humans is open to question.

Mercaptans

Mercaptans are highly toxic volatile thioalcohols, generated largely in the gastrointestinal tract and normally removed by the liver. Whole blood methianol is elevated in HE especially in the presence of coma, and changing levels of methianol correlate with changes in level of coma [26]. Mercaptans, like fatty acids, depress enzymes involved in the detoxification of ammonia via the urea cycle, and in vitro have been demonstrated to inhibit Na/K ATPase and mitochondrial respiration in the liver and brain [27]. The administration of ammonium chloride, dimethyl disulphide (a mercaptan precursor) and octanoic acid to rats in doses that simulated levels seen in experimental coma, may lead to the induction of coma, with VEP resembling those seen in galactoasmine induced HE [28].

Phenols and Fatty Acids

Fatty acids accumulate in FHF with a reduction in the plasma ratio of aceto-acetate to β-hydroxybutyrate. In experimental animals short and medium chain fatty acids and phenols can induce reversible coma, and will act synergistically with ammonia in causing coma [29].

In vitro, even in low concentrations, fatty acids depress Na/K ATPase and glycolytic enzymes and will displace tryptophan from its binding sites on albumin [17], augmenting its uptake by the brain. They will also predispose to hypoglycemia by increasing insulin and depressing glucagon release [20]. Despite lack of direct evidence in humans, the experimental evidence suggests that fatty acids are important in the development of hepatic encephalopathy.

The GABA Hypothesis

The original hypothesis inplicating GABA suggested neural inhibition due to enhanced binding of GABA. This was then modified with the suggestion of increased sensitivity to GABA, increased receptor numbers and the potentiation of the action of GABA, induced by events at the benzodiazepine binding site.

Serum GABA levels in FHF increase significantly before the onset of encephalopathy [30] and the abnormal VEP pattern found in HE is identical to that seen with barbiturates, benzodiazepines or the GABA agonist muscimol [31]. These agents exert their effect by activation of the GABA neurotransmitter system. In coma produced by agents that do not act via the GABA neurotransmitter system the VEP wave forms do not resemble those seen in HE [18, 31].

In liver failure the accumulation of GABA may be partly due to diminished GABA degradation due to porto-systemic shunting and decreased GABA transaminase activity in the diseased liver. Normally GABA does not gain entry to the brain; however in FHF, GABA uptake following intracarotid injection has been shown to be increased [32] consistent with the hypothesis that there is increased permeability of the blood brain barrier. Also inhibition of neuronal Na/K ATPase leads to the release of substances in the neurotransmitter pool, including GABA [33]. Some investigators however, have failed to demonstrate increased levels of brain GABA in laboratory studies, and recent work with dogs could show no evidence of increased brain GABA uptake, brain GABA level or post-synaptic GABA receptors [34]. GABA however undergoes rapid degradation and functional activity of GABA may not be related to total brain levels.

Hepatic coma has been associated with increased density of GABA, glycine and benzodiazepine receptors and decreases in glutinate, aspartate and kainic acid receptor densities, with no changes in density of dopamine, opiate, acetylcholine or muscarinic receptors [35, 36].

GABA and glycine are inhibitory, whilst glutamate, aspartate and kainic acid are excitatory amino acid neurotransmitters. Dopamine, acetylcholine and opiates, although modulators of neuronal events are not as potent at producing neural inhibition or excitation as are the amino acid neurotransmitters. A pattern appears to emerge with the number of inhibitory amino acid neurotransmitters increasing and that of excitatory neurotransmitters decreasing.

If observations with galactosamine-induced HE are specific for encephalopathy, then the changes in GABA status should be found in all studies of encephalopathy regardless of induction method. However this is not the case, and some studies have failed to demonstrate increased levels of GABA in the plasma and cerebrospinal fluid or altered GABA binding.

There are several possible mechanisms for the increase in GABA-ergic tone occurring in liver failure. One possibility is increased sensitivity of the GABA/benzodiazepine receptor system due to increased density or affinity of GABA or benzodiazepine receptors. However, the data are at present inconsistent and it would seem reasonable that such findings are not a prerequisite. Another possible mechanism causing increased GABA-ergic tone could result from increased delivery of GABA to the synaptic clefts (from pre-synaptic neurons or from plasma across the blood brain barrier), but again the evidence is inconclusive. Some of the reported differences in serum GABA levels may well be due to techniques used in the measurement of GABA. A recent paper [37] however, showed good correlation between gas-liquid chromotography and radio-receptor assays in the estimation of GABA. Thus at present, there is still much contoversy regarding GABA, with respect to levels and receptor density and affinity and based on animal experiments the GABA hypothesis must remain somewhat dubious, due to the varied experimental findings. Another initiator of increased GABA-ergic tone relates to the presence of an endogenous ligand potentiating the action of GABA, and recent report demonstrating arousal in HE, after treatment with benzodiazepine antagonists are of great interest [38–44] with respect to alterations in GABA tone, and the role of an endegenous ligand.

Several studies suggest that HE may be associated with increased tone in the GABA neurotransmitter system [30, 31, 36]. Closely associated to the GABA receptor and chloride ionophore are other protein receptors for barbiturates and benzodiazepines [45]. Occupation of any of these sites can modulate transmembrane chloride flux. Increases in neuronal permeability to chloride occur following opening of the chloride channel, and chloride will enter the neuron, resulting in hyperpolarization and depression in neuronal activity. Ultimately, increases in GABA-ergic tone can alter cortical and subcortical function with impairement in conscious level and motor abilities. Endogenous ligands for the benzodiazepine receptor have been looked for, but none have been definitely identified in normal animals, and, as would be expected therefore, the administration of a benzodiazepine receptor antagonist mediates few obvious neurobehavioral effects when given to normal animals [46].

However, the administration of benzodiazepine receptor antagonists, in animal studies of FHF and HE [38–40] causes transient clinical and electrophysiological improvement. The effects of agents acting at the GABA/benzodiazepine receptor on the electrical activity of single neurons in brain slices has also been investigated. The spontaneous firing rate of Purkinje neurons from rabbits with hepatic encephalopathy was found to be 3–5 times more sensitive to depression by the GABA agonist (muscimol) or the benzodiazepine agonist (flunitrazepam) than that of control neurons [47]. Addition of benzodiazepine antagonists (Ro 15-1788, Ro 14-7437) significantly increased the spontaneous activity of Purkinje neurons from rabbits with HE, at concentrations that had no effect on the activity of control rabbit neurons, and the incubation of cerebellar slices from rabbits with HE when pretreated with a benzodiazepine antagonist were resistant to the depression normally seen when exposed to muscimol [47]. Thus there is much evidence to suggest the presence of increased GABA-ergic tone in models of HE and it may be that there is an endogenous substance in the sera of patients with HE, which has benzodiazepine agonist like properties and may contribute to the syndrome of HE by potentiating GABA neurotransmission. Uncontrolled studies in humans with HE [41, 43] have also noted transient improvement in level of coma and in somatosensory evoked potentials after treatment with benzodiazepine antagonists. Traces of benzodiazepine derivatives have been reported in plants and fungi, and also in the brain and plasma of animal models [48, 49]. It may be that because of altered liver metabolism these compounds could accumulate in liver failure and may provide a theoretical basis for the therapeutic action of the benzodiazepine antagonist, Flumazenil. Indeed the presence of a substance, which avidly binds to benzodiazepine receptors, has been suggested in the brains of experimental animals with HE and the cerebrospinal fluid of patients dying with HE [50], with the level of benzodiazepine-like immuno-reactivity in the cerebrospinal fluid of patients with HE being 4 times greater than that in normal controls.

Cerebral Edema in Hepatic Encephalopathy

Although similar biochemical mechanisms appear to be responsible for the development of hepatic encephalopathy in FHF and CLD, and important difference between these two conditions lies in the incidence of cerebral edema. This complication is a major cause of mortality in patients with FHF, but occurs only rarely in hepatic encephalopathy in association with CLD. The reason for this difference is unclear but the rapidity of onset, severity of liver failure and levels of circulating toxins are likely to be relevant factors.

The first report of cerebral edema during FHF was made in 1944 based on post-mortem changes. A report from our unit noted cerebral edema in 81% of patients at post-mortem [51] and elevated levels of intracranial pressure (ICP) were also noted in a similar percentage of patients in clinical studies from this unit [52, 53]. However, elevated ICP may also be related to vascular engorgement due to inappropriate vasodilatation, and it may be difficult to distinguish this form of brain swelling clinically from an increase in water content of the brain.

Factors in the Development of Cerebral Edema and Increased ICP

The impermeability of the BBB allows it to play an important role in regulation of brain volume. In the normal situation the state of the BBB forms the basis of the classification of cerebral edema into vasogenic and cytotoxic forms. Vasogenic edema is characterised by increased permeability of the BBB with leakage of protein rich edema fluid into the extracellular space. The work demonstrating increased permeability of the BBB in FHF would suggest that the cerebral edema is therefore of this type. However the finding that cerebral edema is mitigated by mannitol therapy [52, 53] suggests that it may be of the cytotoxic form, since mannitol is thought to require an intact BBB to exert its osmotic action. It might well be that damage to the BBB is localized to certain areas, accounting for both findings. Studies in the animal model of galactosamine-induced FHF do suggest localized damage to the BBB [8].

Patients with FHF frequently develop systemic lactic acidosis, probably related to poor tissue oxygen extraction [54], and accumulation of lactate within the brain could contribute to the development of cerebral edema [12].

Under normal circumstances cerebral blood flow (CBF) is maintained at a constant level by appropriate vascular responses. This autoregulation occurs independently of the autonomic nervous system, appearing to be dependent on the myogenic response of smooth muscle in the arterioles. Cerebral perfusion pressure should be maintained at 40 mmHg or more to ensure adequate cerebral blood flow. Autoregulation is impaired by a number of factors including hypotension, hypertension, hypoxia, and hypercapnia, and patients with FHF frequently display disturbances in all of these parameters.

Diagnosis

Raised ICP in patients with FHF is suggested by the finding of increased muscle tone progressing to decerebrate posturing. Changes in pupillary responses are a reliable sign of raised ICP even in the patient requiring mechanical ventilation. The results of brain stem function tests should however be interpreted with caution in patients with FHF since transient loss of the occulocephalic reflex has been reported in patients in whom brain stem coning had not occurred [55]. Absence of the oculovestibular reflex would appear to be a more reliable sign of brain stem coning.

The use of an ICP monitor is helpful in patients with signs of cerebral edema and FHF. The standard interventricular catheter is not suitable for monitoring ICP in patients with FHF, due to the risk of hemorrhage and infection. This unit now uses an extradural fiberoptic system with good results. ICP monitors are especially helpful in assessing new treatment methods, and in patients in whom cerebral edema is difficult to control.

Prevention and Treatment

There is little evidence that the use of lactulose will delay or prevent the development of encephalopathy in FHF compared with chronic encephalopathy from cirrhosis. However used in the early stages of encephalopathy it is probably of value in reducing ammonia production, and by its cathartic action in reducing volume of colonic content, thus removing the major source of circulating toxins and inhibitory neurotransmitter substances.

Basic treatment involves maintenance of adequate cardiac filling and perfusion pressures, adequate oxygen delivery and consumption and aggressive treatment of infection. Nursing care in these patients is especially important, including the monitoring for hypoglycemia and pupillary reflexes and ensuring optimization of head position.

Hemoperfusion

A number of different hemoperfusion systems using charcoal and other adsorbent resins have been developed, in an attempt to remove toxic substances that accumulate in FHF. Charcoal is known to be an effective adsorbent for many of the potential toxins, including mercaptans, gamma aminobutyric acid, aromatic amino acids and inhibitors of Na/K ATPase [56]. Initial studies with charcoal hemoperfusion in patients with HE suggested a benefit in terms of survival [51, 56] and incidence of cerebral edema [51]. A more recent controlled trial from this unit [57] has failed to confirm a significant effect of charcoal hemoperfusion, but the possibility of a type II statistical error in this trial would account for a beneficial effect having been missed.

The early institution of renal replacement therapy is important in patients with FHF and HE, renal failure in the past being associated with a very poor prognosis. The institution of hemodialysis in hemodynamically instable patients with cerebral edema can be very difficult. The development of other forms of renal replacement therapy, such as arterio-venous hemofiltration and arterio-venous hemodiafiltration has allowed adequate biochemical control and fluid balance with the additional potential benefit of continuous removal of circulating toxins. Anecdotal evidence suggests that continuous arterio-venous hemodiafiltration may be better than conventional hemodialysis in the unstable patient with FHF, preventing the rapid removal of electrolytes and other solutes and the rapid shifts in osmolarity than can occur during conventional hemodialysis, and which may contribute to worsening of the cerebral edema [58].

Steroids

In animal models of FHF, the institution of steroids immediately following hepatic devascularization appeared to be of benefit in attenuating rises in ICP [53]. However clinical trials using dexamethasone at the onset of grade III coma were unable to demonstrate any benefit [53] (Table 1).

Table 1. Development of cerebral edema in patients with and without dexamethasone. (Reproduced with kind permission from [53])

	Dexamethasone	No dexamethasone
Total number of patients	21	23
Patients developing cerebral edema	16 (%)	18 (%)

Osmotic Diuretics

The use of mannitol to treat cerebral edema in FHF was shown to be beneficial in a randomized controlled trial from this unit, with reversal of the signs of cerebral edema, causing a mean reduction in ICP of 22 mmHg [52, 53] (Table 2). Mannitol infusion should however be used with caution in patients with renal failure since fluid overload may occur and prolonged hyperosmolarity may further damange the BBB and exacerbate cerebral edema. Mannitol infusions may be repeated provided that the plasma osmolarity does not exceed 320 mOsm (Table 3).

Table 2. Effect of mannitol on resolution of cerebral edema. (Reproduced with kind permission from [53])

	Mannitol ICP monitoring	Mannitol No ICP monitoring	No mannitol ICP monitoring	No mannitol No ICP monitoring
No. of patients	9	8	5	12
Episodes of cerebral edema	33	20	5	12
Resolution	27	17	0	1
Survival	3	5	0	1

Table 3. Comparison of dexamethasone and mannitol in the treatment of patients with FHF. (Reproduced with kind permission from [61])

Treatment group	Total No. of patients	No. of patients with raised ICP	No. of survivors
Mannitol	10	10	5 (50%)
Mannitol and dexamethasone	10	7	3 (43%)
Dexamethasone	11	9	1 (11%)
Neither drug	13	8	0 (0%)

Hyperventilation

Variations in CO_2 exert profound effects on the CBF with hypercapnia causing vasodilatation and hypocapnia vasoconstriction. For every mmHg change in PCO_2 there is an approximate 4% change in CBF in normal subjects [60]. Changes in CO_2 also alter the autoregulatory response to blood pressure, with hypercapnia shifting the curve to the left, resulting in a lowering of the upper limit of blood pressure at which autoregulation still occurs.

Studies from this unit have demonstrated elevations in CBF (measured with the xenon washout technique) with up to a 3 fold increase in patients with grade IV coma [61]. Stanley et al. [62] demonstrated decreased cerebral responsiveness to $PaCO_2$ in animal models of FHF, but work from this unit suggests that blood flow is sensitive to changes in CO_2 even in grade IV coma, with reductions in CBF of up to 50% being achieved with hyperventilation techniques [61] (Figs. 6, 7).

Short term hyperventilation has been shown to be of benefit in the treatment of acute rises of ICP in HE and is especially useful in patients in whom mannitol therapy is precluded due to coexistant renal failure. The use of prolonged hyperventilation in HE was recently investigated, but no extra benefit was noted in this group as compared to those receiving hyperventilation during acute rises in ICP only [63] (Fig. 8).

Barbiturate Therapy

Elevation of core temperature increases CBF and cerebral metabolism, and has been shown to increase the cerebral edema associated with cryogenic brain lesions [64], whilst hypothermia has the opposite effect. Animal studies have demonstrated decreases in CBF in association with hypothermia [65]. Pyrexia is common in patients with FHF and HE and our studies have demonstrated that cooling to normal core temperature is associated with a reduction in ICP [66].

CBF is also regulated according to local metabolism, and the tight coupling between cerebral metabolism and CBF forms the basis for the use of drugs such as barbiturates. High dose barbiturates (3-5 mg/kg) reduce ICP by reducing CBF; they also prevent potassium efflux from the cells [67] and quench free radical formation [68]. Their use however is often associated with hemodynamic disturbances and their role in the management of edema in association with FHF awaits the results of controlled trials.

Summary

The increase in GABA-ergic tone in patients with HE is of great interest, but it is likely to be only one of many mediators involved, since if it alone was responsible for the development of HE one might expect to see a return to normal brain function during treatment. In situations in which there is a lack of response, the associated findings of raised ICP, sepsis and renal failure, so often found in HE,

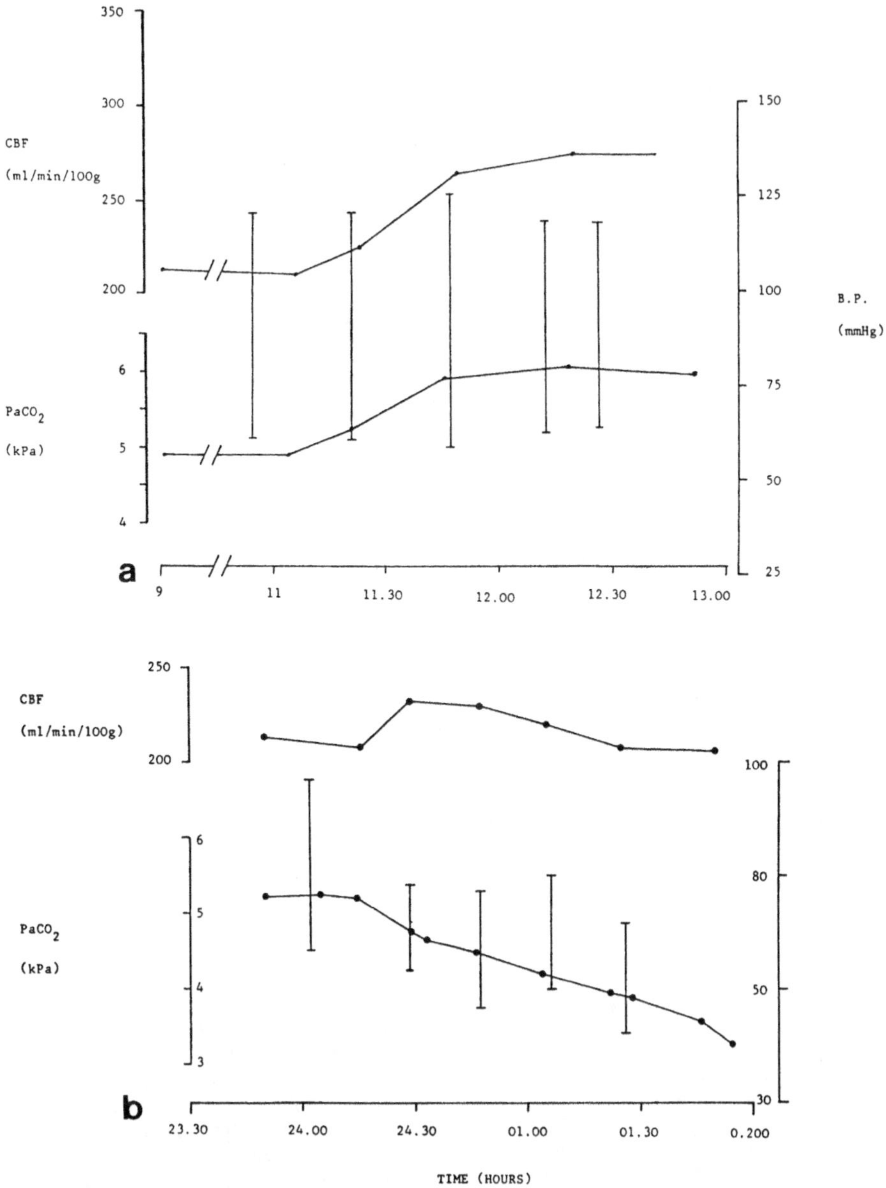

Fig. 6a, b. Relationship between CBF and $PaCO_2$ in a 50-year old woman with FHF due to halothane. **a** 48 h after onset of grade 4 encephalopathy. Response to $PaCO_2$ is intact; **b** 50 h later CBF no longer responds appropriately to changes in $PaCO_2$. The patient died 8 h later. (Reproduced with kind permission from [61])

need to be taken into consideration. The cause of HE therefore remains uncertain and probably multifactorial. Accumulation of toxins secondary to hepatic failure appears to cause neuronal deterioration, possibly due to central nervous

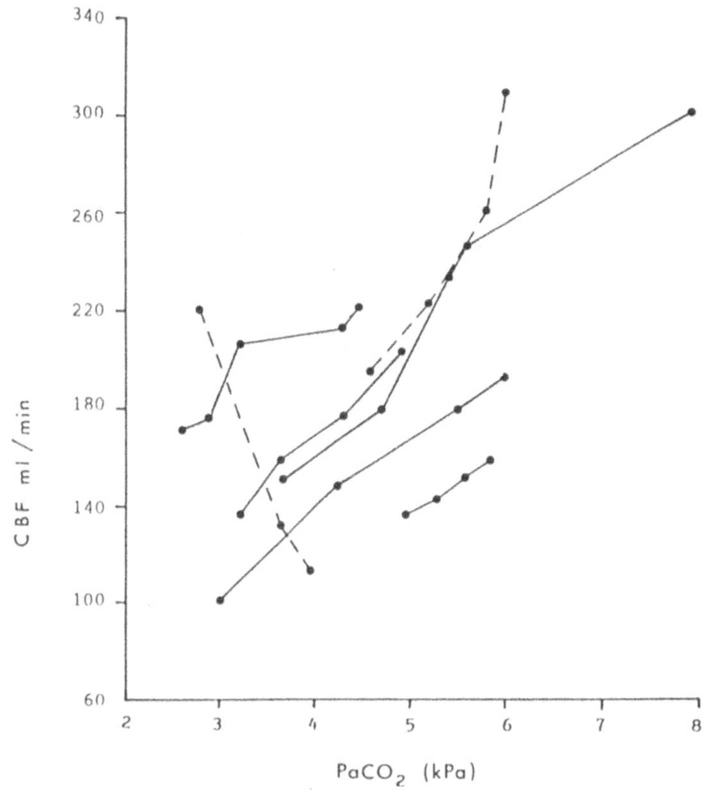

Fig. 7. Relationship between CBF and $PaCO_2$ in patients with grade 4 encephalopathy

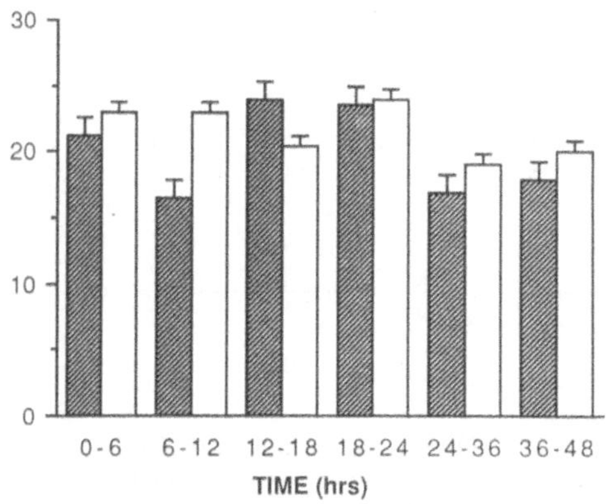

Fig. 8. Intracranial pressure in hyperventilated patients (shaded column, n = 20) and non-hyperventilated patients (unshaded column, n = 16) was calculated for each patient group during the time periods shown following insertion of the ICP monitor. The difference between the groups are not significant (mean ± SEM). (Reproduced with kind permission from [63])

system accumulation of ammonia, formation and efflux of glutamine and an excess of aromatic amino acids within the brain. Increased free tryptophan causes increased levels of serotonin and false neurotransmitters. Intrinsic cell damage from toxins will result in decreased mitochondrial respiration and microsomal Na/K ATPase activity and a consequent reduction in oxidative metabolism. Regardless of the cause of HE, cerebral edema is an important complication, resulting in significant mortality. Thus until a treatment becomes available which alters the natural history of fulminant hepatic failure, management of the cerebral edema will remain a frequent and difficult problem with a high mortality.

Acknowledgements: We are grateful to Drs. Ede, Cannalase, Seda, Gove and Hughes, The Liver Unit, Kings College Hospital, from whose work tables and figures are here reproduced.

References

1. Zieve L (1981) Synergism among toxic factors and other endogenous abnormalities in hepatic encephalopathy. In: Brunner G, Schmidt FW (eds) Artificial liver support. Springer, Berlin Heidelberg New York, pp 18-24
2. Zieve L, Doizaki WM, Lyftot C (1984) Brain methanethiol and ammonia concentrations in experimental hepatic coma induced by injections of various combinations of these substances. J Lab Clin Med 104:655-664
3. Livingstone AS, Potvin M, Goresky CA, et al (1977) Changes in the blood brain barrier in hepatic coma after hepatectomy in the rat. Gastroenterology 73:697-704
4. Zaki AEO, Ede R, Davis M, Williams R (1984) Experimental studies of blood brain barrier permeability. Hepatology 4:359-363
5. Zaki AEO, Wardle EN, Canalese J, Ede RJ, Williams R (1983) Potential toxins of acute liver failure and their effects on blood brain barrier permeability. Experientia 39:988-991
6. Lo WD, Enms SR, Goldstein GW, McNeely DL, Betz A (1987) The effects of galactosamine induced hepatic failure upon blood brain barrier permeability. Hepatology 7:3:452-456
7. Knudsen GM, Poulsen HE, Poulson OB (1988) Blood brain permeability in galactosamine induced hepatic encephalopathy: No evidence for increased GABA transport. J Hepatol 6:187-192
8. Horowitz ME, Schafer DF, Nolnar P, et al (1983) Increased blood brain transfer in the rabbit model of acute liver failure. Gastroenterology 84:1003-1011
9. Dahl DR (1968) Short chain fatty acid inhibition of rat brain Na/K adenosine triphosphatase. J Neurochem 15:815-820
10. Quarforth G, Ahmed K, Zieve L (1976) Action of methanethiol on membrane Na/K ATPase of rat brain. Bioch Pharmacol 25:1039-1044
11. Seda HWM, Gove CD, Hughs RD, Williams R (1984) Inhibition of partially purified rat brain Na/K ATPase by bile acids, phenolic acids and endotoxin. Clin Sci 66:415-420
12. Rehncrona S, Roxi I, Siesjö BK (1980) Excessive cellular acidosis: An important mechanism of neuronal damage in the brain. Acta Physiol Scand 110:435-437
13. Seda HWM, Hughes RD, Gove CD, Williams R (1984) Inhibiton of rat brain Na/K ATPase activity by serum from the patient with fulminant hepatic failure. Hepatology 4:74-79
14. Seda HWM, Hughes RD, Gove CD, Williams R (1984) Removal of inhibitors of brain Na/K ATPase by haemoperfusion in fulminant hepatic failure. Artific Organs 8:174-178
15. Ede R, Gove CD, Hughes RD, Marshall W, Williams R (1987) Reduced brain Na/K ATPase activity in rats with galactosamine induced hepatic failure; a relationship to encephalopathy and cerebral oedema. Clin Sci 72:365-371
16. Lockwood AH, McDonald JM, Reiman RE, et al (1979) The dynamics of ammonia metabolism in man: Effects of liver disease and hyperammonemia. J Clin Invest 63:449-460
17. Zieve L (1987) Pathogenesis of hepatic encephalopathy. Metabolic Brain Disease 2; 3:147-165

18. Pappas SC, Ferenci P, Schafer DF, et al (1984) Visual evoked responses in a rabbit model of hepatic encephalopathy. II Comparison of hyperammonemic encephalopathy: post ictal coma and coma induced by synergistic neurotoxins. Gastroenterol 86:546–551
19. Ferenci P, Pappas SC, Jones EA (1984) Neurotransmitter receptor changes in experimental hyperammonemia in the rabbit. In: Advances in hepatic encephalopathy and urea cycle diseases. Karger, Basel, pp 368–372
20. O'Keefe SJD, Abraham R, El-Zayadi A, Marshall W, Davis M, Williams R (1981) Increased plasma tyrosine concentrations in patients with cirrhosis and fulminant hepatic failure associated with increased plasma tyrosine flux and reduced hepatic oxidative capacity. Gastroenterology 1017–1024
21. James JH, Jeppson B, Ziparo V, Fischer JE (1979) Hyperammonemia, plasma amino acid imbalance and blood brain amino acid transport: A unified theory of portal systemic encephalopathy. Lancet 1:772–775
22. Zieve L, Zoizaki WM, Derr RF (1979) Reversal of ammonia coma in rats by L-Dopa: A peripheral effect. Gut 20:28–38
23. Fahey JC (1957) Toxicity and blood ammonia rise resulting from intra-venous amino acid administration in man. The protective effect of L-arginine. J Clin Invest 36:1647–1655
24. Rossi-Fanelli F, Freund H, Krause R, et al (1982) Induction of coma in normal dogs by infusion of amino acids, and its prevention by the addition of branched chain amino acids. Gastroenterology 83:664–671
25. Borg J, Warter JM, Schleinger JL, et al (1982) Neurotransmitter modifications in human cerebrospinal fluid and serum during hepatic encephalopathy. J Neurol Sci 57:343–356
26. McLain CJ, Zieve L, Doizaki WM, Gilberstadt S, Onstad GR (1980) Blood methanethiol in alcoholic liver disease with and without encephalopathy. Gut 21:318–323
27. Derr RF, Zieve L (1982) Methanethiol and fatty acids depress urea synthesis by the isolated rat perfused liver. J Lab Clin Med 100:585–592
28. Zeneroli ML, Ventura E, Baraldi M, et al (1982) Visual evoked responses in encephalopathy induced by galactosamine, ammonia, dimethylsulphide and octanoic acid. Hepatology 2:532–538
29. Zieve L (1985) Encephalopathy due to short and medium chain fatty acids. In: McCandless CW (ed) Cerebral energy metabolism and metabolic encephalopathy. Plenum Press, New York, pp 163–177
30. Ferenci P, Covell D, Schafer DF, et al (1983) Metabolism of the inhibitory neurotransmitter GABA in a rabbit model of fulminant hepatic failure. Hepatology 3:507–512
31. Schafer DF, Pappas SC, Brody LE, et al (1984) Visual evoked responses in a rabbit model of hepatic encephalopathy I: Sequential changes and comparisons with drug induced comas. Gastroenterology 86:540–545
32. Basset ML, Mullen KD, Schlotz B, et al (1985) Increased brain GABA uptake in pre-coma encephalopathy in the rabbit model of fulminant hepatic failure. Hepatology 5:1032–1036
33. O'Fallen JV, Brosemer RW, Harding JW (1981) The Na/K ATPase: A plausible trigger for voltage independent release of cytoplasmic neurotransmitters. J Neurochem 36:369–378
34. Roy S, Pomier Layrageus G, Butterworth RF, Hoest PM (1988) Hepatic encephalopathy in cirrhotic and portocaval shunted dogs: Lack of changes in brain GABA uptake, brain GABA levels, brain glutamic acid decarboxylase activity and brain post synaptic GABA receptors. Hepatology 8:845–849
35. Schafer DF, Fowler JM, Munson, et al (1983) Gamma aminobutyric acid and benzodiazepam receptors in an animal model of fulminant hepatic failure. J Lab Clin Med 102:870–880
36. Ferenci P, Pappas SC, Munson PJ, et al (1984) Changes in the status of neurotransmitter receptors in the rabbit model of hepatic encephalopathy. Hepatology 4:186–191
37. Levy LJ, Losowsky MS (1987) Evidence for gamma aminobutyric acid as the inhibitor of gamma aminobutyric acid binding in the plasma of humans with liver disease and hepatic encephalopathy. Clin Sci 73:531–534
38. Mullen KD, Martin JV, Bassett ML, et al (1986) Hepatic encephalopathy: A syndrome modulated by an endogenous benzodiazepine ligand. Hepatology 6:1221–1224

39. Baraldi M, Zenerloi ML, Ventura E, et al (1984) Supersensitivity of benzodiazepine receptors in hepatic encephalopathy due to fulminant hepatic failure in the rat: reversal by a benzodiazepine antagonist. Clin Sci 67:167–175
40. Bassett ML, Mullen KD, Skolnick P, Jones EA (1987) Amelioration of hepatic encephalopathy by pharmacological antagonism of the GABA-benzodiazepine receptor complex in a rabbit model of fulminant hepatic failure. Gastroenterology 93:1069–1077
41. Gammal SH, Geller D, Skolnick P, et al (1987) Unequivocal amelioration of hepatic encephalopathy by benzodiazepine antagonists in a rabbit model of fulminant hepatic failure. J Hepatol 4:517–520
42. Scollo-Lavizzar G, Steinmann E (1985) Reversal of hepatic coma by benzodiazepine antagonist (Ro 15-1788). Lancet 1:1320–1324
43. Bansky G, Meier PJ, Reiderer E, Walser H, Zeigler WH, Schmidt M (1987) Effect of a benzodiazepine antagonist in hepatic encephalopathy. Hepatology 7:1103–1105
44. Grimm G, Ferenci P, Katzenschlager L, et al (1988) Improvements in hepatic encephalopathy treated with Flumazenil. Lancet 2:1392–1394
45. Olsen RW, Young J, King RG, Duber SA, Stauber GB, Ransom RW (1986) Barbiturate and benzodiazepine modulation of the GABA receptor and function. Life Sci 39:1969–1976
46. Bonetti EP, Pieri L, Cumm R, et al (1988) Benzodiazepine antagonist Ro 15-1788: neurological and hevaioural effects. Psychopharmacology 78:8–18
47. Basile AS, Gammal SH, Mullen KD, et al (1988) Differential responsiveness of cerebellar Purkinje neurons to GABA and benzodiazepine ligands in an animal model of hepatic encephalopathy. J Neuro Sci 8:2414–2421
48. Wildmann J, Mohler H, Vetter, et al (1987) Diazepam and N-desmethyldiazepam are found in rat brain and adrenal and may be of plant origin. J Neural Transm 70:383–398
49. Sangameswaran L, Fales HM, Freidrich P, et al (1986) Purification of a benzodiazepine from bovine brain and benzodiazepine-like immunoreactivity in human brain. Proc Natl Sci USA 83:9236–9340
50. Mullen KD, Szauter KM, Galloway PG, et al (1986) CSF of patients with hepatic encephalopathy contains significant benzodiazepine binding activity. Correlation with post mortem cortical benzodiazepine binding studies. Hepatology 7:1103–d1106
51. Gimson AES, Braude S, Mellon PJ, et al (1982) Earlier charcoal haemoperfusion in fulminant hepatic failure. Lancet 2:681–683
52. Ede R, Gimson AES, Bihari D, Williams R (1986) Controlled hyperventilation in the prevention of cerebral oedema in fulminant hepatic failure. J Hepatol 2:43–51
53. Canalase J, Gimson AES, Davis C, et al (1982) Controlled trial of dexamethasone and mannitol for the cerebral oedema of fulminant hepatic failure. Gut 23:625–629
54. Bihari D, Gimson AES, Lindridge J, Williams R (1984) Lactic acidosis in fulminant hepatic failure. Crit Care Med 12:255–257
55. Hand MA, Silk DB, Williams R (1978) Prognostic value of oculovestibular reflex in fulminant hepatic failure. Br Med J 1:1029–1030
56. Hughes R, Williams R (1986) Clinical experience with charcoal and resin haemoperfusion. Semin Liver Dis 6:164–173
57. O'Grady J, Gimson AES, O'Brien CJ, et al (1988) Controlled trials of charcoal haemoperfusion and prognostic factors in fulminant hepatic failure. Gastroenterology 94:1186–1192
58. Davenport A, Will EJ, Losowsky MS, Swindels S (1987) Continuous arterio-venous haemofiltration in patient with hepatic encephalopathy and renal failure. Br Med J 295:1028
59. Hanid MA, McKenzie RL, Jenner RE, et al (1974) Intracranial pressure in pigs with surgically induced liver failure. Gastroenterology 76:123–131
60. Skinhoj E, Paulson OB (1969) Carbon dioxide and cerebral circulatory control. Arch Neurol 20:249–252
61. Ede R, Williams R (1986) Hepatic encephalopathy and cerebral oedema. Sem Liver Dis 6:2:107–118
62. Stanley NN, Salisbury BG, McHenry LC, Cherniac NS (1975) Effect of liver failure on the response of ventilation and cerebral circulation to carbon dioxide in man and in the goat. Clin Sci Mol Med 49:157–169
63. Ede R, Gimson AES, Bihari D, Williams R (1986) Controlled hyperventilation in the prevention of cerebral oedema in fulminant hepatic failure. J Hepatol 2:43–51

64. Clasen RA, Pandolfi S, Lang I, Casey D (1974) Experimental study of relationship of fever to cerebral edema. J Neurosurg 41:576–581
65. Michenfelder JD, Theye RA (1968) Hypothermia: Effect on canine brain and whole body metabolism. Anesthesiology 29:1107–1112
66. Ede R, Gimson AES, Canalase J, Williams R (1982) Cerebral oedema and monitoring of intracranial pressure in fulminant hepatic failure. Gastroenterol Jpn 17:163–176
67. Smith AC, Morque JJ (1976) Anaesthetics and cerebral edema. Anesthesiology 45:64–72
68. Desmopoulos HB, Fiamm ES, Seligman ML, et al (1977) Antioxidant effect of barbiturates in model membranes undergoing free radical damage. In: Ingvar DH, Lassen NA (eds) Cerebral blood flow VIII. Cerebral function metabolism and circulation. Copenhagen Munksgaard, pp 152–153

Drug-Induced Encephalopathy

M. Fisher and R. Joffe

Introduction

Adverse effects of drugs and overdosage of drugs as a suicidal attempt are major sources of admission to hospital and intensive care units. Cerebral effects ranging from mild disturbances of memory and disorientation to persistent and protracted coma are often common presenting features. Similarly in hospitalized patients, particularly the elderly, disturbances in cerebral function due to a wide range of causes are common, and drugs may be more than just a superficial component of such adverse events.

Definition

Encephalopathy means disease of the brain. As used in medicine the term usually implies disease which is a disorder of function rather than structure and which will recover when and if the primary disorder resolves. Drugs may be a common cause of encephalopathy in the intensive care unit, but because of the multisystem and complex nature of disorders treated in intensive care units the establishment of a cause and effect relationship between an altered cerebral state and a drug may be difficult to establish. Further, drug induced encephalopathy may be a therapeutic goal. In a patient with tetanus for example, an altered cerebral state is a desirable goal, and is produced with narcotics and sedatives. Prolonged awakening after weeks of such therapy means the desirable effects of the therapy have become undesirable, and the sedation becomes drug induced encephalopathy.

Diagnosis of Drug-Induced Encephalopathy

The diagnosis of drug-induced encephalopathy in the intensive care unit is difficult, as a multitude of factors may lead to altered cerebral function, and in many patients such alteration of function is a desireable goal. Potent drugs are commonly used to alter pain experience, anxiety, seizure threshold, depression and excitable and inappropriate behavior. With such drugs whose primary function is cerebral, in association with other drugs such as neuromuscular blocking agents the physical examination of all aspects of central nervous system function

Table 1. Non pharmacological causes of encephalopathy. (From [1-3])

1. Viral infection - acute toxic encephalopathy
2. Trauma
   a) post-traumatic stupor in children
   b) delayed non-hemorrhagic encephalopathy following mild head trauma
3. Hypoxia
   a) acute
   b) delayed
4. Hypoxic/hypercarbic
5. Hypoglycemic
6. Metabolic
7. Hepatic failure
8. Hypotensive
9. Pulmonary
10. Pancreatic
11. Dialysis
12. Uremia
13. Sepsis
14. Neuropsychiatric syndromes (Intensive Care Syndrome) [5]

is difficult, and with the exception of powerful sedatives and anesthetics the monitoring of electrical activity of the brain rarely provides specific evidence of drug induced encephalopathy. The diagnosis must therefore be dependent on a high index of suspicion based on an understanding of the potential cerebral effects which have been demonstrated in patients who are "less sick" in terms of other disorders with the potential to interfere with cerebral function. Such disorders are summarized in Table 1.

To establish an unequivocal diagnosis of drug-induced encephalopathy would require:

1. An altered cerebral state that was temporally associated with drug therapy.
2. Reversal of that state when the drug is withdrawn.
3. A recurrence of symptoms when the drug was reintroduced.
4. An absence of other factors known to produce encephalopathy.

The diagnosis therefore consists of excluding these disorders, or demonstrating improvement in cerebral function on drug withdrawal in the absence of improvement in underlying disorder. It is unlikely that the pursuit of criterion 3 will appeal to intensivists, and further if the drug is re-introduced in an improving patient, no valuable information may be obtained as the interaction of other processes which are improving may mean the effects are too small to be noticed, or do not occur.

Clinical Signs

Drug-induced encephalopathy presents as do most other metabolic encephalopathies. Cognitive disturbances in these disorders are often the earliest manifestations and disturbances of attention and alertness are the cardinal features. In most instances localizing signs are rare but certain features may be helpful in any given case. Clinically separate from the obvious medical changes, disturbances in respiration often associated with a metabolic acidosis are found. Drugs associated with this include paraldehyde, salicylates in children, methyl alcohol and ethylene glycol. Respiratory acidosis is more usually associated with sedative drugs. Metabolic alkalosis may occasionally be associated with diuretics and hyperkalemia.

In their superb dissertation on stupor and coma, Plum and Posner make the critical observation that the state of the pupils is the single most important criterion distinguishing metabolic encephalopathy from structural disease [1]. It is true that the pupils may be widely dilated in high dose sympathomimetic therapy or in atropine poisoning, constricted after opiates; but if anticholinergic or glutethimide ingestion is ruled out; if there is no pre-existing pupillary disease, and the pupillary light reflex is absent, then the most likely cause of the encephalopathy is structural. Some patients on anticholinergic drugs (especially older patients with Parkinson's disease) may exhibit tachycardia.

In most drug induced encephalopathies eye movements are usually of the random or "ping-pong" type. As coma deepens eye movements will be lost. Cold caloric testing initially may stimulate conjugate eye movements towards the irrigated ear, but ultimately no response will be obtained in severe cases. (While motor disturbances of a focal natura are uncommon in drug induced encephalopathy, primitive reflexes i.e. sucking and grasping may be seen. Tremor, asterixis and myoclonus are frequent accompaniements of metabolic encephalopathies, and of course are seen in the drug induced disturbances.)

Most drugs taken in excess will produce delerium, stupor and even coma. Sedatives ultimately interfere with oxidative enzymes, depressing cellular metabolism. Depressant drugs affect vestibular and cerebellar function, so that nystagmus, ataxia and dysarthria may be early signs of impending problems.

Often respiratory deficiencies are paramount and overshadow motor disturbances. The pupils are usually small and unreactive and later reflex eye movements are lost.

Pathophysiology

Drug function, pharmacokinetics and pharmacodynamics are altered in critically ill patients. Perhaps the best studied example is gentamicin in which the range and dimensions of volume distribution are greatly increased [4]. The blood brain barrier restricts admission of ionized and lipid insoluble drugs into the brain. The capillary endothelial cells restrict passage of both protein bound and lipid insoluble drugs and limit diffusion of drugs in general. Processes from glial cells are in close approximation to the capillary endothelium constitute a further barrier between drugs and the cerebrospinal fluid (CSF). The cells of the choroid plexus also limit drug entry and actively transport organic ions from the cerebrospinal fluid. These processes may be impaired in critical illness, by direct, secondary, or osmotic effects [6, 7]. It is less well appreciated that the blood brain barrier also limits the egress of metabolites and mediators from brain extracellular fluid [8]. A common cause of prolonged coma or encephalopathy is related to cumulative effects, particularly drugs with active metabolites such as diazepam or drugs with high lipid solubility which may be short acting if used in single dose but have greatly increased elimination half lives when used repeatedly or by infusion such as midazolam and propofol. The elimination of drugs such as midazolam may vary 5 fold in intensive care patients [9]. Drugs may affect cerebral function by stabilizing cell membranes such as anesthetic drugs of by interfering with enzyme systems in the cell membrane and intracellular systems. Drugs such as phencyclidine may block the calcium channel and drugs may interfere with receptors for and the enzymatic pathways involving the mediators histamine, serotonin, dopamine, epinephrine and gamma hydroxybutryic acid. Interference with glucose metabolism may produce cerebral hypoglycemia as in aspirin poisoning. The major reported neurotransmitter changes in metabolic encephalopathy have been described by Plum and Posner [3].

Classification and Involvement of Specific Drugs

Direct Therapeutic Effect

This group includes drugs whose primary therapeutic effect is upon the brain.

Anesthetic Drugs

The most common intensive care use is in infusion for sedation or control of seizures or intracranial pressure. All the anesthetic agents commonly used, including thiopentone, midazolam and propofol have cummulative effects. Ketamine may be rarely used in asthma or convulsions and has hallucinogenic properties.

Sedatives

Barbiturates: Barbiturates have increased uptake into the brain in children. Delirium is more common in elderly patients, particularly those with sleep deprivation, and may cause depression. Withdrawal may produce psychological abnormalities.

Benzodiazepines: This group of drugs are commonly taken in overdosage and also may produce psychotic behavior due to acute withdrawal, particularly with oxazepam. A specific antagonist flumazenil exists.

Tranquillizers

Phenothiazines: The primary adverse cerebral effects presenting in intensive care are extrapyramidal features which may be mistaken for psychotic behavior.

Butyrophenones: Extrapyramidal effects, particularly akathisia may be produced. Severe anxiety has described after droperidol premedication. The malignant neuroleptic syndrome which commonly cause coma, is produced by both phenothiazines and butyrophenones.

Toxic Effects of CNS Actions of Therapeutic Agents

Anticholinergic agents: Drugs with anticholinergic effects include antihistaminic agents, belladonna alkaloids, tranquillizers, tricyclic antidepressants and some antiarrhythmic agents. These drugs may produce visual disturbances and psychotic effects ranging from mild aggravation to toxic delirium.

Narcotic analgesics: Withdrawal or reversal with opioid antagonists may produce aggressive behavior and delirium. Encephalopathy occurs in patients with liver disease.

Local anesthesia: Convulsions occur in overdosage. Coma and convulsions may occur with normal doses in patients with liver disease.

Antihistaminic agents [10–12]: Sedation as a side effect of H_1 blockers is well known. The phenothiazines like H_1 blockers may produce extrapyramidal effects. Since the introduction of H_2 blockers for gastric pH control in intensive care confusion and alteration in levels of consciousness have been commonly described. Histamine is found in intracerebral neurones and has vasomotor effects on intracerebral vessels. The effect on extracranial arteries is H mediated but on intracranial arteries is probably not related to a specific receptor. Studies in rats suggest that histamine releasing drugs may produce cerebral vasodilatation by histamine release, but only when the blood brain barrier is disrupted and circulating histamine has access to brain perivascular tissue. Central effects of H_2 blockers are more common in the elderly patients with serious medical illnesses and are dose related. Mental confusion, agitation and coma may occur which reverses on cessation of therapy.

Anticonvulsants: Drowsiness, nystagmus and headaches are common adverse effects.

Toxic Effects of Non CNS Active Drugs

Antibiotics: Antibiotics are a commonly overlooked source of encephalopathy in intensive care. Their effects are summarized in Table 2 [13, 14].

B Agonists: Headache, dizziness and acute anxiety may be precipitated by B agonists.

Table 2. Antibiotic-induced encephalopathies

	Effects	Dose related	Mechanism
Penicillins	- Convulsions - Hallucinations - Loss of alpha rhythms - Encephalopathy (increased in renal failure)	Yes	Interference with gamma-amino-butyric acid (GABA) mediated inhibition
Cephalosporins	- Hallucinations - Nystagmus - Encephalopathy (increased in renal failure)	Yes	?
Sulphonamides	- Ataxia - Hallucinations	?	?
Chloramphenicol	- Psychiatric disturbance	?	?
Aminoglycosides	- Bulging fontanelles - Blurred vision - Psychosis - Encephalopathy		
Tetracyclines	- Pseudotumor cerebri - Raised ICP - Headache - Blurred vision - Papilledema	Yes	
Metronidazole	- Ataxia - Encephalopathy - Seizures	Yes	Interference with GABA
Isonazid	- Vertigo - Hyperreflexia - Reduced epileptigomic threshold - Encephalopathy associated with uremia		?
Rifampicin	- Headache - Drowsiness, fatigue - Dizziness, confusion		
Trimethoprim-Sulfamethoxazole	- Headaches, depression - Hallucinations - Seizures, ataxia		?

Nonsteroidal anti-inflammatory drugs: These agents produce a syndrome of drowsiness, vertigo and confusion.

Steroids: Steroids may produce pseudotumor cerebri.

Vitamin A: Vitamin A in excessive doses may produce pseudotumor cerebri.

Digitalis: Delirium is a sign of digitalis toxicity.

Table 3. Therapy of drug-induced extrapyramidal disorders

Type	Clinical	Cause	Therapy
Parkinsonism	- Akinesia	- Major tranquillizers	- Levodopa
	- Rigidity	- Cholinergic withdrawal	- Cholinergics
	- Tremor	- Rauwolfia alkaloids	
Acute dystonias	- Oculogyric crises	- Aperizic	
		- Prerothiazine	
	- Torscon	- Metoclopramide	- Cholinergic agents (high dose)
	- Dystonia		
	- Torticolies	- Chloroquine	
	- Grimacing	- Levodopa	
Akathisia	- Motor	- Neuroleptics	
	- Restlessness	- Anticholinergics	- Clonazepam
Delirium	- Coma	- Rauwolfa alkaloids	
	- Fever	- Slimming preparations	
	- Tachypnea	- β-Blockers	- Physostigmine
	- Confusion	- Atropine like drugs	
	- Restlessness	- Antihistamines	

Treatment

There are no specific therapeutic maneuvers, apart from the use of the specific antagonists naloxone and flumazenil. Treatment is based upon symptomatic control if the drug cannot be stopped, or ceasing the drug, if the adverse effects of the drug outweigh its potential therapeutic benefit.

In the critically ill patient therapy consits of stopping the drug if the effects are unwanted. Naloxone and flumazenil are specific reversal agents for narcotic and benzodiazepine induced encephalopathy, respectively. In encephalopathy related to overdose general treatment of overdose (lavage, activated charcoal and occasionally forced diuresis) are indicated. Critchley [15] suggests that in drug induced extrapyramidal disorders therapeutic agents such as levodopa and anticholinergics may be helpful (Table 3).

References

1. Plum F, Posner JB (1980) The diagnosis of stupor and coma, 3rd edn. FA Davis Company, Philadelphia
2. Bolton CF (1987) Electrophysiologic studies of critically ill patients. Muscle and Neurone 10:129–135
3. Strillmatter WJ (1988) Altered mental states and coma. In: Civetta JM, Taylor RW, Kirby RR (eds) Critical care. Lippincott, Philadelphia, pp 1199–1207
4. Beckhouse MJ, White JM, Bythe PL, Napier JC, Smith AJ (1988) Altered aminoglycoside pharmacodynamics in the critically ill. Anaesth Intens Care 16:418–424
5. Figge H, Huang V, Kaul AF, Demling RH (1987) The pharmacotherapy of the behavioural manifestations of the ICU syndrome. J Crit Care 2:199–208
6. Edvinsson L, MacKenzie ET (1977) Amine mechanisms in the central circulation. Pharm Rev 28:275–348

7. Robinson PJ (1987) Facilitation of drug entry into the brain by osmotic opening of the blood brain barrier. Clin Exp Pharm Physiol 14:887-901
8. Partride WM (1986) Blood brain barrier: Interface between internal medicine and the brain. Ann Intern Med 105:82-95
9. Oldenhof H, De Jong M, Steehoeck A, Janknegt R (1988) Clinical pharmacokinetics of midazolam in intensive care patients; A wide interpatient variability? Clin Pharm Therap 43:263-271
10. Vesely R, Hoffman WE, Gil KSL, Albrecht RF, Miletich DJ (1987) The cerebrovascular effects of curare and histamine in the rat. Anesthesiology 66:519-523
11. McMillan MA, Ambis D, Siegal JM (1978) Cimetidine and mental confusion. N Engl J Med 298:284-285
12. Fenkelstein W, Isselbacher KJ (1978) Cimetidine. N Engl J Med 299:992-996
13. Snavely SR, Hodges GR (1984) The neurotoxicoty of antibacterial agents. Ann Intern Med 101:92-104
14. Boruck MJU, Matzke DS, Pollard RB (1988) Tremor induced by trimethoprim-sulfamethoxazole in patients with acquired immunodeficiency syndrome (AIDS). Ann Intern Med 77-78
15. Critchley EMR (1988) Neurological emergencies. Saunders, London, pp 470-472

Encephalopathy Associated with Sepsis

D. Bihari

Introduction

Whilst many investigators agree that a 'clouding of consciousness' is perhaps the most common disturbance in organ function associated with septic shock, proven severe systemic sepsis or even the more nebulous 'septic syndrome', it is still not clear exactly what are the relationships between fever, acute confusional states (often described loosely as a form of 'delirium' and most commonly observed in the elderly who may well be hypothermic), stupor and frank coma and how these different disturbances in brain function relate to so-called 'septic encephalopathy' and other organ system dysfunction [1]. One problem that is inherent in all the recent discussions of 'multiple organ failure', 'critical illness' associated with sepsis and trauma etc. has been the unstated supposition that one identifiable mechanism can account for all the metabolic and functional disturbances seen in these patients [2]. This, in my opinion, is patently not the case and when 'septic encephalopathy' is considered in isolation from other organ failure, it becomes apparent that various processes are at work at different times of the illness which can account for the observed disturbances in brain function. Drugs, alcohol and alcohol (or other drug) withdrawal obviously confuse the issue (and the patient!); this subject has been dealt with elsewhere. Drug-induced brain dysfunction is one important factor in the apparent reversibility of 'septic encephalopathy'. It probably accounts fot the majority of patients with severe sepsis and abnormal brain function who also have disturbances in hepatic and renal function and who suddenly 'wake up' as their underlying condition improves. At the same time, their medications are stopped whilst there are spontaneous improvements in hepatic and renal drug clearance. Thus it is difficult to identify patients suffering only from 'septic encephalopathy' and this limits our ability to study the pathogenesis.

However, there may be a real advantage in emphasizing a single conceptual basis for the occurrence of cell injury and organ failure within a septic patient since such an approach may lead to some meaningful therapeutic intervention [3, 4]. When one examines the evidence from carefully performed controlled clinical trials of specific interventions, other than following the basic principles of Intensive Care, i.e. avoid or treat rapidly hypoxia and hypotension, there has been a singular lack of other demonstrable therapeutic successes in this group of patients [5].

The Pathogenesis of Multiple Organ Failure Associated with Sepsis and Trauma - The Prevailing Hypothesis

The more recent publications on this subject have empasized that cell damage and organ dysfunction in sepsis and massive trauma arise initially through two different but interrelated mechanisms [6]. Firstly, the inappropriate and uncontrolled release of the various mediators of the acute inflammatory response may be directly cytotoxic [7-9] whilst also contributing to the second mechanism - the development of a maldistribution of blood flow (and hence the oxygen supply) within the microcirculations of actively respiring tissues [6, 10]. This second process, the consequence of inappropriate vasoconstriction, endothelial cell damage, microembolism, thrombosis and interstitial edema leading directly to hypoxia-related cell dysfunction and death, has been brought to our attention through the description of 'flow dependent oxygen consumption' [11] that often occurs in patients with severe sepsis and respiratory failure despite the presence of an apparently adequate oxygen supply [12-14] and may represent a mitochondrial or extra-mitochondrial oxygen deficiency syndrome [15]. Whether this abnormality in the relationship between the oxygen supply and oxygen demand occurs in the brain is a mute point [16] but we have provided some data to suggest that this may well be the case (see p. 158) [17]. Measurements of blood flow and oxygen uptake, although difficult, are more easily obtained than those of the various different mediators. For this reason, confusion still surrounds the exact role of endotoxin itself together with the activation of the complement system, white cells (neutrophils, monocytes), fixed tissue macrophages, platelets, the coagulation and kinin cascade systems with the release of their various mediators in the pathogenesis of organ failure [18-20].

A third mechanism of importance is the effects of reperfusion on ischemic tissue [3, 4]. There is now considerable evidence to suggest that much of the cellular injury associated with ischemia occurs on reperfusion with the re-establishment of an oxygen supply and a source of extracellular calcium - the so-called 'oxygen and calcium paradox' [21]. Since the severity of the reperfusion injury is most probably related to the length of the ischemic period, and given that tissue survival ultimately depends upon an adequate blood flow, reperfusion must, in principle, be brought about as soon as possible. Thus, whilst the 'no perfusion' injury is more deleterious in the long run than 'reperfusion', and understanding of the various damaging processes that go on during the reperfusion period might allow some further therapeutic intervention aimed at their inhibition [22]. These have been reviewed elsewhere.

The primary stimulus which precipitates activation of the cellular and contact system with the release of mediators in always identified clearly [23]. However, bacterial cell wall products, in particular endotoxin, are the most likely candidates [24, 25] and in the absence of septicemia or a known focus of infection, bacterial/endotoxin translocation through a leaky, ischemic or edematous gut mucosa may account for these phenomena - the so-called 'gut leak - liver prime' hypothesis of multiple organ failure [26]. Why certain organs should be especially susceptible to injury is unknown. The lung and kidneys receive a very high blood flow relative to their weight whilst being unrelated to their metabolic demand. This might contribute to their susceptibility in providing them with a very much greater toxic 'mediator load' compared with other tissues. In the case of the lungs, this 'dosing' effect might be even more important since this organ system is the first to receive the venous effluent from septic of traumatized tissue. Moreover, both these organ systems are at substantial risk in the ICU from injury with an iatrogenic component - oxygen and positive pressure for the lungs, nephrotoxic drugs for the kidneys. This tends not to be the case with the brain in which blood flow is usually tightly controlled and closely related to metabolic demand [27, 28]. Nevertheless, disturbances in the pressure-flow 'Baylis' form of autoregulation have been described in most forms of brain injury [29, 30] and similarly, abnormalities in brain 'metabolic autoregulation' might well occur during severe sepsis and lead directly to global or regional 'supply dependency'.

Other pathogenetic mechanisms accounting specifically for 'septic encephalopathy' have been proposed [1] (Table 1). Direct bacterial invasion of the meninges and brain by circulating micro-organisms with the formation of microabsences undoubtedly occurs in some cases and may be more common than previously thought [31]. The commonly observed abnormalities in liver function together with the preferential metabolism of branched chain amino acids by skeletal muscle leads to a metabolic profile very similar to that seen in hepatic encephalopathy. Fisher's group have championed the hypothesis that brain uptake of aromatic amino acids is increased and leads to the formation of 'false neuro - transmitters' [32, 33]. This may or may not be the case and the observations made in septic animals have never been confirmed in critically ill humans. Moreover, this hypothesis originally proposed to explain the occurrence of hepatic encephalopathy has not stood the test of time and is no longer tenable as an explanation of this latter condition.

Given this rather hazy understanding of the process of cell injury associated with severe sepsis and trauma together with the temporal difficulties in relating mediator release to tissue damage, it is not surprizing that the 'magic bullet' approach to mediator inhibition has been so unsuccessful in preventing or reversing the process [5]. The majority of investigators have demonstrated a surprizing degree of naivety in supposing that a standard, randomized, controlled clinical

Table 1. Proposed mechanisms contributing to the development of septic encephalopathy

1. Direct bacterial invasion of the CNS with the formation of cerebral microabscesses
2. Endotoxin mediated monocyte - macrophage / polymorph / platelet / complement / coagulation / kallikrein-kinin activation with the release of mediators (cytokines, eicosanoids, PAF, proteases and oxygen free radicals)
   - endothelial cell damage within the cerebral microcirculation
   - abnormalities in microcirculatory blood flow leading to ischemic hypoxia
   - mediator and hypoxia induced increases in blood brain barrier permeability
   - direct mediator cytotoxicity
3. Abnormalities in the plasma profile of aminoacids together with a change in the permeability of the blood brain barrier resulting in an increased cerebral uptake of aromatic aminoacids and the formation of 'false neurotransmitters' (e.g. octopamine)

trial of a single compound is likely to demonstrate a positive effect on survival in such a complex, unstandardized condition. Therefore, the less than critical introduction of individual forms of anti-inflammatory therapy (steroids [34, 35] or non-steroidal anti-inflammatory drugs (NSAIDs) and/or vasodilatory prostaglandins) [36, 37] in an attempt to reduce the severity of the tissue injury was almost bound to lead to disappointment. The same concern now surrounds the structure of the various clinical trials which have been proposed, and in some cases, initiated, to examine the protective effects of calcium channel antagonists, by themselves, in episodes of cerebral ischemia.

Nevertheless, there have been, recently, some interesting studies of the mechanisms and treatment of other encephalopathies, related to sepsis, perhaps in a seemingly tenuous fashion – i.e. those associated with bacterial meningitis, cerebral malaria and cardiopulmonary bypass – but which throw some light on septic 'brain failure', and suggest some possibilities for treatment.

Encephalopathy Associated with Bacterial Meningitis

A recent workshop on bacterial meningitis emphasized a number of features associated with the condition in various animal models [38, 39]. Firstly, there is a profound microangiopathic element to the disease with histological and functional abnormalities affecting the blood brain barrier reflected endothelial cell damage [40, 41]. These are similar to the more generalized endothelial cell injury associated with severe sepsis. In the case of meningitis, brain edema readily occurs but may be reduced in part, in animal models, using dexamethasone. This may reflect the role of the 'activated neutrophil' in potentiating brain edema since superoxide dismutase appears also to reduce its severity. Moreover, a reduction in brain edema can be achieved by pretreating the animals with indomethacin but this is not necessarily related to a fall in intracranial pressure (ICP) [42]. More importantly, perhaps, changes in cerebral blood flow in these animals can be observed following manipulations of their blood pressure suggesting a loss of cerebrovascular autoregulation. Increased cerebral blood flow appears to be associated with an increase in ICP reflecting the importance of intracranial blood volume in a relatively noncompliant system, presumably a consequence of the increased brain water. These findings are classic of the raised ICP associated with the 'hyperemic' form of head injury and the hyperemia (CBFs often of 200 ml/min per 100 g brain tissue) that occurs in patients with acute liver failure (Ede and Williams, personal communication). Raised in meningitis might also develop as a function of CSF outflow obstruction but this is apparently unusual.

The questions that arise from this workshop fall into 2 groups: firstly, how common is raised ICP in children and adults with meningitis and does this reflect hyperemia? Similarly, do patients with severe systemic sepsis presenting with a high cardiac output/low systemic vascular resistance state exactly the same hemodynamic disturbance as seen in acute liver failure – do these patients also develop brain edema, cerebral hyperemia and a raised ICP? Obviously, the answer to these questions is an aggressive approach to ICP monitoring and simultaneous measurements of cerebral blood flow, mean arterial pressure and cardiac output. The second question surrounds attempts to improve the compliance of the intracranial tissues. Are corticosteroids beneficial in bacterial meningitis? A recent controlled clinical trial from McCracken's group suggests that dexamethasone (0.15 mg/kg six hourly for four days) may reduce the incidence of bilateral sensorineural hearing loss, thus reducing morbidity from the condition [43]. An accompanying editorial expressed some concern over this conclusion but within the last paragraph, its author capitulated and stated that he 'would probably administer it (dexamethasone) to a severely ill child ...'! [44].

Sadly, like our 'Irish Question' in the U.K. we have not found the solution to the use of steroids in intensive care and we may have to wait some few years more for the answers. In the face of the dogma generated from two poorly designed controlled clinical trials [32, 33], and some animal evidence which suggests that glucocorticoids might potentiate ischemic injury to neurons [45], when considering acute confusional states, one has to remember the study of Hoffman et al. which demonstrated that in delirious patients with severe typhoid fever, high dose dexamethasone reduced mortality from 56% to 10% [46]. What is the relevance of all this to 'septic encephalopathy'? Interestingly, when attempting to understand how steroids might exert their effects in these infective conditions (i.e. meningitis and typhoid), most authors cite those processes which I have outlined above as being the most likely mechanisms of the widespread cellular injury and organ failure associated with severe systemic sepsis! As usual, as a clinician, one remains sceptical, asking the question 'how does a controlled trial of dexamethasone in meningitis, in children, performed by Texas physicians affect one's own prescribing habits in all adult ICU's?'. The answer is – it doesn't; further studies with a wider population base are required before a definitive answer becomes available. All that remains is to re-emphasize the importance of maintaining cerebral perfusion pressure in infants, children and adults with infections of the CNS. Certainly, outcome in the pediatric age group seems to be most closely related to this particular hemodynamic variable [47].

The Encephalopathies Associated with Cerebral Malaria and Cardiopulmonary Bypass

Whilst it might not be immediately obvious why these two forms of brain dysfunction should be grouped together and compared with 'septic encephalopathy', it is worthwhile considering the underlying mechanisms in both conditions since they give some insight into the 'microangiopathic' component accompanying a metabolic encephalopathy.

Cerebral malaria has been extensively investigated in the past few years by the Oxford/Bangkok group. Their studies have demonstrated a number of important features of the encephalopathy. Cerebral edema as a cause of coma in this condition is rare if one accepts that CT-scanning is a sensitive means of detecting an increase in brain water [48]. This may account for the observation that high dose dexamethasone (3 mg/kg loading dose; total 11.4 mg/kg per 48 h) has no effect in this condition [49] and may even be deleterious by promoting the incidence of pneumonia and gastrointestinal bleeding in treated patients [50].

Cerebral blood flow appears to range widely (23–70 ml/100 gm/min) with a normal mean (52/100 gm/min) in comatose patients but cerebral vascular resistance is increased, perhaps reflecting cytoadherence and uneven obstruction of the microcirculation by infested red cells [51]. Moreover, since the majority of these patients had fever and a reduced arterial oxygen content, one might have predicted an increase in flow and metabolism by 15–30%. These vascular changes are associated with evidence of cerebral anaerobic glycolysis and lactate production as in Robertson's head injured patients who had a frank infarct on the CT-scan [52]. During coma associated with cerebral malaria, in the presence of fever, the cerebral oxygen consumption is apparently low (1.9 ± 0.23 ml/100 gm/min) with a reduced cerebral oxygen extraction ratio and a normal or raised jugular venous bulb oxygen tension (5.7 ± 0.2 kPa). Normal (or increased) flow, reduced oxygen uptake, reduced extraction ratio, increased lactate production together with a raised venous oxygen tension smacks of the systemic hemodynamic disturbance associated with sepsis and the patchy, heterogenous and often covert tissue hypoxia that contributes to organ dysfunction [5, 10]. This is the disturbance that results in 'supply dependency' and although Warrell and his group did not assess their 12 patients in coma from cerebral malaria for this abnormality of oxygen transport, it is highly likely that it was present in the brain leading to coma.

Whilst there is argument concerning the relevance of the finding that early neuropsychological changes are found in 60% of patients undergoing cardiopulmonary bypass surgery [53], there is no doubt that a small number of patients (2–5%) 'stroke out' during the procedure and are left with major neurological abnormalities [54]. Retinal microembolism with microocclusion has been described [55] but the cerebral consequences of bypass appear to be most strongly associated with a low cerebral perfusion pressure and a prolonged bypass time [56]. Hypocapnia and reduced cerebral blood flow immediately before the onset of bypass followed by a period of relative hypercapnia not surprizingly increases the likelihood of brain ischemia and subsequent neurological deficits [57]. Measurements of cerebral blood flow before, during and 8 days after bypass suggest that a low CBF is the underlying problem and that CBF may stay low in some patients for some time after the procedure [56]. Thus, this form of encephalopathy establishes quite an interesting group of individuals to pretreat with 'brain protection' regimens providing any analysis of collected data takes into account, a priori, age, perfusion pressure and bypass time.

Abnormalities in Cerebral Blood Flow and Metabolism in Patients with Severe Sepsis

In our studies of septic encephalopathy, we have attempted to measure cerebral blood flow (CBF) (radiolabelled xenon; Novocerebrograph 10a) and cerebral oxygen uptake ($CMRO_2$) simultaneously in eight patients with severe sepsis and acute respiratory failure in order to assess the presence or absence of metabolic autoregulation within the brain. We have compared the relation of systemic hemodynamics and cerebral oxygen transport in these cases with 8 other head injury patients (Glasgow coma score on admission < 8) who required treatment in the Middlesex Hospital ICU. Our aim was to try and identify those factors regulating CBF and $CMRO_2$ in these groups of patients and to determine whether those abnormalities of oxygen transport occurring systemically in severe sepsis [58], also occur regionally within the brain itself and so underlie the development of septic encephalopathy. Obviously, all the patients we studied had been resuscitated and were hemodynamically stable. All patients were sedated. Five patients had required mechanical ventilation for the management of their cerebral edema.

Table 2 gives the values (medians with ranges) for the various hemodynamic and oxygen transport measurements obtained in the two groups of patients. Given the heterogenous nature of the populations studied, it was not surprizing to see a such wide range in cardiac index and whole body oxygen delivery and uptake. Nevertheless, patients with sepsis appeared to have a slightly higher whole body oxygen uptake than head injured cases (perhaps partly related to an elevation in core temperature) and this, in the presence of a slightly lower systemic oxygen delivery, gave the septic group a statistically significant greater oxygen extraction ratio than in the head injured group (medians 30 an 20% respectively, $p < 0.05$). Similarly, the cerebral circulation mirrored these systemic events with septic patients having a slightly greater $CMRO_2$ with a lower CBF and cerebral oxygen delivery thus giving a greater cerebral oxygen extraction ratio. However, as a consequence of the small numbers of patients studied in

Table 2. Systemic hemodynamics and oxygen transport variables in the 16 patients studied

	Head injured group	Septic group
Mean arterial pressure (mm Hg)	87 (66-95)	99 (72-128)
Cardiac index ($L/min \cdot m^2$)	3.6 (2.5-4.2)	3.2 (2.5-4.6)
Cerebral blood $flow_{isi}$ (no units)	36 (14-64)	36 (24-62)
Cerebral blood $flow_{f1}$ (ml/min per 100 g)	75 (22-160)	70 (48-112)
Arterial oxygen delivery (ml $O_2/min \cdot m^2$)	482 (353-720)	412 (349-667)
Cerebral oxygen delivery (ml O_2/min per 100 g)	10.7 (3.2-22.3)	9.4 (5.0-12.2)
Oxygen uptake index (ml $O_2/min \cdot m^2$)	89 (72-140)	123 (83-209)
Cerebral oxygen uptake (ml O_2/min per 100 g)	2.9 (0.9-4.5)	3.7 (2.4-5.9)
Systemic oxygen extraction ratio (%)	20 (15-26)	30 (18-36)*
Cerebral oxygen extraction ratio (%)	26 (9-39)	34 (25-49)

* $p<0.05$

each group, and the wide range of values observed, these changes did not reach statistical significance.

The relations of CBF to arterial CO_2, mean arterial pressure and cardiac index in these 16 patients were most interesting. While CBF_{f1} was unrelated to $PaCO_2$ (r_s [Spearman rank correlation coefficient] = 0.25, p NS) and mean arterial pressure (r_s = 0.18), overall, it was correlated most closely with the cardiac index, r_s = 0.51, $p<0.05$ (Figs. 1 and 2). This was rather surprizing since most investigators emphasized the importance of maintaining cerebral perfusion pressure (Mean arterial pressure - ICP or cerebral venous pressure, which ever the greater) as the major determinant of cerebral blood flow. Our finding might be interpreted in two ways; firstly, one might assume that as a group, pressure related autoregulation was intact so that values of CBF were independent of individual blood pressure as one might find in the normal population. In this situation, arterial pressure is held constant (as the most tightly regulated variable of the cardiovascular system) and CBF changes as a consequence of variations in regional vascular resistance and total flow. This seems unlikely given the presence of a substantial head injury in eight patients and severe systemic sepsis in the others. Perhaps a more likely explanation might be that in this group of critically ill patients, mean arterial pressure, on its own, was an inaccurate guide to cerebral perfusion pressure so that measurements of systemic flow were more helpful in assessing the adequacy of cerebral perfusion. Given that CBF is usually 15% of the cardiac output, if the cardiac output is very high (as in some patients with severe sepsis, acute liver failure or associated with the massive sym-

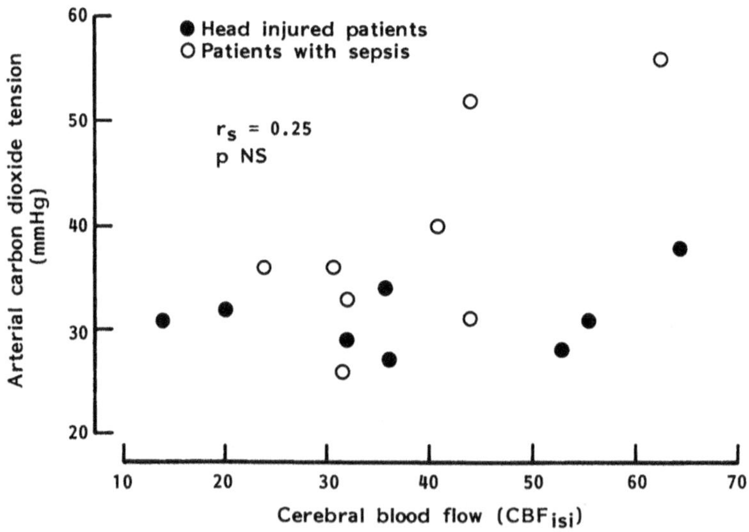

Fig. 1. The relation of cerebral blood flow to arterial carbon dioxide tension in the 16 patients studied.

Whilst there was no overall statistically significant relation between these two variables (r_s = Spearman rank correlation coefficient), patients with sepsis and higher $PaCO_2$ values tended to have slightly higher cerebral blood flows

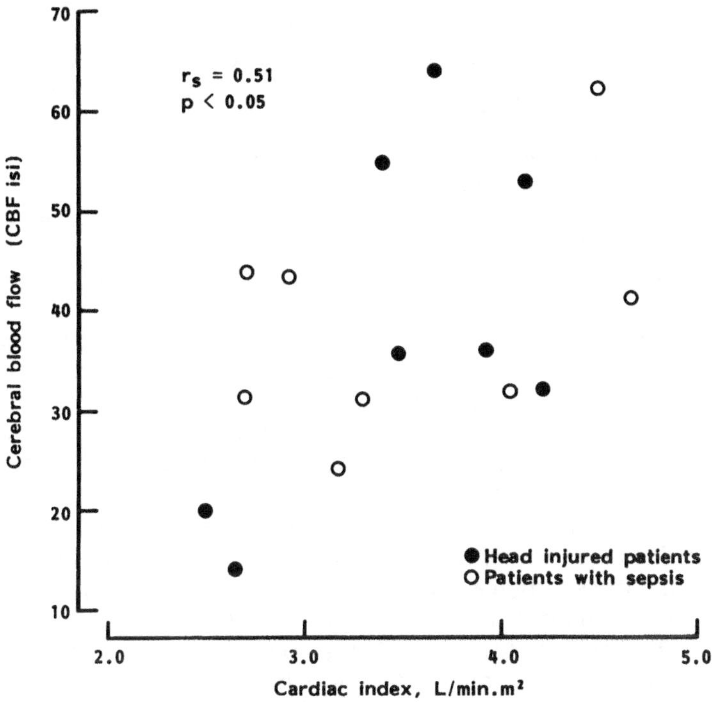

Fig. 2. The relation of cerebral blood flow to the cardiac index in the 16 patients studied. In this group of patients, there was a statistically significant relation between these two variables (r_s = Spearman rank correlation coefficient). Patients with a high cardiac index tended to have a high cerebral blood flow

pathetic surge occurring after a severe head injury), and in the absence of any strict autoregulation of blood flow, cerebral blood flow is likely to be high and may contribute to a rise in ICP. Certainly, it begs the question of whether cardiac output along with arterial pressure and ICP should be monitored in head injured patients in the ICU when measurements of CBF are unavailable.

A physiological principle that is generally accepted by most investigators is that the level of oxygen uptake of an organ or the whole organism is set by the metabolic demands of that system [11, 16]. Oxygen demand is usually related to the rate of ATP utilization, the production of which through the process of oxidative phosphorylation accounts for 85% of the oxygen consumed in a normal aerobic system. It may also reflect the activity of other extra-mitochondrial oxygen requiring reaction (usually only 10–15% of whole body oxygen consumption but which may rise in hypermetabolic states); in the brain, these reactions are particularly important in the synthesis of neurotransmitters (see section on reversible hypoxic/ischemic encephalopathy [15]).

Theoretically, there are two ways an individual can maintain their set level of oxygen uptake in the brain as in any other organ or as in the whole organism; firstly, the oxygen demand of the brain can be met by an increase in cerebral oxygen delivery. Since PaO_2, arterial saturation and hemoglobin cannot be adjusted internally from moment to moment, this mechanism depends upon a rise in CBF. This might occur, as previously mentioned, as in health, through a redistribution of the cardiac output by the tight control of the various regional vascular resistances, in the absence of a change in perfusion pressure. In situations in which the regulation of blood flow to the various organs is deranged, e. g. sepsis and trauma, the proportion of the cardiac output going to a particular organ bed might well be fixed, reflecting passive opening and closing of short, low resistance blood vessels within the various regional circulations as the cardiac output changes.

The second mechanism by which an increase in oxygen demand can be met is through an increase in the oxygen extraction ratio, this could occur as a result in right shifts in the hemoglobin oxygen dissociation curve or as a consequence of an increase in the number of perfused capillaries and a reduction in diffusion distance from capillaries into cells within the organ under consideration (Fig. 3). Figure 4 shows the relationships of $CMRO_2$ to cerebral oxygen delivery and extraction ratio in these patients. The data suggest that the second mechanism, an increase in oxygen extraction ratio, may be more important in supporting brain oxygen uptake and this would certainly be the case in situations in which flow was limited to any extent by brain swelling, hypocapnia, a relatively low cardiac output etc.. Again, the question arises that if an elevation in cerebral oxygen extraction ratio is the more important mechanism in maintaining brain oxygenation (and evidence from PET scanning would seem to confirm this suggestion), surely then it is more appropriate to monitor continuously cerebral oxygen extraction rather than CBF in patients with or at risk of a brain injury? This can be done with the various 'new technologies' – near infra-red spectroscopy

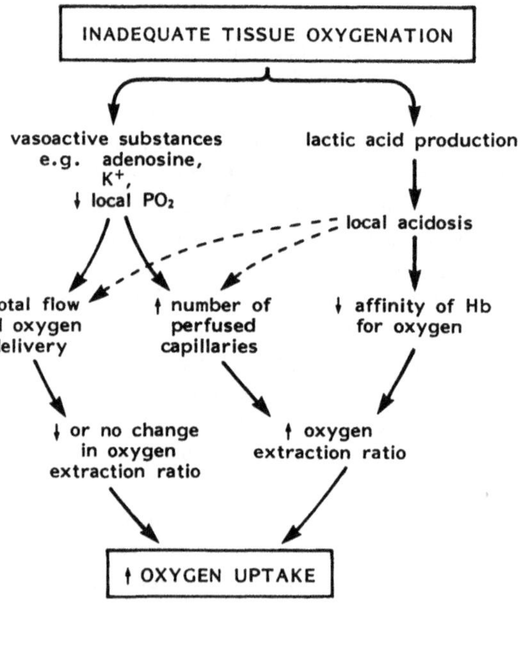

Fig. 3. Mechanisms by which an increase in tissue oxygen demand may be matched by an increase in the oxygen supply. There are only two mechanisms which can bring about the resolution of inadequate tissue oxygenation. Firstly, total flow may increase as a consequence of a reduction in local vascular resistance. Secondly, the efficiency of oxygen transport can be improved by increasing the proportion of the oxygen convectional supply actually utilized, i.e. by increasing the oxygen extraction ratio

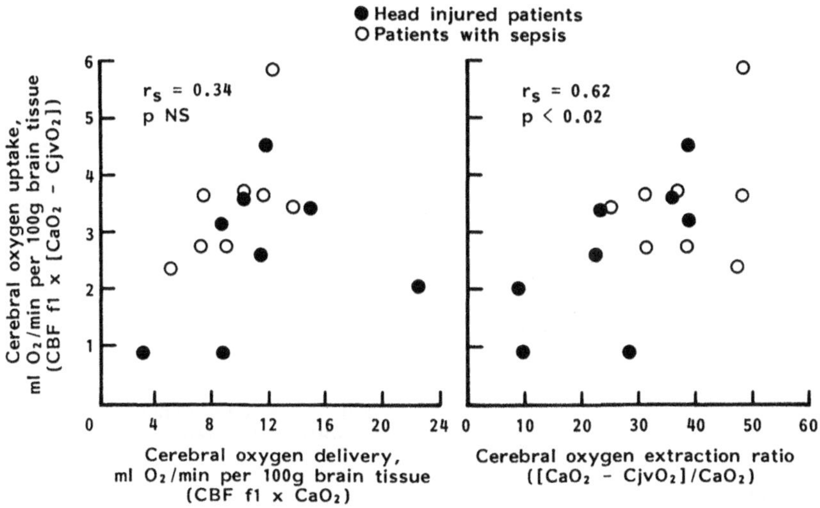

Fig. 4. The relation of cerebral oxygen uptake ($CMRO_2$) to cerebral oxygen delivery (left hand panel) and cerebral oxygen extraction ratio (right hand panel) in the 16 patients studied. In this group of patients, there was no relation between cerebral oxygen delivery and uptake as might have been predicted. By contrast, there was a statistically significant correlation between $CMRO_2$ and cerebral OER. This suggests that inadequate oxygenation within a damaged brain is primarily compensated for by an increase in extraction ratio rather than an increase in flow

or PET scanning [59, 60] – but more importantly, it can be done at the bedside in the general ICU with a pulse oximeter (arterial saturation) and an 'Oximetrix' (Abbott Laboratories) fiberoptic catheter inserted in a retrograde direction into the jugular bulb (jugular venous saturation) [17]. Using the 'dual oximeter' theory of Rasanen and Downes [61], a–v/a gives a continuous measure of extraction ratio and forms a powerful tool for assessing changes in brain oxygenation.

Finally, when attempting to define a group of patients as being 'hyperemic' or 'ischemic', measurements of flow on their own are useless! Our systemic studies of oxygen transport in sepsis have led us to emphasize the importance of relating flow to metabolism before and after some manipulation to increase blood flow (and hence oxygen delivery), thereby assessing the presence of 'delivery dependency' – the so-called oxygen flux test [58]. Similarly, within the brain, it is difficult to interpret 'on – off' measurements of flow or metabolism in isolation. Obviously, it the CBF is very low (less than 20 ml/min.m^2), life threatening ischemia may be present; alternatively, if it is very high (more than 100 ml/min.m^2) it may contribute to raised ICP. These are clear cut situations, rarely observed in our experience in the ICU.

On the other hand, by relating cerebral blood flow to the cardiac output (CBF_{f1} as a % of CO: normal value 15%) and comparing this with the $CMRO_2$ as a percentage of the total body oxygen uptake (normally around 20%), one can get some idea of whether perfusion and metabolism are matched. This relation for our patients is shown in Fig. 5 with an overall Spearman correlation coeffi-

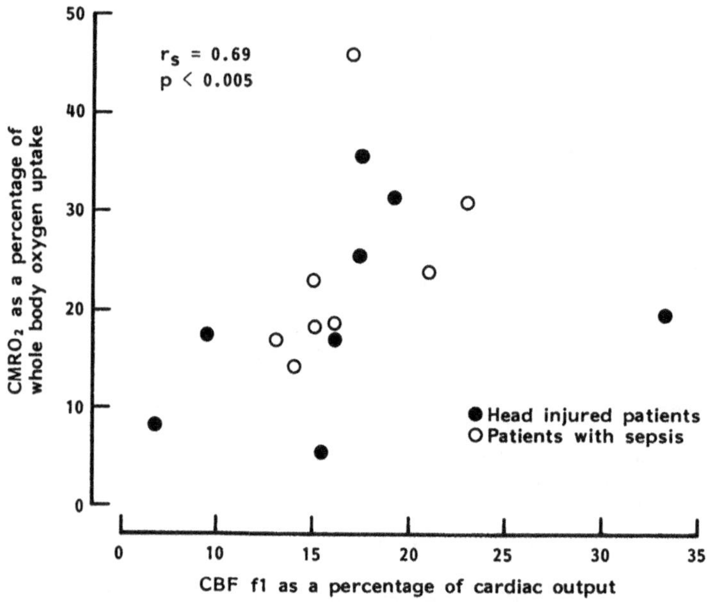

Fig. 5. The relation of cerebral oxygen uptake as a percentage of whole body oxygen consumption to the cerebral blood flow as a percentage of cardiac output in the 16 patients studied. (r_s = Spearman rank correlation coefficient. See text for details)

cient of 0.69. From this scattergram, one can see that there was one head injured patient who was markedly hyperemic with a CBF (160 ml/min per 100 g brain tissue) that was 33% (twice normal) of the cardiac output whilst his $CMRO_2$ (2.03 ml O_2/min per 100 g brain tissue) was only 21% (normal) of the total oxygen uptake. There was a second head injured patients who was also relatively hyperemic with a CBF that was 16% of the cardiac output whilst the $CMRO_2$ in this case was only 6% of whole body oxygen utilization. This patient had a CBF_{f1} of 67 ml/min per 100 g brain tissue which many would have considered to be 'normal' but in this setting is frankly hyperemic. Both these cases did badly, developing severe raised ICP that was difficult to control. The third head injured patient of note was a young girl receiving a barbiturate infusion for the control of raised ICP. Her CBF_{f1} was only 22 ml/min per 100 g brain tissue – that is 8% of her cardiac output. This might seem very low tending towards the 'ischemic penumbra' but her $CMRO_2$ was only 0.9 ml O_2/min per 100 g brain tissue, exactly 8% of her whole body oxygen consumption. Metabolism and flow were low but they were matched. This patient survived to make a good recovery although she did have a prolonged in-hospital course.

Of the septic patients, seven had apparent matching of perfusion with metabolism but the eighth (with a severe encephalopathy) had a $CMRO_2$ (5.9 ml O_2/min per 100 g brain tissue) that was 46% of whole body oxygen uptake supported by a CBF_{f1} (76 ml/min per 100 g brain tissue – supposedly normal!) that was only 17% of the cardiac output. This is quite obviously inappropriate, although the numbers on their own might have convinced the attending clinicians that brain oxygenation was adequate.

In a preliminary study, we did manage to obtain CBF, cerebral oxygen delivery and cerebral oxygen uptake together with the systemic measures of oxygen transport in 6 patients (4 septic and 2 head injured patients) before and during an inotropic vasodilator (dopamine or dopexamine) infusion. We chose to examine patients with apparently normal CBF and $CMRO_2$ and our aim was to increase the cardiac output by 20%. We found that the increase in cardiac output was associated with increases in CBF in 5 of the 6 patients, and in 4 of these (three septic and one head injured patients), $CMRO_2$ also increased suggesting the presence of 'delivery dependency'. In this small number of patients, the presence of cerebral 'delivery dependency' occurred in those cases who also had systemic 'delivery dependency' so that it may be that this abnormality of oxygen transport occurs not only in the periphery of septic patients but also within the brain itself, and could underly in some cases, the development of encephalopathy. There are many problems in the interpretation of these data, not least the fact that the dopamine or dopexamine might have caused a primary increase in $CMRO_2$ and the changes in flow were in fact, secondary phenomena. This subject requires further investigation.

In the meantime, our approach has changed somewhat. We recognize the difficulty and expense in obtaining accurate and reproducible measurements of CBF before and after an intervention to increase cerebral oxygen flux. Now we tend to rely on thermodilution cardiac output for assessing changes in flow whilst monitoring continuously cerebral oxygen extraction ratio by dual oximetry. Thus, following an intervention to increase systemic oxygen delivery, providing there is no fall in cerebral perfusion pressure, CBF and cerebral oxygen delivery probably increase proportionately. Providing the brain is well oxygenated and 'delivery dependency' is not present, cerebral oxygen extraction ratio will decrease and one will observe a rise in the jugular venous saturation. On the other hand, should the jugular venous saturation not change in the presence of an increased systemic flow, two explanations are possible. Firstly, CBF may not have risen in association with the increase in cardiac output, (this suggests either intact autoregulation - unlikely in the critically ill - or, much more likely and very importantly, the presence of clinically significant brain edema limiting any potential increase in blood flow). Secondly, an unchanged jugular venous saturation together with a rise in CBF is a marker of 'delivery dependency'. Both situations require treatment, and as usual we tend to do 'all things to all patients' - sedation, osmotherapy with attempts to increase further CBF if cerebral oxygen extraction is raised ($>$ 35%) and cerebral hyperemia as a cause of raised ICP unlikely.

The jugular venous saturation, like the mixed venous saturation, is only a loose guide to what is happening in the brain. Changes in saturation are more useful to monitor than absolute values. There are many problems in its interpretation, both technical and physiological. The heterogeneity of the distribution of blood flow within the brain might often be such that areas of relative ischemia exist with areas of relative hyperemia so that the global venous effluent has a PO_2 and hemoglobin saturation that is normal ($P_{jv}I_2$ 32–35 mmHg, saturation

65–70%) but only an average, not reflecting disturbances in regional flow and metabolism. An oxygen flux test may get over some of these problems but the results of increasing flux will reflect the method used to achieve this end. Sympathomimetics may be metabolic stimulants (especially in the absence of an intact blood-brain barrier) whereas vasodilators, whilst increasing cardiac output, may drop cerebral perfusion pressure and reduce CBF and so may not achieve the required increase in flux. We have been particularly interested in the effects of prostacyclin in sepsis and have demonstrated that this compound can recruit capillaries and does indeed increase whole body oxygen extraction ratio [58]. These are areas for further study.

Reversible Hypoxic/Ischemic Encephalopathy As It Might Occur in Sepsis

Finally, it is the impression of many clinicians that patients who develop abnormal cerebral function associated with sepsis usually have a completely reversible condition. Providing that there is effective treatment of the primary underlying septic problem, most patients make a full recovery once renal and hepatic function improve and any contributing drugs withdrawn. Occasionally, an elderly patient with widespread atherosclerosis will 'stroke out' during their critical illness and this becomes apparent with time. But in the absence of frank infarction, what then might be the mechanism by which patients are at one moment psychotic, confused with markedly distrubed cognitive functions and which may progress eventually to rigidity and coma (often with frank extrapyramidal motor signs) and yet at the next moment, responding appropriately to verbal questioning with a reasonably intact sensorium? The clinical picture is not like the brain failure associated with a head injury or following a cardiac arrest – and it is unlikely that severe ischemia (leading to ATP depletion within neurones, with the subsequent ionic pump failure, cellular swelling and death) accounts for the majority of cases with readily reversible disturbances in cerebral function. Yet I have suggested that 'delivery dependent oxygen consumption' does occur in the brain of septic patients and might lead to functional disturbances in the absence of structural change.

This hypothesis of 'hypoxia – related neurotransmitter failure' is relatively mature having been first proposed by Davies and Siesjö back in 1972 [62]. Essentially, it suggests that in times of relatively mild hypoxia (cerebral venous PO_2 25–50 mmHg, saturations 45–80%), extra-mitochondrial oxygen requiring reactions (e.g. those controlled by the hydroxylases of tyrosine and tryptophan, the rate limiting enzymes in the synthesis of dihydroxyphenylalanine [DOPA], (and hence dopamine and the other catecholamines) and 5-hydroxytryptophan [5-HTP] (and hence serotonin) respectively) will be inhibited at oxygen tensions well above the so-called Pasteur point, the oxygen tension at which mitochondrial aerobic respiration (and efficient ATP production) ceases and cytoplasmic anaerobic respiration with lactate accumulation begins [62–64].

The theoretical Pasteur point, i.e. the mitochondrial PO_2 at which oxidative phosphorylation is inhibited by a deficiency of the substrate, oxygen, is thought to be around 0.5–1.0 mmHg, reflecting the very low measurement, made in vitro, of the K_mO_2 for cytochrome oxidase $_{aa3}$, the rate limiting enzyme of oxidative phosphorylation. In vitro, cytochrome oxidase $_{aa3}$ appears to have a very high affinity for oxygen, fully oxidized at these very low PO_2s but studies in vivo using the technique of near infra-red spectroscopy have suggested that a certain proportion of the enzyme (5–20%, depending upon the organ studied) may be in the reduced form under normoxic conditions [65]. This may reflect a higher K_mO_2 in vivo or it may be related to the structure and function of the microcirculation such that areas of marked hypoxia can occur under resting conditions. This is a very contentious field of investigation. While this may or may not be the case in vivo, Davies has demonstrated a substantial fall in both DOPA (K_mO_2 for tyrosine hydroxylase 7.6 mmHg) and 5-HTP (K_mO_2 for tryptophan hydroxylase > 200 mmHg) synthesis in hypoxic rat brains long before there is any accumulation of lactate or change in the energy charge of the cell. Others have suggested that hypoxia might also exert its effects by disturbing the rate of turnover of the intermediates of the citric acid cycle, thus changing the rate of synthesis of aspartate, glutamate, GABA and acetylcholine. Thus, a plausible explanation for the reversible disturbances in brain function observed during critical illness are hypoxia related changes in neurotransmitter synthesis and this may account for the rapid recovery seen in some patients. Moreover, this hypothesis which relates to the early and reversible functional effects of ischemia negates many of the suppositions surrounding the application of the 'new technologies' in this field. To wait for an intracellular acidosis, a fall in cellular ATP levels or even an increase in the reduced cytochrome oxidase$_{aa3}$ (as detected by NMR spectroscopy or near infra-red spectroscopy) as a consequence of cerebral ischemia is too long. The reversible disturbance in brain function occurs earlier at a higher cerebral PO_2.

This hypothesis also gains support from observations made in mountaineers, climbing at high altitudes without oxygen, who are obviously hypoxemic and demonstrate quite marked cognitive defects (which can lead to terrible tragedies, e.g. the K2 disaster) long before they loses consciousness or sustain a major permanent brain injury [66]. Subtle abnormalities of brain function can be found in climbers upto one year after their descent to more normal altitudes [67] but as yet there have been few if any, follow-up studies of patients with septic encephalopathy which have carefully looked for these minor abnormalities and compared their frequency with those of a control group. It seems likely that these persisting neuropsychological abnormalities, described in climbers and similar to those occurring after cardiopulmonary bypass also pertain to patients recovering from septic encephalopathy. A prolonged septic illness with swings in the cerebral perfusion pressure and arterial saturation does most likely lead to some permanent disability but as yet, this has not been identified.

Conclusion

Disturbances in cerebral function associated with sepsis, whether it be localized to the CNS or systemic, frequently occur and probably arise through the same mechanisms by which cellular injury and organ dysfunction/failure develop in other systems. Studies of cerebral blood flow and cerebral oxygen uptake suggest that the brain, to a greater than lesser degree, follows the whole body by demonstrating a similar abnormality of oxygen transport within the cerebral circulation which has been well described systemically in patients with severe sepsis and respiratory failure. Cerebral oxygen uptake that is dependent upon the convectional oxygen supply is in marked contrast to the usual matching of supply to demand. Flow dependency in the early stages may produce a reversible form of cerebral dysfunction, the most likely explanation of which is a disturbance in synthesis and breakdown of neurotransmitters. If this flow dependency remains uncorrected for a prolonged period of time, then it is likely that life threatening ischemia/hypoxia will develop. This may be detected in the comatose patients by an increase in cerebral oxygen extraction ratio associated with cerebral lactate production. In this setting, irreversible brain damage is at hand and attempts must be made to correct the underlying ischemia/hypoxia. Treatment will depend upon the relative contributions of hypotension or hypertension, low or high cardiac output, arterial hypoxemia, raised ICP, cerebral hyperemia, abnormal cerebral microcirculatory blood flow and high cerebral oxygen demand to the clinical problem. Until these variables are measured regularly in the ICU, it will be difficult to tailor available therapy (and new cytoprotective cocktails) in an appropriate fashion.

References

1. Bolten C, Young G (1986) Sepsis and septic shock: central and peripheral nervous systems. In: Sibbald W, Sprung C (eds) Perspectives on sepsis and septic shock, new horizons, vol 1. Society of Critical Care Medicine, Fullerton, California, pp 157–171
2. Cerra F, West M, Keller G, Mazuski J, Simmons R (1988) Hypermetabolism and organ failure – the role of the activated macrophage as a metabolic regulator. In: Bond R, Adams H, Chaudry I (eds) Perspectives in shock ressearch, progress in clinical and biological research, vol 264. Liss, New York, pp 27–42
3. Cheung J, Bonventre J, Malis C, Leaf A (1986) Calcium and ischaemic injury. N Engl J Med 314:1670–1676
4. Krause G, White B, Aust S, Nayini N, Kumar K (1988) Brain cell death following ischaemia and reperfusion: a proposed biochemical sequence. Crit Care Med 16:714–726
5. Bihari D, Tinker J (1988) The therapeutic value of vasodilator prostaglandins in multiple organ failure associated with sepsis. Intensive Care Med 15:2–7
6. Bihari D, Cerra F (eds) (1988) Multiple organ failure, new horizons, vol 3. Society of Critical Care Medicine, Fullerton, California
7. Movat H, Cybulsky M, Colditz I, Chan M, Dinarello C (1987) Acute inflammation in gram negative infection: endotoxin, interleukin 1, tumor necrosis factor and neutrophils. Fed Proc 46:97–104
8. Beutler B, Cerami A (1987) Cachectin: more than a tumor necrosis factor. N Engl J Med 316:379–385
9. Weiss S (1989) Tissue destruction by neutrophils. N Engl J Med 320:365–376
10. Bihari D (1987) Mismatch of the oxygen supply and demand in septic shock. In: Vincent JL, Thijs LG (eds) Septic shock – an european view. Springer, Berlin New York Tokyo, pp 148–160
11. Cain S (1984) Supply dependency of oxygen uptake in the adult respiratory distress syndrome – myth or reality? Am J Med Sci 288:119–124

12. Schumacker P, Cain S (1987) The concept of a critical oxygen delivery. Intensive Care Med 13:223–229
13. Gutierrez G, Pohil R (1986) Oxygen consumption is linearly related to the oxygen supply in critically ill patients. J Crit Care 1:45–53
14. Astiz M, Rackow E, Falk J, Kauman B, Weil M (1987) Oxygen delivery and consumption in patients with hyperdynamic septic shock. Crit Care Med 15:26–28
15. Bihari D (1988) Oxygen delivery and consumption in the critical ill; their relation to the development of multiple organ failure. In: Kox W, Bihari D (eds) Shock and the adult respiratory distress syndrome. Springer, Berlin Heidelberg New York Tokyo, pp 95–124
16. Bryan-Brown C (1988): Blood flow to organs: parameters for function and survival in critical illness. Crit Care Med 16:170–178
17. Garlick R, Bihari D (1987) The use of intermittent and continuous recordings of jugular venous bulb oxygen saturation in the unconscious patient. Scand J Clin Lab Invest (Suppl 188):47–52
18. Westaby S (1986) Mechanisms of membrane damage and surfactant depletion in acute lung injury. Intensive Care Med 12:2–5
19. Hyers T, Gee M, Andreadis N (1987) Cellular interactions in the multiple organ injury syndrome. Am Rev Respir Dis 135:952–953
20. Demling R (1988) The role of mediators in human ARDS. J Crit Care 3:56–72
21. Farber J (1982) Membrane injury and calcium homeostasis in the pathogenesis of coagulative necrosis. Lab Invest 47:114–123
22. Patt A, Harken A, Burton L, et al (1988) Xanthine oxidase derived hydrogen peroxide contributes to ischaemia reperfusion induced edema in gerbil brains. J Clin Invest 81:1556–1562
23. Carrico C, Meakins J, Marshall J, Fry D, Maier R (1986) Multiple organ failure syndrome. Arch Surg 121:196–208
24. Goris R, te Boekhorst T, Nuytinck J, Gimbrere J (1985) Multiple organ failure: generalized autodestructive inflammation. Arch Surg 120:1109–1115
25. Brigham K, Meyrick B (1986) Endotoxin and lung injury. An Rev Respir Dis 133:913–927
26. Baker J, Deitch E, Berg R, Specian R (1988) Hemorrhagic shock induces bacterial translocation from the gut. J Trauma 28:896–906
27. Kuschinsky W, Wahl M (1978) Local chemical and neurogenic regulation of cerebral vascular resistance. Physiol Rev 58:656–689
28. Siesjö B (1984) Cerebral circulation and metabolism. J Neurosurg 60:883–908
29. Siesjö B (1987) Critical degrees of hypoxia and ischemia when cerebral function and metabolism are perturbed. In: Bryan-Brown C, Ayres S (eds) Oxygen transport and utilisation, new horizons, vol 2. Society of Critical Care Medicine, Fullerton, California, pp 293–310
30. Procter H, Palladino G, Fillipo D (1988) Failure of autoregulation after closed head injury; an experimental model. J Trauma 28:347–352
31. Pendlebury W, Perl D, Karibo R, et al (1983) Disseminated microabscesses of the central nervous system. Neurology 33:223
32. Fischer J, Funovies J, Aguirre A (1975) The role of plasma aminoacids in hepatic encephalopathy. Surgery 78:276–283
33. Jeppson B, Freund H, Gimmon Z, et al (1981) Bloodbrain barrier in sepsis. Cause of septic encephalopathy? Am J Surg 141:13
34. Bone R, Fisher C, Clemmer T, Slotman G, Metz C, Balk R and the Methylprednisolone severe sepsis study group (1987) A controlled clinical trial of high dose methylprednisolone in the treatment of severe sepsis and septic shock. N Engl J Med 317:653–658
35. Veterans Administration Systemic Sepsis Cooperative Study Group (1987) Effect of high-dose glucocorticoid therapy on mortality in patients with clinical signs of systemic sepsis. N Engl J Med 317:659–665
36. Hallenbeck J, Leiitch D, Dutka A, Greenbaum L, McKee A (1982) Prostaglandin I_2, indomethacin and heparin promote postischemic neuronal recovery in dogs. Ann Neurol 12:145–156

37. Kochanek P, Dutka A, Hallenbeck J (1987) Indomethacin, prostacyclin and heparin improve cerebral blood flow without affecting early post-ischaemic granulocyte accumulation. Stroke 18:634–637
38. Klein J, Feigin R, McCracken G (1986) Report of the task force on diagnosis and treatment of meningitis. Paediatrics 78 (suppl):959–982
39. Sande M, Scheld W, McCracken G (1987) Summary of a workshop: pathophysiology of bacterial meningitis, implications for new management strategies. Pediatr Infect Dis J 6:1167–1171
40. Tauber M, Brooks-Fournier R, Sande M (1986) Experimental models of CNS infections – contributions to concepts of disease and treatment. Neurol Clin 4:249–264
41. Scheld W (1987) Morphofunctional alterations of the blood brain barrier during experimental meningitis. Pediatr Infect Dis J 6:1145–1146
42. Tureen J, Stella F, Clyman R, Mauray F, Sande M (1987) Effect of indomethacin on brain water content, cerebrospinal fluid white blood cell response and prostaglandin E_2 levels in cerebrospinal fluid in experimental meningitis in rabbits. Pediatr Infect Dis J 6:1151–1153
43. Lebel M, Freij B, Syrogiannopoulos G, et al (1988) Dexamethasone therapy for bacterial meningitis – results of two double-blind, placebo controlled trials. N Engl J Med 319:964–971
44. Smith A (1988) Neurologic sequelae of meningitis. N Engl J Med 319:1012–1014
45. Sapolsky R, Pulsinelli W (1985) Glucocorticoids potentiate ischemic injury to neurons – therapeutic implications. Science 229:1397–1400
46. Hoffman S, Punjabi N, Kumala S, et al (1984) Reduction of mortality in chloramphenicol treatment severe typhoid fever by high dose dexamethasone. N Engl J Med 310:82–88
47. Goitein K, Tamir I (1983) Cerebral perfusion pressure in central nervous system infections of infancy and childhood. J Paediatrics 103:40–43
48. Locareesuwan S, Warrell D, White N, et al (1983) Do patients with cerebral malaria have cerebral oedema? A computed tomography study. Lancet 1:434–437
49. Hoffman E, Punjabi N, Sanjaya B, McKee K, Cambell J, Laughlin L (1988). High dose dexamethasone in quinine treated patients with cerebral malaria – a double-blind, placebo controlled trial. J Inf Dis 158:325–331
50. Warrell D, Looaressuwan S, Warrell M, et al (1982) Dexamethasone proves deleterious in cerebral malaria: a double-blind trial in 100 comatose patients. N Engl J Med 306:313–319
51. Warrell D, White N, Veall N, et al (1988) Cerebral anaerobic glycolysis and reduced cerebral oxygen transport in human cerebral malaria. Lancet 2:534–538
52. Robertson C, Grossman R, Goodman J, Narayan R (1987) The predictive value of cerebral anaerobic metabolism with cerebral infarction after head injury. J Neurosurg 67:361–368
53. Shaw P, Bates D, Cartlidge N, Heaviside D, Julian D, Shaw D (1985) Early neurological complications of coronary artery bypass surgery. BMJ 291:1384–1387
54. Gilston A (1986) Brain damage after cardiac surgery. Lancet 1:1323
55. Blauth C, Arnold J, Kohner E, Taylor K (1986) Retinal microembolism during cardiopulmonary bypass demonstrated by fluorescein angiography. Lancet 2:837–839
56. Smith P, Treasure T, Newman S, Joseph P, Ell P, Schneidau A, Harrison M (1986) Cerebral consequences of cardiopulmonary bypass. Lancet 1:823–825
57. Nevin M, Colchester A, Adams S, Pepper J (1987) Evidence for the involvement of hypocapnia and hypoperfusion in aetiology of neurological deficit after cardiopulmonary bypass. Lancet 2:1493–1495
58. Bihari D, Smithies M, Gimson A, Tinker J (1987) The effect of vasodilatation with prostacyclin on oxygen delivery and uptake in critically ill patients. N Engl J Med 317:397–403
59. Frackowiak R, Lenzi GL, Jones T, et al (1980) Quantitative measurement of regional cerebral blood flow in man using $^{15}0$ and positron emission tomography: Theory, procedure and normal values. J Computer Assisted Tomography 4:727–736
60. Reynolds E, Wyatt J, Azzopardi D, et al (1988) New non-invasive methods for assessing brain oxygenation and haemodynamics. Br Med Bull 44:1052–1075
61. Rasanen J (1988) Dual oximetry. In: Vincent JL (ed) Update in intensive care and emergency medicine, vol 5. Springer, Berlin Heidelberg New York Tokyo, pp 436–441

62. Davis J, Carlsson A, MacMillan V, Siesjö B (1973) Brain tryptophan hydroxylation: dependence on arterial oxygen tension. Science 182:72–74
63. Davis J, Carlsson A (1973) Effect of hypoxia on tyrosine and tryptophan hydroxylation in unanaesthetized rat brain. J Neurochem 20:913–915
64. Gibson G, Pulsinelli W, Blas J, Duffy T (1981) Brain dysfunction in mild to moderate hypoxia. Am J Med 70:1247–1254
65. Epstein F, Balaban R, Ross B (1982) Redox state of cytochrome aa_3 in isolated perfused rat kidney. Am J Physiol 243:F356–F363
66. West J (1982) Man at extreme altitude. J Appl Physiol 52:1393–1399
67. West J (1986) Do climbs to extreme altitude cause brain damage? Lancet 2:387–388

Energy Metabolism in Brain Injury

R. L. Chiolero, N. de Tribolet, and Y. Schutz

Introduction

Brain failure is associated with extensive physiological changes, involving circulation, respiration, metabolism, endocrine and immunological systems. These changes have been well studied in patients with non cranial trauma and less extensively in patients with head trauma. In the latter, these responses can be so severe as to threaten the outcome. Most of the studies on energy metabolism in patients suffering from acute brain failure have been carried out in head-injured patients; very few have been published concerning other kinds of brain failure. In this paper, some of the basic information regarding the changes in energy metabolism in patients suffering from head injury will be reviewed.

Hormonal Responses

The endocrine response to trauma is characterized by stimulation of the hypothalamic nuclei, with increase in pituitary hormone secretion, activation of the sympathoadrenal system and elevation in counterregulatory hormone secretion [1]. Severe head injury produces alterations in the hypothalamo-pituitary response to trauma, particularly in the patients with poor outcome [2]. Such patients present a decrease in pituitary hormone secretion, associated with various hypothalamic dysfunctions, which are correlated with the severity of head injury, in particular the Glasgow coma score on admission, the intracranial pressure (ICP) level and the outcome [2]. By contrast, they exhibit a normal response of the counterregulatory hormones, with elevation of the urine catecholamine levels as well as of the plasma levels of cortisol and glucagon [3]. Counterregulatory hormones play important metabolic roles: catecholamines increase lipolysis and hepatic glucose production, decrease the response to insulin, whereas glucagon and cortisol promote protein catabolism for neoglucogenesis. In patients with severe brain injury or multiple injury, a negative correlation has been found between nitrogen balance and both urinary catecholamine excretion and plasma glucagon levels [3].

Metabolic Responses

The metabolic responses to injury are characterized by complex and integrated changes involving the rate of energy expenditure, substrate mobilization, and utilization, the hepatic synthesis of acute phase proteins, changes in the distribution of plasma trace elements, and various biochemical processes [4]. These metabolic changes are often called "acute phase" responses. Numerous mediators have been described, among which lymphokines and hormonal mediators seem to play key roles [5].

Increased proteolysis and muscle amino acid mobilization occur following any severe trauma, including head injury [4, 6]. This produces the well known elevation in nitrogen urinary excretion. In addition, carbohydrate and fast metabolisms are profoundly altered. Increase in plasma glucose level results mainly from elevated glucose production by the liver secondary to catecholamines and counterregulatory hormones action. Furthermore, there is a marked resistance to insulin. Free fatty acids are mobilized in traumatized patients, under the combined action of the sympathoadrenergic system and other counterregulatory hormones. The physiologic suppression of lipolysis in response to glucose administration is reduced. Ketone body production and utilization are diminished.

In addition to host factors, exogenous factors may modify the metabolic responses to injury. Catecholamine administration as previously mentioned induces wide metabolic responses. Steroids produce significant increase in nitrogen losses, associated with marked changes in carbohydrate metabolism but no apparent effect on resting metabolic rate [12].

Energy Expenditure

Energy expenditure (EE) can be assessed in critically ill patients by indirect calorimetry. This determines the heat released by the oxidative processes from the measurement of O_2 consumption ($\dot{V}O_2$) and CO_2 production ($\dot{V}CO_2$) [7]. Two methods are available in ICU patients: the gas exchange technique or the Fick method using a Swan-Ganz catheter [8]. The former is a continuous and more accurate method, which allows prolonged measurements, even in patients on mechanical ventilation. The accuracy of indirect calorimetry using an open-circuit technique in patients breathing room air is high, usually 1–2%. However, in patients on mechanical ventilation or receiving oxygen therapy, many factors can reduce the accuracy which is usually around 5–10% or more.

Total EE of a normal subject can be partitioned into three major components: basal EE, thermogenesis, i.e. increases in EE over basal values due to various physiological stimuli, and EE due to physical activity. In children, the energy cost of growth must be taken into account. In injured and critically ill patients two additional components must be considered: the effects of illness (which usually increases EE) and the influence of drugs.

Basal EE is defined as the rate of heat production of a healthy subject measured under highly standardized conditions: 12–14 h fast, complete rest without previous physical activity, thermoneutrality, awake, emotionally undisturbed state. Sixty to 70% of basal EE is devoted to the function of the vital organs: liver, brain, kidney, heart.

Thermogenesis refers to the various conditions that increase basal EE, like nutrition and cold. Diet-induced thermogenesis is produced by the processes of digestion, absorption, storage and transformation of the nutrients ("obligatory" thermogenesis). In addition, overfeeding, particularly with carbohydrates, induces an adrenergic stimulation, which elevates the metabolic rate ("adaptive" component). Diet-induced thermogenesis is related to the type of nutrients: the thermogenesis of fat averages 2–3%, carbohydrates 5–10% and proteins 20–30% of the energy administered. In patients receiving hyperalimentation with elevated glucose loads or with unbalanced nutrient supply, the diet-induced thermogenesis may markedly increase and is associated with deleterious metabolic and systemic effects such as respiratory failure and fatty liver.

Cold-induced thermogenesis is related to the maintenance of body temperature, which is actively regulated by the balance between total heat production and heat losses. Two processes increase EE during cold exposure, shivering-and non-shivering thermogenesis.

Effect of Head Injury

Numerous factors may influence the EE of patients with brain injury and modify all the components of EE (Table 1). Basal conditions are never present with brain failure. In clinical conditions, the EE measured in resting condition is called the resting EE. It includes the basal EE, different thermogenic stimuli, variation in muscular tone, as well as illness and drug effects. Resting EE of patients with head injury varies widely according to the data reported in the literature, including ours! [9–17]. A hypermetabolic response is commonly reported but the variability between studies and between subjects is high. Individual values of EE in the literature range from 43% to 280% of normal reference value (Fig. 1). Such differences may be related to the large number of confounding factors which are known to either elevate or decrease the metabolic rate (Ta-

Table 1. Factors influencing energy expenditure in patients with head injury

1. *Resting energy expenditure*
   - Basal EE: body weight and composition, height, age, sex
   - Temperature: fever, hypothermia, shivering
   - Diet: fast, fed (maintenance), overfeeding
   - Effect of trauma: adrenergic activity, hormones, lymphokines
   - Level of consciousness
   - Pain
   - Drugs
   - Respiration and ventilation: Mechanical vs spontaneous, respiratory work
   - Muscular tone
2. *Physical activity*
   - Muscular activity: postures, agitation, immobile coma

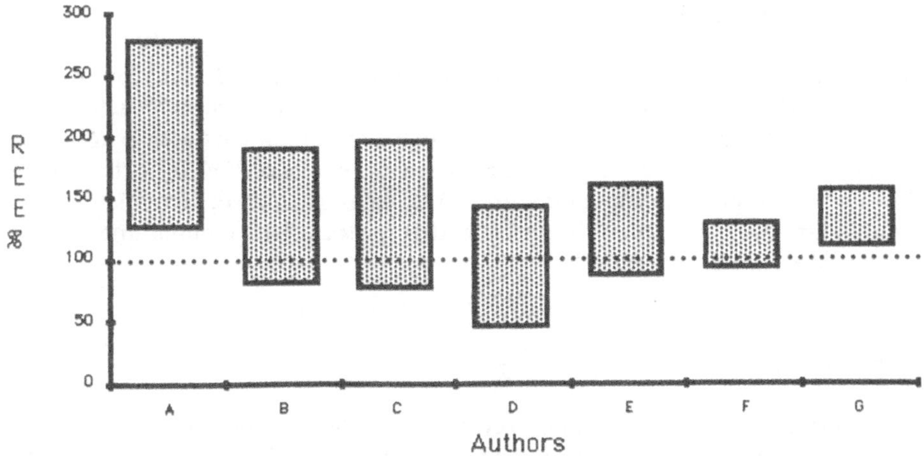

Fig. 1. Range of resting energy expenditure (REE) (% of normal values) in patients following head injury according to various authors: A) Haider et al. 1985 [9], B) Clifton et al. 1984 [10], C) Dempsey et al. 1985 [11], D) Dempsey et al. 1985 [11], E) Clifton et al. 1986 [14], F) Clifton et al. 1986 [14], G) Chiolero et al. 1989 [17]

ble 1). In addition the methods of measurement (indirect calorimetry with a Douglas bag or a ventilated hood, Tissot spirometer, reverse Fick equation) as well as the technique and conditions of measurements (duration of measurement, ventilatory status, supplementary oxygen) may also influence the results and their accuracy [8].

We have studied resting EE in 12 extubated non septic patients with head injury, in resting postabsorptive conditions [17]. Indirect calorimetry was performed on days 3 to 14, i.e. during the early recovery phase. Resting EE was normal (90–110% of predicted values) in one patient and increased (112–156%) in 11 patients. Mean resting EE was $126 \pm 14\%$ of normal reference values. This study showed that head injured patients, in standard conditions, are moderately hypermetabolic during the recovery period following intensive treatment.

Effects of Adrenergic Activity

Trauma induces a state of sympathoadrenal hyperactivity with elevation in catecholamine secretion. This state of adrenergic hyperactivity is particularly pronounced following head injury [18]. We have evaluated the importance of adrenergic activity on energy metabolism in patients following severe head injury by inducing progressive β-blockade with i.v. propranolol [17]. The 24-h urinary catecholamine excretion was elevated in these patients (adrenaline: $420 \pm 240\%$ of normal values; noradrenaline: $413 \pm 259\%$ of normal values). Propranolol produced a rapid decrease in resting EE, heart rate, and systemic arterial blood pressure. The decrease in metabolic rate corresponded to $26 \pm 12\%$ of the excess metabolic rate, i.e. about a quarter of the net hypermetabolism.

Effect of Temperature

The regulation of temperature is affected in traumatized and many severely ill patients under the influence of catecholamines and "acute phase" reaction mediators. Fever can be observed in a large proportion of patients with head injury during the "acute phase". Resting EE increases by about 10% for each degree Celsius elevation in body temperature. We have calculated, in patients with brain injury using the Dubois's equation, that fever explained about one quarter of the excess metabolic rate [17].

Drug Effects

Many drugs which are commonly prescribed in the treatment of patients with brain failure may significantly influence resting EE (Table 2). Catecholamines increase $\dot{V}O_2$ and $\dot{V}CO_2$ via their β-adrenergic action. By contrast, β-blockers, as previously mentioned, decrease these parameters. Barbiturate sedation and coma markedly reduce resting EE [11]. In patients with acute pain, opiates produce moderate decrease in metabolic rate [23]; these agents together with muscle relaxants may dramatically diminish both $\dot{V}O_2$ and $\dot{V}CO_2$ in shivering patients [24].

Effect of Neurological State

There is no simple relationship between the level of consciousness, the neurological status and the level of energy expenditure. An inverse relationship between the Glasgow coma score and the resting EE was found by Clifton et al. in both comatose and non-comatose patients during the first two weeks post injury [14]. There was a mean increase in resting EE of 42% (range 28–66%) above normal values in comatose patients with Glasgow coma scores of 4–5, and of 20% (range 7–82%) in comatose patients with Glasgow coma scores of 6–7. By contrast, the same group [10] and ourselves [17] failed to find such a correlation. Normal, decreased or increased metabolic rate have been found in comatose patients.

Table 2. Some important drugs influencing resting energy expenditure in patients following head injury

Agents	Action	Order of magnitude	Ref.
Catecholamines	Increase	5–30%	[22]
Beta-blockers	Decrease	5–30%	[17]
Barbiturates (high doses)	Decrease	15–30%	[11]
Opiates for analgesia	Decrease	5–10%	[23]
Opiates against shivering	Decrease	50–300%	[24]
Relaxants	Decrease	20–40%	[14]

This can be explained by the numerous factors which can influence EE in addition to the level of consciousness, particularly muscular tone and physical activity (Table 1).

Effect of Physical Activity

The proportion of EE which is due to physical activity is highly variable in neurosurgical patients. It can be negligible in curarized patients on mechanical ventilation, but it can largely exceed resting EE in posturing or agitated patients (Fig. 2a–c). Moderately increased to moderately decreased resting EE are usually found in curarized patients, illustrating the importance of physical activity on metabolic rate [14]. By contrast, flexion or extension postures produce sharp and prolonged increases in EE, ranging between 50 and 150% of the reference values [14, 17].

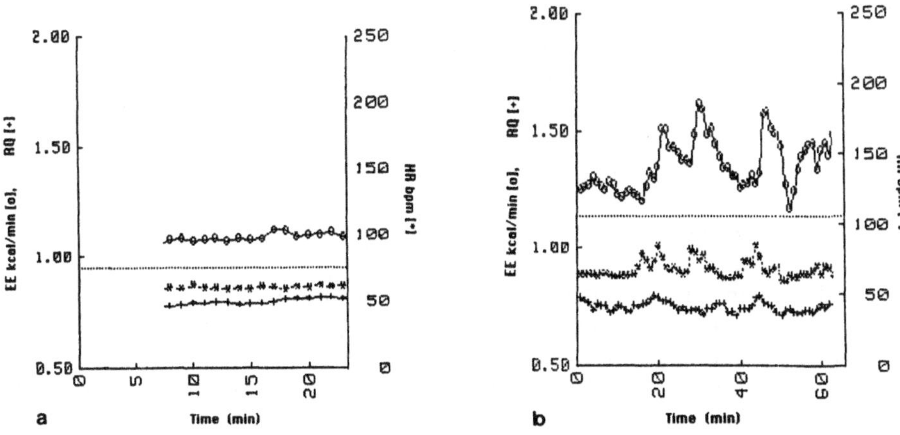

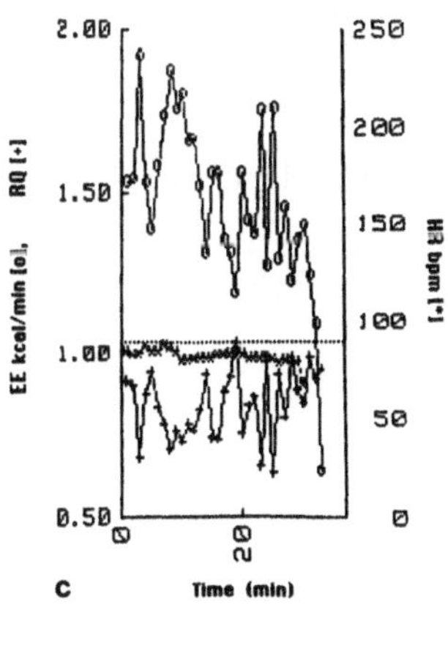

Fig. 2a–c. Resting energy expenditure (EE), respiratory quotient (RQ), and heart rate (HR) in 3 patients after head injury. **a** Comatose, immobile; **b** with some muscular activity; **c** agitated

Muscular or neuromuscular dysfunction in patients with neurological diseases, may influence the rate and efficiency of physical work. Work capacity is decreased, while the energy cost of exercise and/or breathing may increase in parallel [19].

Substrate Oxidation

Trauma induces marked protein and fast mobilization and modified substrate and nutrient utilization [4]. Very high urinary nitrogen excretion, in the range of 10 to 30 g nitrogen per day have been described following brain injury, associated with marked negative nitrogen balance despite high protein and energy intakes, lasting usually from 2 to 4 weeks [9, 10, 12, 14, 17].

The protein energy contribution represents the fraction of the expended energy which is covered by protein oxidation. It is mainly influenced by the nutritional status, the endocrine and metabolic conditions as well as the energy level and the diet composition. In normal post-absorptive conditions, the protein energy contribution is in the range of 10–15%. It is elevated in patients with brain injury. In 12 post-absorptive head-injured patients, we found a value of 21 ± 10% [17] (Table 3), whereas Clifton et al. observed a values of 24 ± 7% in fed patients receiving high levels of proteins [14]. Thus patients with brain injury oxidize large quantities of proteins. Fat oxidation is also elevated: fat covered 65% of EE in head-injured patients in fasting conditions [17] (Table 3).

Nutritional Consequences

Elevated protein and fat catabolism resistant to nutritional support is usually observed in patients following severe head injury [10]. These metabolic changes are prolonged during 2 to 4 weeks and may adversely affect the nutritional state of the patient [10, 13, 14]. The systemic consequences of prolonged catabolism are well known and include loss of lean body mass, impaired wound healing and decreased immune responses. Indeed a high rate of systemic infection is known to occur in patients after head injury [20]. Recent studies suggest that early nutritional support using parenteral supply may improve the outcome of such pa-

Table 3. Energy expenditure (EE) and substrate oxidation in 12 patients following head injury. (From [17])

Resting EE (kcal/min)	1.40 ± 2.7
(% reference)	126 ± 14
Oxidation of protein (mg/min)	72 ± 35
(% of EE)	21 ± 10
- of lipids (mg/min)	96 ± 21
(% EE)	66 ± 14
- of glucose (mg/min)	43 ± 37
(% EE)	13 ± 11

tients [21]. Thus, an adequate and early nurtitional support constitutes a therapeutic priority in patients with severe head injury.

These patients require large protein and highly variable energy supplies. Twenty to 30% of the energy intake should be provided by proteins or amino acids due to the elevated protein energy contribution. Lipid utilization is enhanced in these patients. In addition, the administration of large quantities of glucose may disturb brain metabolism. Thus nutritional intake should contain a sufficient amount of lipids to cover a large portion of the metabolic rate.

There is no simple mean to estimate the energy requirements at the bedside. Both prolonged over- or undernutrition are undesirable. Indirect calorimetry using commercial systems (when available to the clinician) may provide useful indications. For other patients, normograms and various recommendations have been proposed: Clifton et al. have developed a normogram to estimate energy expenditure from heart rate and simple neurological findings in comatose patients during the first 2 weeks after brain injury [14]. The same authors have developed equations allowing a prediction of resting EE in comatose and noncomatose patients from heart rate, Glasgow coma score and duration of illness. We found high linear correlations between resting EE and both 24 h urinary nitrogen excretion and heart rate in small sample of head injured patients [17]. The value of such estimations of EE for nutritional supply is still unknown.

References

1. Frayn K (1986) Hormonal control of metabolism in trauma and sepsis. Clin Endocrinol 24:577-599
2. Chiolero RL, Lemarchand TH, Schutz Y, et al (1988) Plasma pituitary hormone levels in severe trauma with or without head injury. J Trauma 28:1368-1374
3. Chiolero R, Schutz Y, Lemarchand TH, et al (1989) Hormonal and metabolic changes following severe head injury or non cranial injury. JPEN 13:5-12
4. Gelfand RA, de Fronzo RA, Goldberg R (1983) Metabolic alterations associated with major injury or infection. In: Kleinberger G, Deutsch E (eds) New aspects of clinical nutrition. Karger, Basel, pp 247-270
5. Pomposelli JJ, Flores EA, Bistrian B (1988) Role of biochemical mediators in clinical nutrition and surgical metabolism. JPEN 12:212-218
6. Elwyn DH (1987) Protein metabolism and requirements in the critically ill patient. Crit Care Clin 3:57-69
7. Jequier E, Acheson K, Schutz Y (1987) Assessment of energy expenditure and fuel utilization in man. Ann Rev Nutr 7:187-208
8. Damask MC, Schwarz Y, Weissman C (1987) Energy measurements and requirements of critically ill patients. Crit Care Clin 3:71-96
9. Haider W, Lackner F, Schlick W, et al (1975) Metabolic changes in the course of severe acute brain damage. Eur J Intensive Care Med 1:19-26
10. Clifton GL, Robertson CS, Grossman RG, et al (1984) The metabolic response to severe head injury. J Neurosurg 60:687-696
11. Dempsey DT, Guenter P, Mullen JL, et al (1985) Energy expenditure in acute trauma to the head with and without barbiturate therapy. Surg Gynecol Obstet 160:128-134
12. Robertson CS, Clifton GL, Goodman JF (1985) Steroid administration and nitrogen excretion in the head-injured patient. J Neurosurg 63:714-718
13. Young B, Ott L, Norton J, et al (1985) Metabolic and nutritional sequelae in the non-steroid treated head injury patient. Neurosurgery 17:784-790

14. Clifton GL, Robertson CS, Choi SC (1986) Assessment of nutritional requirements of head-injured patients. J Neurosurg 64:895–901
15. Fruin AH, Taylon C, Pettis MS (1986) Caloric requirements in patients with severe head injuries. Surg Neurol 25:25–28
16. Ott L, Young B, McClain C (1987) The metabolic response to brain injury. JPEN 11:488–493
17. Chiolero RL, Breitenstein E, Schutz Y, et al (1989) Effects of propranolol on resting metabolic rate after severe head injury. Crit Care Med (in press)
18. Clifton GL, Robertson CS, Kyper K, et al (1983) Cardiovascular response to severe head injury. J Neurosurg 59:447–454
19. Sanjak M, Paulson D, Sufit R, et al (1987) Physiologic and metabolic response to progressive and prolonged exercise in amyotrophic lateral sclerosis. Neurology 37:1217–1220
20. Hemmer M (1987) Non-neurological management of head injury. In: Vincent JL (ed) Update in intensive care and emergency medicine, vol 3. Springer, Berlin Heidelberg New York Tokyo, pp 402–406
21. Rapp RP, Young B, Twyman D, et al (1983) The favorable effects of early parenteral feeding on survival in head-injured patients. J Neurosurg 58:906–912
22. Sjöström L, Schutz Y, Gudinchet F, et al (1983) Epinephrine sensitivity with respect to metabolic rate and other variables in women. Am J Physiol 245 (8):E431–E442
23. Swinaher DL, Phang PT, Jones RL, et al (1988) Effect of routine administration of analgesia on energy expenditure in critically ill patients. Chest 92:4–10
24. Macintyre PE, Pavlin EG, Dwersteg JF (1987) Effect of meperidine on oxygen consumption, carbon dioxide production and respiratory gas exchange in postanesthesia shivering. Anesth Analg 66:751–755

Perspectives in Aneurysmal Subarachnoid Hemorrhage: Present and Future

D. Chyatte

Introduction: Early Strides

Intracranial aneurysms have been a source of human illness for centuries. Human remains excavated at Nubia dating back to the Byzantine period show pathological changes compelling us to believe that the people were affected by intracranial aneurysms. Despite this, surviving medical writings rarely describe patients who may have suffered a subarachnoid hemorrhage. It was not until the 18th century when Morgagni (1761) and Biumi (1778) first described cerebral aneurysms and showed that their rupture might lead to subarachnoid hemorrhage. Future evaluation of their observations did not occur until 1859 when Sir William Gull recognized the pathologic nature of aneurysms with his now famous statements, "Whenever young persons die with ingravescent apoplexy, and after death a large effusion of blood is found, especially if the effusion be over the surface of the brain, in the meshes of the pia mater, the presence of an aneurysm is probable." As refinements in clinical neurology were made in the 19th century, several autopsy series described giant intracranial aneurysms which presented during life because of mass effect. However, understanding the clinical syndrome of aneurysmal subarachnoid hemorrhage awaited Quincke's description of the technique for lumbar puncture in 1872.

By the early part of the 20th century, the clinical syndrome of subarachnoid hemorrhage was well recognized and it was possible to confirm the diagnosis using lumbar puncture. In the absence of a localizing neurological finding, however, the exact source of the subarachnoid hemorrhage could not be determined before death. In 1927, Egas Moniz introduced cerebral angiography. Refinement of this technology finally allowed clinicians not only to make the diagnosis of subarachnoid hemorrhage anti-mortem, but also localize its source. Despite these advances, surgical attitudes toward treatment of symptomatic intracranial aneurysms remained nihilistic. In 1923, Harvey Cushing described intracranial aneurysms as "... a lesion having such remote surgical bearing ... whether there are surgical indications such as ligation of the internal carotid artery only further experience can tell." Ayer commented in 1934 "Can surgery offer anything? The possibility of clipping off a small Berry aneurysm on one of the communicating branches might be considered, but would be a most formidable procedure and exceedingly dangerous, and the writer feels, quite impractical." Despite this, reports of deliberate efforts to directly repair intracranial aneurysms with surgery began to appear. In 1933, Dott reported a series of eight patients, all of whom had undergone angiography with the diagnosis of subarachnoid hemorrhage. He described the location of their aneurysms and reported his operative results. Later that decade, Dandy was the first to use a metallic clip to directly repair an intracranial aneurysm and thus, launched the modern era of aneurysm surgery. Since that time, an increased understanding of the pathophysiology of aneurysmal subarachnoid hemorrhage, refined surgical techniques, the use of the operating microscope, and advanced neuroanesthetic techniques have all worked together to improve the overall management outcome of patients who suffer an aneurysmal subarachnoid hemorrhage. Despite these improvements, it is estimated that with modern techniques, less than half of the patients who survive to hospital admission will have a favorable outcome [1].

Modern Management Results: Too Little, Too Late

Although the incidence of and death rate from thrombo-embolic stroke has been decreasing over the last three decades a similar decline in the incidence and mortality associated with aneurysmal subarachnoid hemorrhage has not occurred [2]. Intracranial aneurysms are found in approximately 5% of all autopsies performed on patients over the age of 10 years [3]. It is estimated that in the United States the incidence of non-traumatic subarachnoid hemorrhage from any cause is approximately 25 out of 100000 people. Intracranial aneurysms are the most common cause of spontaneous non-traumatic subarachnoid hemorrhage being responsible for approximately 11 out of 100000 people. Extrapolation of this data indicates that nearly 30000 Americans suffer an aneurysmal subarachnoid hemorrhage each year.

One third to one half of all patients who suffer an aneurysmal subarachnoid hemorrhage will not survive to hospital admission. Analysis of long term management result of the patients who reach medical attention show that despite modern surgical and medical treatment an unacceptably poor morbidity and

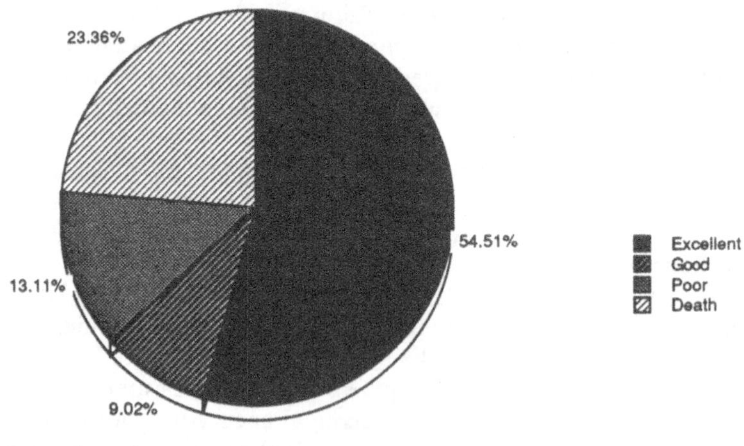

Fig. 1. Overall management results of aneurysmal SAH 1979–1985

mortality occurs [1, 4–17]. Figure 1 shows our recent overall management results for patients who survived to hospital admission. Overall 22% of all patients died. Half of these deaths occurred before surgery could be performed and the other half of these deaths occurred after surgery. Only 64% of all patients survived and had normal employment, normal mentation and little or no neurological deficit in follow up (excellent or good result). Long term outcome was closely linked to neurological function at the time of admission with "poor grade" patients fairing

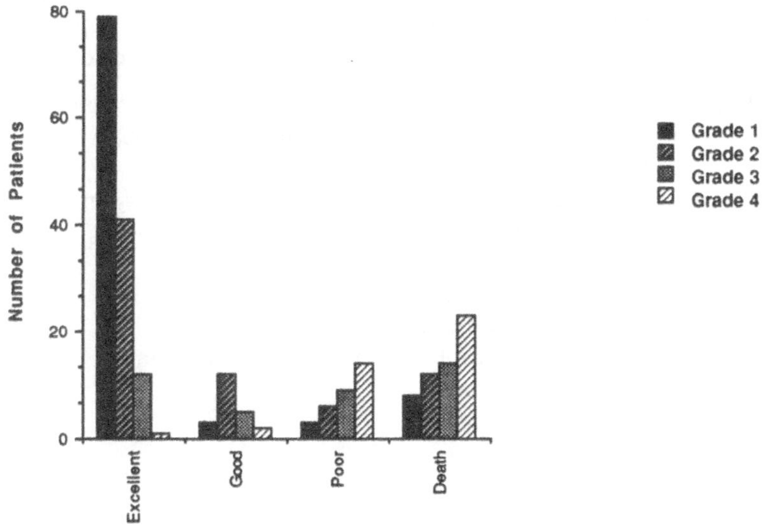

Fig. 2. Overall management results by admitting grade. "Good" grade patients do better than poor grade patients

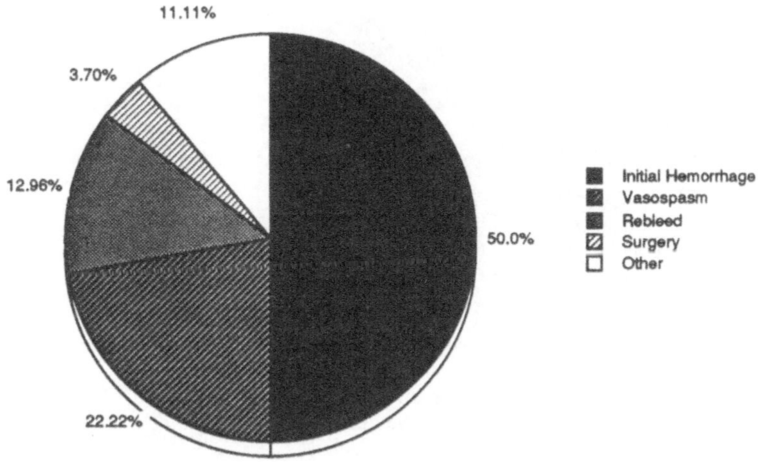

Fig. 3. The cause of death in all patients admitted with the diagnosis of aneurysmal SAH 1979–1985. Most mortality occurs as a direct result of the initial hemorrhage

substantially worse than "good grade" patients as shown in Fig. 2. Overall, the most common cause of mortality and morbidity were the direct effects of a severe initial hemorrhage as shown in Fig. 3. In those patients that survived to surgery delayed cerebral ischemia ascribed to "vasospasm" was the most common cause of mortality and morbidity as shown in Fig. 4. These results show that management morbidity and mortality occur *primarily* as a direct result of the initial hemorrhage. Although aneurysmal rebleeding and delayed cerebral ischemia ascribed to "vasospasm" are responsible for a poor outcome in some patients, their overall impact on management outcome is substantially less than the direct effect of the initial hemorrhage. It is clear, then, that if the dismal outcome following subarachnoid hemorrhage is to be improved in the future efforts and resources must be focused in the following directions:

1. Prevention of subarachnoid hemorrhage from intracranial aneurysm.
   - Diagnosis of asymptomatic intracranial aneurysms.
   - Natural history of asymptomatic aneurysms.
   - Risks and benefits of treating asymptomatic aneurysms.
2. Prevention and treatment of delayed cerebral ischemia.
   - Identification of patients at risk.
   - Diagnosis of delayed cerebral ischemia.
   - Prevention of delayed cerebral ischemia.
   - Treatment of established delayed cerebral ischemia.
   - Monitoring treatment.
3. Prevention of rebleeding.

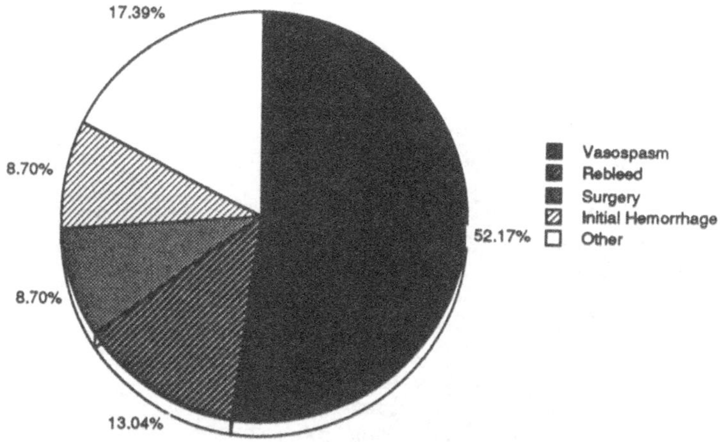

Fig. 4. Cause of death in patients surviving to surgery. Vasospasm is the leading cause of the death

Prevention of Aneurysmal Subarachnoid Hemorrhage

Because most morbidity and mortality occurs as a direct effect of a severe initial hemorrhage, prevention of aneurysmal subarachnoid hemorrhage would appear to be the best way to improve the overall management results. Successful application of this strategy requires the ability to identify people at risk for the development and rupture of cerebral aneurysms from the general population. Once identified, the risk of hemorrhage in these high risk patients should be eliminated by specific treatment or modification of risk factors. The treatment given or modification of risk factors should be less risky than the natural history of the disease alone.

At the present time no method exists to identify individuals at risk for developing and rupturing cerebral aneurysms. Most patients remain entirely asymptomatic until aneurysm rupture occurs. Occasionally a patient will present with a focal neurological deficit or seizure related to mass effect associate with the aneurysm and the correct diagnosis can be made before rupture. This, however, is an unusual situation and in the overwhelming majority of cases no clinical features can be used to identify individuals at high risk before hemorrhage has occurred. Similarly, although there are a few families whose members appear to be at high risk for subarachnoid hemorrhage, family history is not particularly useful in identifying high risk individuals.

Diagnostic testing, although able to identify high risk individuals is impractical for other reasons. At the present time there is no safe, reliable, quick screening test that can be applied to large segments of the population. Anatomical demonstration of intracranial aneurysms requires cerebral angiography. This procedure is associated with some risks (about a 1% risk of stroke), and is time consuming and costly. Magnetic Resonance Imaging (MRI), unlike Computerized Tomography has the potential to show cerebral blood vessels in fine detail. In brief, MRI works by transiently perturbing the resting energy levels of tissues by exposing them to electromagnetic radiation. As these tissues "relax" and return to their normal resting energy states energy is giving off. This emitted energy is used to construct images of the tissue. Blood, because it is flowing within the cerebral blood vessels, has already moved away from the area of interest before it "relaxes" and gives off its energy. Structures that contain flowing blood, such as cerebral vessels, aneurysms and arteriovenous malformations, appear as a signal void on the formatted image. In the near future it may be possible to routinely demonstrate cerebral aneurysms in exquisite detail using MRI. Despite these technological advances MRI is both costly and time consuming. Anatomical demonstration of intracranial aneurysms by both angiography and MRI, therefore will not be a practical way to screen large segments of the population for aneurysm disease.

The cause or causes of aneurysm formation and rupture remain unknown. Since no uniformly accepted hypothesis exists to explain the genesis and subsequent rupture of aneurysms, no clinical, physiological or biochemical methods exist to identify high risk asymptomatic individuals that may require further evaluation and possible treatment. Some recent work regarding the origin of cerebral aneurysms may eventually lead to a practical screening test and deserves mention. Typically, aneurysms arise at branch points where the elastic lamina fragments and the medial layer is the thinnest [18]. Histological examination of cerebral and somatic arteries points to a generalized abnormality in the arterial bed of some patients with ruptured saccular aneurysms [19, 20]. Specifically a 35% reduction in histologically apparent reticular fibers has been found in both cerebral and somatic arteries of aneurysm patients. Most authorities today suspect that inborn errors in the vessels wall, influenced by acquired abnormalities such as hypertension, artheriosclerosis, cigarette smoking, oral contraceptive use, and the relative lack of vessel wall support in the central nervous system are responsible for aneurysm production [18, 19, 21–39]. The fact that intracranial aneurysms:

1. are associated with genetically transmitted diseases (Type IV Ehlers-Danlos syndrome, Marfan's syndrome, pseudoxanthoma elasticum and polycystic kidney disease);
2. occur in identical twins; and
3. are reported in familial clusters [40]

led to the hypothesis that these errors in the vessel wall may be the result of a genetic abnormality.

Pope [41] was the first to provide direct chemical evidence suggesting that aneurysm patients may have an inborn error in the vessel wall. This work suggested that most patients with intracranial aneurysms have a relative deficiency of Type III collagen, the major type of collagen in cerebral blood vessels. Cell culture experiments suggested that this abnormality may be the result of a depressed synthesis in Type III collagen. Since Pope's original observations this work has been repeated a number of times [42–44] and all but one group have confirmed their original observations. Further analysis has shown that both cerebral arteries and somatic arteries taken from aneurysm patients show an increased extensibility at stresses corresponding to blood pressures of 100–200 mmHg when compared to arteries taken from control patients. Patients who exhibit these abnormal mechanical properties are also Type III collagen deficient. These works have led to the "collagen hypothesis". Type III collagen accounts for approximately 70% of the collagens in cerebral blood vessels [41]. A primary abnormality in Type III collagen synthesis directly interferes with the mechanical properties of the arterial wall in such a way as to promote aneurysm formation and rupture. Conversely, patients with Type III collagen abnormalities are at high risk for developing and rupturing cerebral aneurysms. Work to test this hypothesis is currently underway and may ultimately lead to a simple, safe, reliable and cheap screening test to identify patients at risk for aneurysmal subarachnoid hemorrhage (i.e. the molecular diagnosis of aneurysm disease).

Delayed Cerebral Ischemia: "Vasospasm"

Perspectives

Cerebral vasospasm after subarachnoid hemorrhage was originally described in 1951 by Ecker and Riemenschneider [45]. Initially the very existence of this phenomenon was disputed, but today it is recognized as the most important cause of morbidity in survivors of an acute subarachnoid hemorrhage. After more than 30 years of clinical and experimental research, its pathophysiological features, cause or causes, and treatment remain controversial. In part, this controversy has been due to confusion about what cerebral vasospasm actually is, and in part, it has been due to simplistic and poorly constructed studies.

Frequency of Occurrence and Related and Unrelated Clinical Features

Depending on the criteria used to define it, cerebral vasospasm has been reported to occur in 21 to 78% of all patients after a subarachnoid hemorrhage [12, 46–56] although most studies estimate its frequency of occurrence to be between 40 and 60%. In our experience 33% of patients develop delayed cerebral ischemia ascribed to vasospasm. In most instances the delayed ischemia is reversible with permanent ischemia occurring in only 13% of all patients. Most often angiographic vasospasm occurs in cerebral arteries near the source of the subarachnoid hemorrhage and tends to occur in the segments of cerebral arteries that are intimately related to the densest collections of subarachnoid blood [47, 57]. Distant focal or diffuse global vasospasm does occur but is considerably less common.

The frequency and severity of cerebral vasospasm increase with increasing volumes of subarachnoid blood, as judged by cranial computed tomography [58, 59]. Fisher et al. found that 23 of 24 patients with subarachnoid clots judged to be 5 by 3 mm or larger on initial computed tomographic scan subsequently had symptomatic chronic cerebral vasospasm in the corresponding arterial territories, whereas only 1 of 18 patients with no or diffusely distributed subarachnoid blood on initial computed tomographic scan subsequently had symptoms of vasospasm [59]. The presence of intraventricular or intraparenchymal blood did not correlate with the frequency of occurrence of vasospasm.

Similarly, the frequency and severity of vasospasm increase with worsening initial clinical grade [14, 47, 60] and plurality of bleeding episodes [61]. Vasospasm also appears to be more common in patients with severe meningeal signs than in those without such signs. Although several report have suggested that the frequency of vasospasm may vary with the location of the aneurysm, those sites identified as being associated with a high frequency of vasospasm differ from study to study. Other reports suggest that the frequency of vasospasm does not vary with anatomic position [14, 47, 57, 60–63]. In our experience the risk of developing symptomatic vasospasm does not vary with aneurysm location. The age and sex of the patient and the size of the aneurysm do not seem to be related to the frequency of vasospasm [47, 60, 61].

Temporal Profile

Experimental cerebral vasospasm after subarachnoid hemorrhage seems to be a biphasic event [64, 65]. In dogs, arterial narrowing begins immediately after subarachnoid hemorrhage and reaches maximal intensity by 30 min. Within 2 days, this early phase of vasospasm reverses spontaneously. Early spasm, however, has been difficult to substantiate in humans [66, 67]. Although this difficulty may reflect the transient nature of acute vasospasm, the fact that human cerebral arteries contract less strongly when challenged with blood than do vessels from other species suggest that acute vasospasm may be attenuated in humans [68].

Late or chronic vasospasm begins approximately 48 h after experimental subarachnoid hemorrhage and lasts from days to weeks. Unlike early vasospasm, chronic spasm clearly has a counterpart in humans and is the major cause of delayed neurological deterioration [6, 69]. The onset of chronic vasospasm in humans has been reported to occur anytime from the first day to several weeks after subarachnoid hemorrhage [47, 56, 57, 70], however it most commonly becomes apparent 5 to 7 days after a subarachnoid hemorrhage and rarely becomes symptomatic after 2 weeks. When symptoms occur, they usually develop insidiously over hours and are heralded by signs and symptoms of a generalized reduction in cerebral blood flow (such as drowsiness, stupor, and semicoma). Later, focal abnormalities (for example, speech dysfunction, monoparesis, monoplegia, and hemiplegia) may appear as a result of the localized reduction in blood flow in the distribution of affected arteries. Rarely, patients will have focal symptoms in the absence of generalized changes in consciousness.

The relationship of early vasospasm to late vasospasm is uncertain. Whether they share common mechanisms or whether the events occurring during early vasospasm lead to chronic vasospasm is unknown.

Hemodynamic Consequences

Differences in hemodynamic properties facilitate classification of cerebral arteries into at least two types: proximal large conducting vessels on the surface of the brain and distal small penetrating arterioles. In normal subjects, cerebral arterial resistance and, consequentially cerebral blood flow are primarily regulated at the level of the penetrating arterioles rather than by the conducting arteries. With modification of resistance in this arteriolar bed, cerebral blood flow is maintained at a relatively constant level over a wide range of systemic blood pressures through a process referred to as autoregulation. After a subarachnoid hemorrhage, as chronic cerebral vasospasm narrows the lumen of conducting arteries, the relative contribution that these vessels make to intracranial arterial resistance increases. When severely spastic, conducting vessels may be the major site of intracranial resistance that results in depressed cerebral blood flow. Because of this shift in the site of the major arterial resistance, the capacity for autoregulation is lost and cerebral blood flow varies greatly with systemic arterial pressure and intravascular volume [71].

Efforts to demonstrate the hemodynamic importance of cerebral vasospasm have not always been successful. This result is not surprising when one considers that multiple mechanisms may alter cerebral perfusion after a subarachnoid hemorrhage. Vasospasm, increased intracranial pressure, decreased mean arterial blood pressure, altered responsiveness of small cerebral resistance vessels, abnormal cerebral metabolism, intravascular dehydration, and altered blood viscosity [72–74] can all impede cerebral perfusion, whereas recruitment of collateral vascular channels, hypervolemia, and arterial hypertension may augment it. Thus, the hemodynamic importance of vasospasm will be a function of its severity and the summated influence of these modifying factors.

Fisher et al., in a study of 25 patients with subarachnoid hemorrhage, were able to correlate the site and temporal profile of vasospasm with the location and time of appearance of cerebral infarcts [75]. Other investigators have reported similar findings [76]. Kelly et al. studied 90 patients and concluded that cerebral infarction after subarachnoid hemorrhage is related to angiographic vasospasm in some cases but can occur even in its absence [77]. In a clinicopathologic study, Schneck and Kricheff found a poor correlation between vasospasm and cerebral infarction [50].

Global cerebral blood flow in humans is decreased after subarachnoid hemorrhage [78–80]. In addition, this decrease in global cerebral blood flow worsens with worsening clinical grade [78–80]. The cause of this global change is unknown and does not seem to be related to angiographic vasospasm [81]. Measurement of regional cerebral blood flows in the distribution of vasospastic arteries in humans has produced differing results. Although many authors have reported that the regional cerebral blood flow is depressed in the distribution of vasospastic arteries [79, 82, 83], others have found no correlation [84]. Interestingly, cerebral blood volume is elevated in regions supplied by severely spastic vessels, a finding that suggests that distal small penetrating arterioles may dilate and lose their capacity fo autoregulation in an effort to decrease intracranial arterial resistance [85]. Measurement of regional cerebral blood flows in experimentally induced early as well as late vasospasm has also produced divergent results [86–89].

Electroencephalographic abnormalities suggestive of focal cortical dysfunction routinely appear in the distribution of vasospastic arteries in humans after the occurrence of subarachnoid hemorrhage [90, 91]. Similarly, the findings on radionuclide cerebral perfusion scintigraphy suggest that at least severe spasm is associated with perfusion abnormalities in humans who have had a subarachnoid hemorrhage [92].

Vascular Pathological Features

Both vasospastic arteries taken from human subarachnoid hemorrhage victims and chronic experimental situations show histological and electron microscopic changes suggestive of a vasculopathy. Severe degenerative changes and necrosis of smooth muscle cells predominate and may persist for more than one year. Extracellular debris is abundant in all layers of the affected cerebral artery. In places, endothelial cells are elevated from the underlying internal elastic lamina or are frankly denuded. Leukocytes, mast cells, and erythrocytes are present in the arterial wall during the first few days of chronic vasospasm, and macrophages appear several weeks later [93].

Functional Abnormalities of Vasospastic Arteries

Despite the fact that numerous investigators have successfully prevented or treated experimental vasospasm with a wide variety of dilatation drugs, clinically the final result has been disappointing [94]. Lack of a reliable animal model of chronic vasospasm prompted many investigators to study acute in vitro or in vivo vasospasm; consequently, these observations were irrelevant to the human situation. With improvements, animal models were developed which showed the same refractory pharmacological changes to vasodilatory drugs seen in humans. In addition, the contractile responses of these arteries to cells surface receptor mediated agonists, those which directly depolarize the cell surface membrane, and those which act directly on the contractile proteins themselves is markedly depressed [95]. The fact that chronically spastic arteries are refractory to pharmacological dilatation or contraction and show myonecrotic changes on histological examination suggests that chronic cerebral vasospasm represents a structural derangement of the blood vessel wall which leads to its narrowing, rather than a sustained contraction of vascular smooth muscle.

Pathogenesis of Vasospasm

Although the mechanism responsible for these vascular changes remains unknown, circumstantial evidence is consistent with several possibilities:

Prolonged active contraction: A wide variety of amine, lipid, polypeptide and protein agents are known to cause active contraction of cerebral vessels [96]. After a subarachnoid hemorrhage, exposure of the cerebral vessels to many of these agonists may result in acute arterial narrowing. Evidence, however, linking these agents to the chronic phase of vasospasm is less clear.

Although chronic vasospasm has been produced by the intrathecal injection of some contractile agonists, efforts to reproduce these results by injection of doses simulating the concentrations present in the cerebral spinal fluid after subarachnoid hemorrhage have been unsuccessful [93]. Others have argued that, because contractile agonists may be trapped in subarachnoid clot, cerebral vessels may be exposed to higher concentrations of contractile agonists than those reflected in the cerebral spinal fluid [97]. Objective data addressing this issue are not currently available.

Depressed vessel respiration: Unlike systemic arteries, cerebral arteries lack vaso vasorum. Scanning electron micrographs have demonstrated adventitial openings or pores in cerebral vessels [98]. It has been postulated that these adventitial channels may act as nutritional or waste disposal pathways. After a subarachnoid hemorrhage, erythrocytes or other blood elements may block these channels and interfere with normal vessel respiration. Although hypoxia or hypoglycemia may be expected to produce rigor in a previously contracted vessel, inasmuch as relaxation and contraction are energy dependent processes, in vitro studies suggest that these conditions lead to vessel relaxation and decreased calcium uptake [99]. Whether prolonged interference with vessel respiration can lead to the structural and functional changes associated with chronic vasospasm is not known.

Inflammatory vasculopathy: An inflammatory response appears to occur in the subarachnoid space after a subarachnoid hemorrhage [100]. Linking this occurrence to the vascular changes associated with chronic vasospasm, however, is a novel concept. Neutrophils, which are present in the cerebral arterial wall several days after a subarachnoid hemorrhage, are capable of producing vascular damage when activated by C5a, a complement activation product. In addition, platelets, mediated through the prostaglandin metabolite thromboxane A_2, are also capable of damaging cerebral blood vessels. Aside from these possible cellular and thrombocytic mechanisms, the conversion of oxyhemoglobin to methemoglobin releases an activated form of oxygen which is capable of producing free radical reactions that result in the synthesis of various lipid peroxides. Hematin, a degradation product of hemoglobin, can catalyze the auto-oxidation of lipids, and similar products will be produced. Spinal fluid concentrations of these lipid peroxides appear to correlate with the occurrence of cerebral vasospasm in humans who have had a subarachnoid hemorrhage. Although these lipid peroxides may exert a toxic effect by directly acting on cerebral vessels, many of them resemble metabolic products of arachidonic acid formed after enzymatic oxidation by lipoxygenase and consequently may act by recruiting other inflammatory elements [101].

Both steroidal and nonsteroidal agents prevent or reduce angiographic vasospasm and improve neurological outcome in dogs after experimental subarachnoid hemorrhage. In addition, treatment with these drugs preserves the ultrastructural integrity of the vascular smooth muscle cells and their ability to respond to contractile agonists [95]. Preliminary experience with these drugs in human patients at high risk for vasospasm suggests that these drugs may improve overall management outcome [102].

Diagnosis and Treatment

The diagnosis of symptomatic vasospasm or delayed cerebral ischemia remains a clinical diagnosis of exclusion. In symptomatic patients, other causes of delayed neurological deterioration should be investigated and excluded. A computed tomographic scan can be used to investigate the possibility of hydrocephalus, increased intracranial pressure due to mass lesions and the presence of brain infarctions. An electroencephalogram can be used to investigate the possibility of seizures. Measurement of serum electrolytes and arterial blood gases eliminate fluid and electrolyte disturbances and abnormal respiration and ventilation as a cause for delayed neurological deterioration. If no other cause for delayed neurological deterioration is apparent and if the temporal profile is consistent, delayed cerebral ischemia from vasospasm is the most likely diagnosis. Transcranial Doppler examination can be used to estimate the blood flow velocities in the large conducting arteries at the base of the brain. Flow velocity should be distinguished from flow volume, the latter being the actual measurement of cerebral blood flow. Flow velocities tend to increase as vessel luminal narrowing occurs. Worsening neurological function associated with increasing flow velocity as measured by the transcranial Doppler is suggestive evidence of delayed cerebral ischemia due to vasospasm [103, 104]. Cerebral blood flow velocity can be affected by parameters other than vessel diameter and these factors should be kept in mind when interpreting transcranial Doppler results [105]. Direct measurement of regional cerebral blood flow can be made by a variety of methods. Although these studies provide different information than transcranial Doppler, application of these techniques tends to be more cumbersome and more difficult to apply at the bedside of an ill patient. At one time, angiography was commonly used to make the diagnosis of vasospasm. The risk of angiography in a patient with fluctuating cerebral ischemia is substantial and today angiography is used only in selected situations.

Treatment of symptomatic vasospasm today relies on efforts directed at enhancing cardiac output, inducing arterial hypertension, and expanding the intravascular volume in an attempt to increase cerebral perfusion and promote cerebral blood flow [93]. The specifics of the techniques used tend to vary from clinic to clinic. Major differences in the treatment protocols focus on the ideal hematocrit needed to optimize oxygen delivery but not hinder cerebral blood flow by increasing blood viscosity and on the issue of whether induced arterial hypertension is needed in addition to volume expansion. At our institution, initial treatment consists of expanding the intravascular volume by transfusing blood or appropriate fluids while monitoring the central venous pressure or pulmonary wedge pressure. Because hyponatremia and also hypovolemia frequently occur after subarachnoid hemorrhage, electrolyte balance must be meticulously maintained. If symptoms persist, hemodynamics are further augmented by the administration of ionotropes and pressors. Such treatment, although helpful in many instances, is not always effective and may be complicated by pulmonary edema or rebleeding from untreated aneurysms. Efforts to mechanically dilate vasospastic cerebral arteries using endovascular balloon angioplasy has recently met with some success, however, these techniques should still be considered experimental [106].

Recent efforts have been directed at preventing the occurrence of delayed cerebral ischemia due to vasospasm. Calcium channel blockers have been associated with improved management outcome following subarachnoid hemorrhage [107–109]. The mechanism of action of these class of drugs in lessening or improving delayed cerebral ischemia is not certain. They do not appear to act directly on the vasospastic large conducting arteries. Whether these agents act by dilating parenchymal arterioles and thereby promoting collateral circulation, improving red cell deformability, or improving neuronal and glial cell calcium homeostasis remains unclear. Regardless of their mechanism of action, these drugs appear to

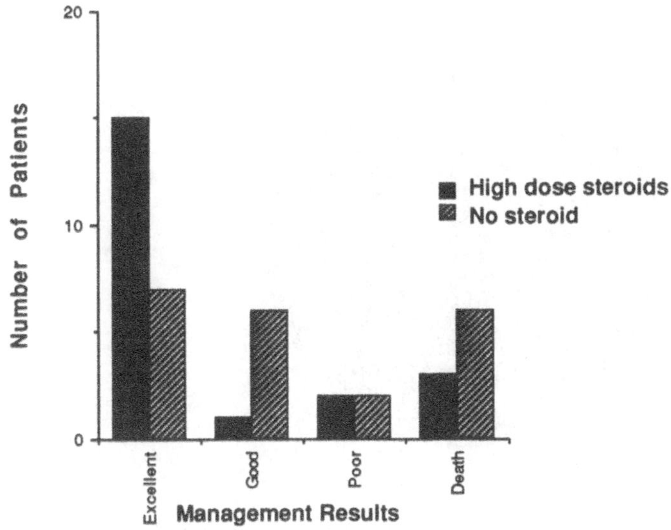

Fig. 5. Improved management results with high dose steroids in high risk patients

be useful in preventing or lessening delayed cerebral ischemia due to vasospasm. The rational for the use of anti-inflammatory agents has been discussed previously. They appear to be of some benefit, at least in peliminary human trials, as shown in Fig. 5. Further evaluation, however, is necessary before their safety and efficacy can be established [102]. Early surgery coupled with through irrigation of the subarachnoid space has been advocated as a method of decreasing delayed cerebral ischemia. Early surgery alone, at least in our hands, has not been associated with a decreased incidence of delayed cerebral ischemia. Complex efforts to irrigate the subarachnoid space and hopefully decrease the risk of delayed cerebral ischemia have been associated with some complications and therefore are not widely performed.

Prevention of Rebleeding

Rebleeding, although contributing to the poor outcome in some patients, has less of an impact on overall management results than does the direct effects of the initial hemorrhage and vasospasm. Nevertheless, rebleeding can dramatically alter the outcome in otherwise salvageable patients. For this reason, interest in early surgical repair of intracranial aneurysms has been renewed. With modern techniques, early aneurysm surgery is technically feasible. In the hands of skillful neurosurgical teams, the risk of direct surgical repair of ruptured cerebral aneurysms is quite small as shown in Fig. 6. Surgical misadventures today are largely limited to those patients who have large or giant aneurysms that require complex repair [6]. Endovascular balloon obliteration of intracranial aneurysms may be an alternative to open surgery in high risk patients [106]. Regardless of

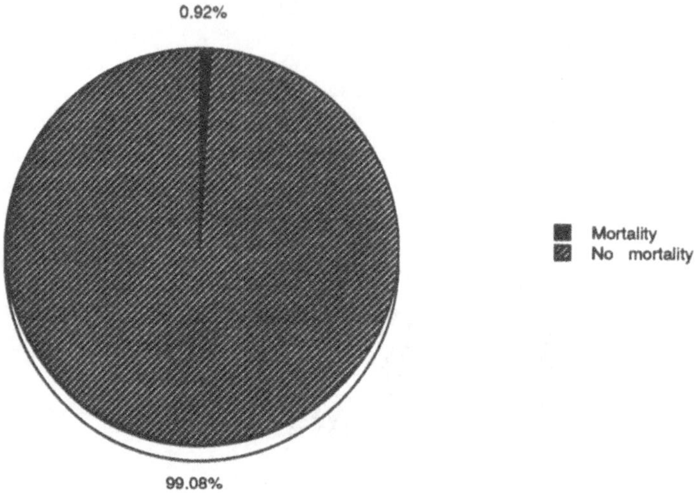

Fig. 6. The risk of intracranial surgery for aneurysmal SAH

the therapeutic strategy selected for aneurysmal obliteration differences in management outcomes will likely be small as most morbidity and mortality occurs as a direct result of the initial hemorrhage.

References

1. Kassel N, Adams H, Torner J, et al (1981) Influence of timing of admission after aneurysmal subarachnoid hemorrhage on overall outcome. Report of the Cooperative Aneurysm Study. Stroke 12:620–623
2. Goldstein M (1986) Cerebrovascular research: The opportunity has never been better. Stroke 17:1067–1068
3. Stehbens W (1963) Aneurysms and anatomical variation of cerebral arteries. Arch Path 75:45–64
4. Auer L (1984) Acute operation and preventive nimodipine improve outcome in patients with ruptured cerebral aneurysms. Neurosurg 15:57–66
5. Bolander H, Kourtopoulos H, West K (1984) Retrospective analysis of 162 consecutive cases of ruptured intracranial aneurysms. Acta Neurochir 70:31–41
6. Chyatte D, Fode N, Sundt T (1988) Early vs. late intracranial aneurysm surgery in subarachnoid hemorrhage. J Neurosurg 69:326–331
7. Hori S, Suzuki J (1979) Early intracranial operation for ruptured aneurysms. Acta Neurochir 46:93–104
8. Hunt W, Hess R (1968) Surgical risk as related to time of intervention in the repair of intracranial aneurysms. J Neurosurg 28:14–20
9. Ljunggren B, Brant L, Sundbarg G, et al (1982) Early management of aneurysmal subarachnoid hemorrhage. J Neurosurg 62:547–551
10. Ljunggren B, Saveland H, Brandt G, et al (1985) Early operation and overall outcome in aneurysmal subarachnoid hemorrhage. J Neurosurg 62:547–551
11. Ropper A, Zervas N (1984) Outcome 1 year after SAH from cerebral aneurysm. Management morbidity, mortality, and functional status in 112 consecutive good-risk patients. J Neurosurg 60:909–915

12. Sano K, Saito I (1978) Timing and indication of surgery for ruptured intracranial aneurysm with regard to cerebral vasospasm. Acta Neurochir 41:49-60
13. Sundt TJ, Whisnant J (1978) Subarachnoid hemorrhage from intracranial aneurysms. Surgical management and natural history of disease. N Engl J Med 299:116-122
14. Sundt TJ, Kobayashi S, Fode N, et al (1982) Results and complications of surgical management of 809 intracranial aneurysms in 722 cases. Related and unrelated to grade of patient, type of aneurysm, and timing of surgery. J Neurosurg 56:753-765
15. Suzuki J, Onuma T, Yoshimoto T (1979) Results of early operations of cerebral aneurysms. Surg Neurol 11:407-412
16. Weir B, Aronyk K (1981) Management mortality and the timing of surgery for supratentorial aneurysms. J Neurosurg 54:146-150
17. Whisnant J, Phillips LI, Sundt TJ (1982) Aneurysmal subarachnoid hemorrhage. Timing of surgery and mortality. Mayo Clin Proc 57:471-475
18. Glynn L (1940) Medical defects in the circle of Willis and their relation to aneurysm formation. J Path Bact 51:213-222
19. Ostergaard J, Reske-Nielsen E, Oxlund H (1987) Histological and morphometric observations on the reticular fibers in the arterial beds of patients with ruptured intracranial saccular aneurysms. Neurosurg 20:554-558
20. Hegedus K (1984) Some observations on reticular fibers in the media of the major cerebral arteries. Surg Neurol 22:301-307
21. Housepian E, Pool J (1958) A systematic analysis of intracranial aneurysms from the autopsy file of the Presbyterian Hospital, 1914 to 1956. J Neuropathol Exp Neurol 17:409-423
22. Sacco R et al (1984) Subarachnoid and intracerebral hemorrhage: Natural history, prognosis, and precursive factors in the Framingham study. Neurology 34:847-854
23. Sekhar L, Heros R (1980) Origin, growth and rupture of saccular aneurysms: A review. Neurosurg 8:248-260
24. Bremer J (1943) Congenital aneurysms of the cerebral arteries. Arch Pathol 35:819-831
25. Forbus W (1930) On the origin of miliary aneurysms of the superficial cerebral arteries. Bull Johns Hopkins Hosp 47:239-284
26. Eppinger H (1887) Pathogenesis (histogenesis and aetiology) der aneurysmen einschliesslich des aneurysmen equi verinosum. Arch Klin Chir 35(Suppl):1-563
27. McCormick W, Schmalstieg E (1977) The relation of arterial hypertension to intracranial aneurysms. Arch Neurol 34:285-287
28. Walker A, Allegre G (1954) The pathology and pathogenesis of cerebral aneurysms. J Neuropathol Exp Neurol 13:248-259
29. Stehbens W (1962) Hypertension and cerebral aneurysms. Med J Aust 2:8-10
30. Black B, Hicks S (1952) The relation of hypertension to arterial aneurysms of the brain. US Armed Forces Med J 3:1813-1818
31. Handa H, Hashimoto N, Nagata I, et al (1983) Saccular aneurysms in rats: A newly developed animal model of the disease. Stroke 14:857-886
32. Kwak R, Mizoi K, Katakura R, et al (1979) The correlation between hypertension in past history and the incidence of cerebral aneurysms. In: Suzuki J (ed) Cerebral aneurysms. Neuron, Tokyo, pp 20-24
33. Andrews R, Spiegel P (1979) Intracranial aneurysms: Age, sex, blood pressure, and multiplicity in an unselected series of patients. J Neurosurg 51:27-32
34. Ostergaard J, Hog E (1985) Incidence of multiple intracranial aneurysms. Influence of arterial hypertension. J Neurosurg 63:49-55
35. Bell B, Symon L (1979) Smoking and subarachnoid hemorrhage. Br Med J 1:577-578
36. Bell B, Ambrose J (1982) Smoking and the risk of stroke. Acta Neurochir (Wien) 64:1-7
37. Crawford T (1959) Some observations on the pathogenesis and natural history of intracranial aneurysms. J Neurol Neurosurg Psychiatry 22:259
38. Weibers D, Whisnant J, O'Fallon W (1981) The natural history of unruptured intracranial aneurysms. N Engl J Med 304:696-698
39. Keller A (1970) Hypertension, age and residence in the survival with subarachnoid hemorrhage. Am J Epidemiol 91
40. Fox J (1983) Intracranial aneurysms. Springer, Berlin Heidelberg New York Tokyo

41. Pope F et al (1981) Some patients with cerebral aneurysms are deficient in type III collagen. Lancet 1:690–696
42. Leblanc R, Lozano A: Absence of collagen deficiency in familial cerebral aneurysms. J Neurosurg (in press)
43. Neil-Dwyer G, Bartlett J, Nicholls A, Narcisi P, Pope F (1983) Collagen deficiency and ruptured cerebral aneurysms. A clinical and biochemical study. J Neurosurg 59:16–20
44. Ostergaard J, Oxlund H (1987) Collagen type III deficiency in patients with rupture of intracranial saccular aneurysms. J Neurosurg 67:690–696
45. Ecker A, Riemenschneider P (1951) Arteriographic demonstration of spasm of the intracranial arteries: with special reference to saccular arterial aneurysms. J Neurosurg 8:660–667
46. Weir B (1980) The incidence and onset of vasospasm after subarachnoid hemorrhage from ruptured aneurysm. In: Wilkins R (ed) Cerebral arterial spasm. Williams and Wilkins, Baltimore, pp 302–305
47. Saito I, Sano K (1980) Vasospasm after aneurysm rupture: incidence, onset, and course. In: Wilkins R (ed) Cerebral arterial spasm. Williams and Wilkins, Baltimore, pp 294–301
48. DuBoulay G (1963) Distribution of spasm in the intracranial arteries after subarachnoid hemorrhage. Acta Radiol (Diagn) (Stockh) 1:257–266
49. Fletcher T, Taveras J, Pool J (1959) Cerebral vasospasm in angiography for intracranial aneurysms: incidence and significance in one hundred consecutive angiograms. Arch Neurol 1:38–47
50. Schneck S, Kricheff I (1964) Intracranial aneurysm rupture, vasospasm, and infarction. Arch Neurol 11:668–680
51. Allcock JM, Drake C (1965) Ruptured intracranial aneurysms – the role of arterial spasm. J Neurosurg 22:21–29
52. Wilkins R, Alexander J, Odom G (1968) Intracranial arterial spasm: a clinical analysis. J Neurosurg 29:121–134
53. Ohta T, Kawamura J, Osaka K, Kajikawa H, Handa H (1969) Angiographic classification of so-called cerebral vasospasm – correlation between existence of vasospasm and postoperative prognosis in subarachnoid hemorrhage. No To Shinkei 21:1019–1027
54. Heilbrun M (1973) The relationship of neurological status and the angiographic evidence of spasm to prognosis in patients with ruptured intracranial aneurysms. Stroke 4:673–679
55. Milikan C (1975) Cerebral vasospasm and ruptured intracranial aneurysm. Arch Neurol 32:433–449
56. Kwak R, Niizuma H, Ohi T, Suzuki J (1979) Angiographic study of cerebral vasospasm following rupture of intracranial aneurysms. Surg Neurol 11:257–262
57. Kim H, Mizukami M, Kawase T, Takemae T, Araki G (1979) Time course of vasospasm – its clinical significance. Neurol Med Chir (Tokyo) 19:95–102
58. Mizukami M, Takazawa T, Tazawa T, Kawase T, Matsuzaki T (1980) Value of computed tomography in the prediction of cerebral vasospasm after aneurysm rupture. Neurosurg 7:583–585
59. Fisher C, Kistler J, Davis J (1980) Relation of cerebral vasospasm to subarachnoid hemorrhage visualized by computerized tomographic scanning. Neurosurg 6:1–8
60. Saito I, Sano K (1979) Vasospasm following rupture of cerebral aneurysms. Neurol Med Chir (Tokyo) 19:103–107
61. Graf C, Nibbelink D (1974) Cooperative study of intracranial aneurysms and subarachnoid hemorrhage: report on a randomized treatment study. III. Intracranial surgery. Stroke 5:559–601
62. Post K, Flamm E, Goodgold A, Ransohoff J (1977) Ruptured intracranial aneurysms: case morbidity and mortality. J Neurosurg 46:290–295
63. Niizuma H et al (1978) Angiographical study of cerebral vasospasm following rupture of intracranial aneurysm (2nd report). Relation between the site of aneurysm and the occurrence of the vasospasm. No Shinkei Geka 6:863–869
64. Kuwayama A, Zervas N, Belson R, Shintani A, Pickren K (1972) A model for experimental cerebral arterial spasm. Stroke 3:49–56
65. Brawley B, Strandness D, Kelly W (1968) The biphasic response of cerebral vasospasm in experimental subarachnoid hemorrhage. J Neurosurg 28:1–8

66. Wilkins R (1976) Aneurysm rupture during angiography: does acute vasospasm occur? Surg Neurol 5:299–303
67. Odom G (1974) Cerebral vasospasm. Clin Neurosurg 22:29–58
68. Wellum G, Irvine TJ, Zervas N (1980) Dose response of cerebral arteries of the dog, rabbit and man to human hemoglobin in vitro. J Neurosurg 53:486–490
69. Peerless S (1979) Pre- and postoperative management of cerebral aneurysms. Clin Neurosurg 26:209–231
70. Weir B, Grace M, Hansen J, Rothberg C (1978) Time course of vasospasm in man. J Neurosurg 48:173–178
71. Davis D, Sundt TJ (1980) Relationship of cerebral blood flow to cardiac output, mean arterial pressure, blood volume, and alpha and beta blockade in cats. J Neurosurg 52:745–754
72. Watanabe H, Hasegawa T, Ishii S (1980) Studies on intravascular factors of cerebral ischemia in vasospasm after rupture of cerebral aneurysm. In: Wilkins R (ed) Cerebral arterial spasm. Williams and Wilkins, Baltimore, pp 378–384
73. Wood J, Snyder L, Simeone F, Golden M, Fink EA (1981) Cerebrovascular and cardiac responses to intravascular volume expansion following focal cerebral ischemia (abstract). Stroke 12:130
74. Wood J, Simeone F, Kron R, Snyder L, Litt M (1981) Relationship of cortical blood flow and cardiovascular responses to alteration in fresh blood viscosity as determined by capillary step-response viscometry. J Cereb Blood Blow Metab 1(Suppl 1):233–234
75. Fisher C, Roberson G, Ojemann R (1977) Cerebral vasospasm with ruptured saccular aneurysm-the clinical manifestations. Neurosurg 1:245–248
76. Kodama N, Mizoi K, Sakurai Y, Suzuki J (1980) Incidence and onset of vasospasm. In: Wilkins R (eds) Cerebral arterial spasm. Williams and Wilkins, Baltimore, pp 361–365
77. Kelly P, Gorten R, Rose J, Grossman R (1980) Cerebral infarction and ruptured intracranial aneurysms. In: Wilkins R (ed) Cerebral arterial spasm. Williams and Wilkins, Baltimore, pp 366–371
78. Kagstrom E, Greitz T, Hanson J, Galera R (1966) Changes in cerebral blood flow after subarachnoid hemorrhage. Excerpta Medica International Congress Series 110:629–633
79. James I (1968) Changes in cerebral blood flow and systemic arterial pressure following spontaneous subarachnoid hemorrhage. Clin Sci 35:11–22
80. Heilbrun M, Olesen J, Lassen N (1972) Regional cerebral blood flow studies in subarachnoid hemorrhage. J Neurosurg 37:36–44
81. Grubb R, Raichle M, Eichling J, Gado M (1977) Effects of subarachnoid hemorrhage on cerebral blood volume, blood flow, and oxygen utilization in humans. J Neurosurg 46:446–453
82. Heilbrun M, Olesen J, Lassen N (1980) Regional cerebral blood flow studies in subarachnoid hemorrhage. In: Wilkins R (ed) Cerebral arterial spasm. Williams and Wilkins, Baltimore, pp 314–319
83. Symon L et al (1972) The use of the xenon clearance method in subarachnoid hemorrhage: post operative studies with clinical and angiographic correlation. Eur Neurol 8:8–14
84. Zingesser L, Schechter M, Dexter J, Katzman R, Scheinberg L (1968) On the significance of spasm associated with rupture of a cerebral aneurysm: the relationship between spasm as noted angiographically and regional blood flow determinations. Arch Neurol 18:520–528
85. Pitts L et al (1980) Effects of vasospasm on cerebral blood flow after subarachnoid hemorrhage. In: Wilkins R (ed) Cerebral arterial spasm. Williams and Wilkins, Baltimore, pp 333–337
86. Simone F, Trepper P, Brown D (1972) Cerebral blood flow evaluation of prolonged experimental vasospasm. J Neurosurg 37:302–311
87. Petruk K, Weir B, Marriott M, Overton T (1973) Clinical grade, regional cerebral blood flow and angiographic vasospasm in the monkey after subarachnoid and subdural hemorrhage. Stroke 4:431–445
88. Hashi K, Meyer J, Shinmaru S, Welch K (1972) Hemodynamic and metabolic changes in experimental subarachnoid hemorrhage in monkeys. Eur Neurol 8:32–37

89. Yamaguchi T, Waltz A (1971) Effects of subarachnoid hemorrhage from puncture of the middle cerebral artery on blood flow and vasculature of the cerebral cortex in cats. J Neurosurg 35:664–671
90. Parkes J, James I (1971) Electroencephalographic and cerebral blood flow changes following spontaneous subarachnoid hemorrhage. Brain 94:69–76
91. Rumpl E, Bauer G, Gertenbrand F, Stampfel G (1980) Focal electroencephalographic changes associated with vasospasm after subarachnoid hemorrhage. In: Wilkins R (ed) Cerebral arterial spasm. Williams and Wilkins, Baltimore, pp 356–360
92. Kelly P, Gorten R, Grossman R, Eisenberg H (1977) Cerebral perfusion, vascular spasm, and outcome in patients with ruptured intracranial aneurysms. J Neurosurg 47:44–49
93. Chyatte D, Sundt TJ (1983) Cerebral vasospasm after subarachnoid hemorrhage. Mayo Clin Proc 59:498–505
94. Wilkins R (1980) Attempted prevention or treatment of intracranial arterial spasm: a survey. In: Wilkins R (ed) Cerebral arterial spasm. Williams and Wilkins, Baltimore, pp 542–555
95. Chyatte D, Rusch N, Sundt TJ (1983) Prevention of chronic experimental cerebral vasospasm using ibuprofen and high dose methylprednisolone. J Neurosurg 59:925–932
96. White R (1980) Overview of the pharmacology of vasospasm. In: Wilkins R (ed) Cerebral arterial spasm. Williams and Wilkins, Baltimore, pp 229–236
97. Ohta T et al (1980) Cerebral vasospasm and hemoglobins: clinical and experimental studies. In: Wilkins R (ed) Cerebral arterial spasm. Williams and Wilkins, Baltimore, pp 166–172
98. Zervas N, Liszcak T, Mayberg M (1982) Cerebral spinal fluid may nourish cerebral vessels through pathways in the adventitia that may be analogous to systemic vaso vasorum. J Neurosurg 56:475–481
99. Simone F, Vinall P (1980) Effect of oxygen and glucose deprivation on vasoactivity and calcium movement in isolated middle cerebral arteries. In: Wilkins R (ed) Cerebral arterial spasm. Williams and Wilkins, Baltimore, pp 223–228
100. Hammes EJ (1944) Reaction of the meninges to blood. Arch Neurol Psychiatry 52:505–514
101. Chyatte D, Sundt T (1988) Cerebral vasospasm: evidence supporting an inflammatory etiology. In: Wilkins R (ed) Cerebral vasospasm. Raven Press, New York, pp 357–365
102. Chyatte D, Fode N, Nichols D, Sundt T (1987) Preliminary report: effects of high dose methylprednisolone on delayed cerebral ischemia in patients at high risk for vasospasm after aneurysmal subarachnoid hemorrhage. Neurosurg 21:157–160
103. Sekhar L, Weschler L, Yonas H, Luyckx K, Obrist W (1988) Value of transcranial Doppler examination in the diagnosis of cerebral vasospasm after subarachnoid hemorrhage. Neurosurg 22:813–821
104. Compton J, Redmond S, Symon L (1987) Cerebral blood velocity in subarachnoid hemorrhage: a transcranial Doppler study. J Neurol Neurosurg Psychiatry 50:1499–1503
105. Brass L, Pavlakis S, De Vivo D, Piomelli S, Mohr J (1988) Transcranial Doppler measurements of the middle cerebral artery. Effect of hematocrit. Stroke 19:1466–1469
106. Heishima G et al (1986) Balloon embolization of a large distal basilar artery aneurysm. J Neurosurg 65:413–416
107. Flamm E, Adams H, Beck D et al (1988) Dose-escalation study of intravenous nicardipine in patients with aneurysmal subarachnoid hemorrhage. J Neurosurg 68:393–400
108. Ohman J, Heiskanen O (1988) Effect of nimodipine on the outcome of patients after aneurysmal subarachnoid hemorrhage and surgery. J Neurosurg 69:683–688
109. Petruk P, West M, Mohr G (1988) Nimodipine treatment in poor-grade aneurysm patients. J Neurosurg 68:505–517

Influence of Mechanical Ventilation on Brain Circulation and Function

D. M. Payen and C. Lamer

Introduction

Whatever the technique used for ventilatory support, positive pressure breathing (PPB) elevates intrathoracic pressure. Local circulations can be altered by different mechanisms acting all together or separately [1]. These mechanisms consist in:

1. a reduction in systemic arterial pressure (SAP);
2. an impairment of local venous return and an increase in venous pressure;
3. an intrinsic or extrinsic modification of local vasoactive status.

The final result differs according to the physiological properties of the considered local circulation. Before analyzing the consequences of an increase of intrathoracic pressure on brain circulation and function, two concepts should be remembered. The first one concerns the autoregulation of cerebral blood flow (CBF). For many years, it has been generally accepted that CBF remains constant when cerebral perfusion pressure (CPP) changes between low and high pressure limits. Beyond these limits CBF varies linearly with CPP. The CBF plateau corresponds to vasoactive modifications parallel to CPP variations.

The second concept is known as the "waterfall" phenomenon. This concept concerns circulations in which the pressure surrounding the vessels cannot be neglected and may actually collapse the vessels. In this case, flow becomes dependent on the level of this external pressure referred to local venous pressure. The waterfall mechanism was first demonstrated in the pulmonary circulation and was thereafter confirmed in other circulations especially for venous brain drainage.

To understand the effects of an elevation of intrathoracic pressure on brain circulation it should be mentioned that CBF has been shown to vary differently from cerebral venous return measured in jugular vein. Consequently venous drainage of the brain appears to be the most important determinant of the effect of positive pressure breathing on CBF and function.

Anatomical and Physiological Aspects of Brain Venous Drainage

The anatomy and physiology of venous drainage of the brain, especially in humans, are not yet well described and understood. This system basically includes

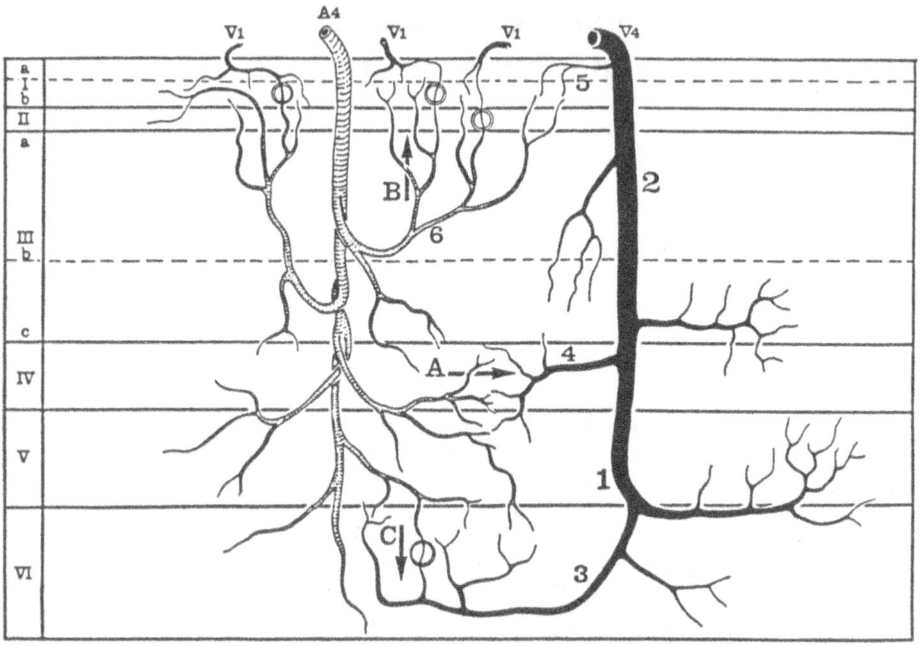

Fig. 1. Morphological features of typical intracortical artery and deep cortical veins (group 4: A4 and V4). On the left the scale represents the disposition of cortical cellular layers. Circles correspond to possible precapillary arterio-venous anastomoses. A: middle intracortical blood pathway; B: superficial intracortical blood pathway collected by intracortical veins; C: deep intracortical blood pathway collected by deep branches of large cortical veins. (From [1])

the parenchymal cerebral veins drained by deep cerebral veins, and the venous sinuses [2].

Parenchymal veins: Superficial cortical veins or pial veins form a dense network covered by arterial ramifications. Blood seems to flow freely into these veins and could only be impaired by compression resulting from arterial hypertension. Although still debated, the existence of venous anastomoses seems likely, even if these anastomoses vary in size and number. Conversely, at this level there is no arterio-venous anastomosis.

Intracortical or deep veins are divided in five groups according to their degrees of cortical penetration. The deeper veins (group 5) are remarkable by their important diameter and their large drainage territory. They seem to be disposed in a regular fashion and form cortical vascular units in association with the arteries which surround them.

Ultrastructure of the veins [2]: According to the size and the localization of the vein, ultrastructure differs between post capillary venules and collecting venules. The structure of endothelium does not differ in either type of venule and is similar to that of capillaries. Cells surrounding venous endothelium are not smooth muscle cells and are called periendothelial cells. These cells are in close contact with nervous tissue. In collecting veins, periendothelial cells are not yet smooth muscle cells even if they show some ramifications. Conversely venous containing smooth muscle are found cells in relation with unmyelinated fibers.

In summary, if parenchymal venules seem to be distended passively by the contained blood volume, the collecting veins might be influenced by sympathetic stimulation modifying the capacitance and hydraulic hydrance.

Venous brain drainage: Brain is drained by two series of veins:

1. the deep or great cerebral vein (Galenic) system which functions as a single unit system and receives tributaries from the entire brain in a neurovascular pattern similar to that provided by the arteries;
2. the second system drains blood from suprasegmental cerebral or cerebellar cortices into the overlying venous sinuses. Moreover, extensive collaterals exist between the veins of these two systems.

The pattern of blood flow in the dural sinuses in equally variable. This leads to the suggestion that sampling blood from the internal jugular vein could produce erroneous conclusions concerning the area of brain drained. It is clear that venous blood can leave the skull by a number of routes other than the internal jugular veins. However for human investigators, the most serious difficulty to measure cerebral venous drainage arise from anastomoses outside the skull between jugular and vertebral venous systems. The size of vertebral veins varies considerably and precise knowledge of the proportion of intracerebral blood drained into vertebral veins in unavailable.

Cerebral Hemodynamic Effects of Positive Pressure Breathing

Due to the unique location of the brain within the rigid skull, the effects of elevated cerebral venous pressure (CVP) or intracranial pressure (ICP) must be considered. However the relationship between CVP and ICP and the precise way in which these two pressures interact to modify CBF are relatively poorly understood.

Evidence for a Starling Resistor Regulating Cerebral Venous Outflow

Luce et al. demonstrated in dogs the presence of a Starling resistor between the sagittal sinus and the cerebral veins which regulates cerebral venous outflow when pressure in the sagittal sinus (Pss) is increased [3]. The waterfall mechanism maintained CVP and ICP at normal levels when Pss was reduced. Even if this study had some limitations (including the absence of CBF and $PaCO_2$ measurements, a lack of arterial pressure and cardiac output control), it seems clear that although ICP and CVP varied with Pss, these changes were somewhat limited. Figure 2 represents a schematic illustration of the intra-cranial space during modifications of ICP. The waterfall concept can be summarized as follows. The

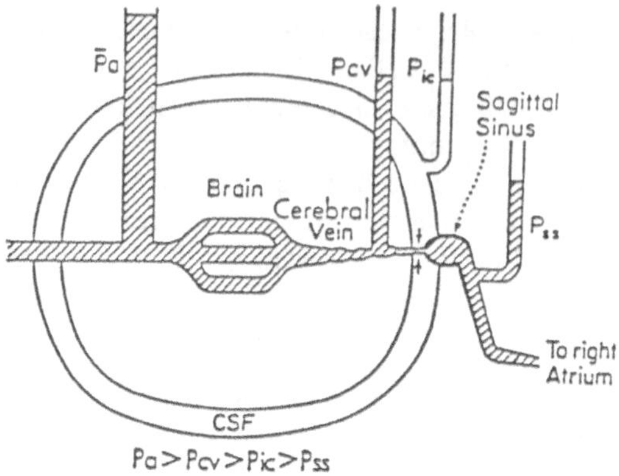

Fig. 2. Schematic representation of the waterfall between cerebral vein and sagittal sinus (arrow). Pa = systemic arterial pressure; Pic = intracranial pressure superior than sagittal pressure (Pss). For explanation see the text. (From [2])

ICP represents the effective outflow pressure from the brain when ICP exceeds Pss, because in this circumstance ICP reflects CVP more closely than does Pss. When intrathoracic pressure increases, Pss increases to an extent related to the duration of increase of intrathoracic pressure. A transient increase as produced by a cough, only slightly modifies Pss in comparison with PPB during which Pss elevation is more pronounced, especially with the introduction of PEEP [3]. In the latter case, the increase in Pss impairs cerebral venous return and increases ICP, preserving the pressure gradient between ICP and Pss and thus maintaining venous return. Because ICP increases, CVP rises above ICP and the gradient for cerebral venous outflow is maintained. Cerebral perfusion pressure then becomes the major determinant for CBF because SAP can be maintained or decreased during PEEP.

When intracranial hypertension exists, the gradient between ICP and Pss is large and an increase in Pss secondary to an increase in intrathoracic pressure causes only a relatively small increase in ICP and then a small decrease in CPP and CBF. However, this situation could be deleterious if SAP is concomitantly reduced, especially during ventilation with PEEP, leading to a reduction in CBF.

On the other hand, when right atrial pressure decreases as it might occur in hypovolemia, the decrease in Pss is only small. This limitation in reduction of Pss relative to the fall in right atrial pressure may also be due to a waterfall effect in the external jugular vein. This hypothesis explains the maintenance of cerebral venous outflow when a person sits up.

Relationship Between Cerebral Venous Pressure and CBF

The impact of increases in Pss on cerebral venous outflow and regional and global CBF has been recently demonstrated in anesthetized dogs using microspheres [4]. As shown in Fig. 3, when Pss was elevated to approximately 16 mmHg, cerebral venous outflow decreased to 40% of control while total and regional cerebral blood flow remained unchanged; this global and regional re-

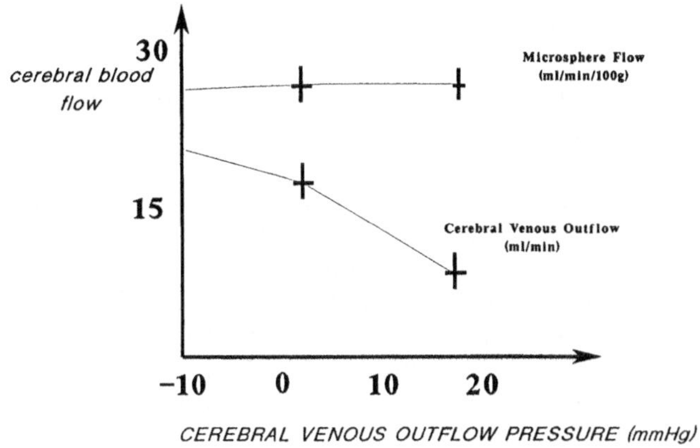

Fig. 3. Evolution of cerebral blood flow and venous outflow during venous pressure elevation. (From [3])

sistance decreased. Moreover this study demonstrated that the decrease in cerebral venous outflow during Pss elevation was not due to a concomitant increase in ICP, since the same results were observed when ICP was maintained constant. The maintenance of CBF in the presence of a fall in CPP was interpreted as a manifestation of autoregulation. The relative discrepancy between the maintenance in CBF and the reduction in cerebral vein blood flow suggests that cerebral venous blood drainage is diverted to other sites away from the measured venous blood flow. The same group of investigators have also shown that an independant increase in ICP has no effect on cerebral venous outflow until the ICP is increased to levels higher than those measured (16 mmHg). Only when ICP is so increased that CPP falls below the lower limit of cerebral autoregulation, does CBF fall.

Thus, the effects of an increase in CVP on CBF is a direct consequence of venous pressure elevation to a level resulting in a CPP below the lower limit of CBF autoregulation. Above this limit, CBF remains unchanged whereas cerebral venous outflow may decrease. In this case, it appears that elevation in cerebral venous pressure diverts venous drainage from the confluence to other intracranial veins that can drain into the cavernous sinus. While autoregulation of CBF seems to be important for the adaptation to an increase in CVP, it is interesting to study the mechanism by which blood flow is maintained despite a rise in CVP. Recently, this question was answered in a cat model in which a stable increase in venous pressure consistently induced arteriolar vasodilation, which occurred when arterial pressure was normal [5]. It also occurred irrespective of whether ICP was kept constant or was allowed to increase during venous hypertension.

In addition to changes in the CVP, positive pressure ventilation may also result in a fall in cardiac output and arterial blood pressure and the relative role of these factors in the relationship between mechanical ventilation and CBF is debated. Doblar et al. have attempted to define these relative roles using a goat model [6]. They measured CBF and ICP during PPB (PEEP of 5, 10 and 15 cmH_2O) in three groups of animals: Group I: with no fluid administration; Group II: normal saline fluid infusion to maintain blood pressure, and Group

III: mannitol 20% solution. In Group I, SAP decreased by about 30%, whereas ICP increased by about 40%, with a fall in CBF of 22%. In Group II, SAP was maintained with an increase in ICP of about 84% and a decrease in CBF of around 32%. In Group III, SAP was also maintained, but ICP increased only by about 14% and CBF did not change. It should be noted that right atrial pressure increased to a similar extent in both situations, demonstrating the absence of direct transmission of venous pressure. This study showed differences between the saline-infused group compared with the mannitol-infused group, suggesting that another mechanism than venous pressure elevation accounted for the increase in ICP during PEEP. This mechanism may be related to an increase in brain interstitial fluid pressure resulting from the extravasation of a fraction of the fluid given for volume expansion, which is reduced if this fluid is hyperosmotic.

Nevertheless, the role of increases in venous pressure during ventilation with PEEP had been stressed in many other studies. Using a dog model, Luce et al. have investigated the possible mechanisms by which PEEP might increase cerebrospinal fluid pressure [7]. They concluded that PEEP increases ICP primarily by increasing superior vena cava pressure and decreasing cerebral venous outflow. This effect was augmented if cerebral arterial inflow was increased as well.

Positive Pressure and Cerebral Function

Despite the crucial importance of this question for patients suffering from severe head injury or intracranial mass lesion, clinical data are relatively scarce. This is related primarily to the extreme difficulty to assess brain function, expecially in patients with other neurological disease. From the previous discussion, two types of responses to PEEP could be expected: ICP can increase more or less than the amount of PEEP applied. If ICP increases greatly, PEEP could impair neurological function. However, it is not easy to determine in which patients this detrimental response might occur. Apuzzo et al. [8] found that 10 cmH_2O PEEP increased ICP only in 12 out of 25 patients studied after a severe head injury. These 12 patients manifested a reduction in cerebral compliance. A small variation of cerebral blood volume led to a large increase in ICP. Among these patients with a reduction in compliance, only 50% had a decrease in cerebral perfusion pressure below the lower limit of autoregulation. Although CBF was not measured, it may have been impaired by the PEEP with the possible generation of cerebral ischemia. This study strongly suggests that accurate monitoring of ICP is required especially in patients with reduced cerebral compliance, if PEEP should be applied.

Conclusion

From the previous analysis it can be concluded that PEEP or PPB impaired cerebral venous return by an elevation in right atrial pressure, which is dependent on lung compliance. This venous drainage impairment induces an increase in ICP which is influenced by the presence of a waterfall phenomenon between cerebral veins and sinuses. Thus, an increase in ICP at the same level of PEEP will be more pronounced proportionally when ICP is normal than it is high. Because PEEP will be more pronounced proportionally when ICP is normal than it is high. Because PEEP frequently alters SAP, CPP can be reduced to a such level than it exceeds the lower limit of CBF autoregulation leading to a decrease in CBF. Moreover, the maintenance of SAP may worsen ICP increase during PEEP at least by two mechanisms:

1. an increase in cerebral blood volume which shifts the cerebral compliance to a steeper part;
2. a possible extravasation of fluid increasing interstitial edema and shifting also the brain compliance curve.

References

1. Payen DM, Beloucif S (1987) Circulatory effects of mechanical ventilation. In: Vincent JL, Suter PM (eds) Update in intensive care and emergency medicine, vol 2. Springer, Berlin Heidelberg New York Tokyo, pp 135–145
2. Auer LM, Loew F (eds) (1983) The cerebral veins. An experimental and clinical update. Springer, Berlin Heidelberg New York Tokyo, pp 3–38
3. Luce JM, Huseby JS, Kirk W, Butler J (1982) A Starling resistor regulates cerebral venous outflow in dogs. J Appl Physiol 53:1496–1503
4. Wagner EM, Traystman RJ (1983) Cerebral venous outflow and arterial microsphere flow with elevated venous pressure. Am J Physiol 244:H505–H512
5. Wei EP, Kontos HA (1982) Responses of cerebral arterioles to increased venous pressure. Am J Physiol 243:H442–H447
6. Doblar DD, Santiage TV, Kahn AU, Edelman NH (1981) The effect of positive end-expiratory pressure ventilation (PEEP) on cerebral blood flow and cerebrospinal fluid pressure in goats. Anesthesiology 55:244–250
7. Luce JM, Huseby JS, Kirk W, Butler J (1982) Mechanism by which end-expiratory pressure increases cerebrospinal fluid pressure in dogs. J Appl Physiol 52:231–235
8. Apuzzo MLJ, Weiss MN, Petersons V, Small RB, Kurze T, Heiden JS (1977) Effect of positive end-expiratory pressure ventilation on intracranial pressure in man. J Neurosurg 46:227–232

Cerebral Blood Flow in Head Injury

K. Gunning and A. Forster

Introduction

For the past 10 years it has been possible to measure cerebral blood flow (CBF) at the bedside in head-injured patients. Many clinical studies have been performed which have improved our understanding of the pathophysiological processes that occur after a severe head injury. These studies are complex and summarized in Table 1. Care must be taken when comparing results from different centers, as head injured patients do not form a homogeneous group with regard to age, mechanism and severity of injury. Differences in technique or in timing of CBF measurement after the acute event must be taken into account as well as the effects of different therapeutic regimens. Severe head injuries rarely occur in isolation; shock and hypoxia due to concomitant multiple trauma will be superimposed on the initial damage caused by the head injury.

In this chapter, the results of these studies will be reviewed and the potential use of CBF measurement in evaluating and applying the various therapeutic regimens used in the management of head injuries will be discussed.

Acute Studies

In contrast to the relative homogenous reduction of CBF in patients with only mild disturbances of consciousness [1], one of the most consistent findings in

Table 1. Problems in the interpretation of CBF studies after head injury may be due to differences in

1. Type of study: experimental versus clinical
2. Glascow coma scale
3. Associated trauma
4. Mechanisms of trauma
5. Therapeutic regimens
6. Technique of CBF measurement
7. Timing of CBF measurements
8. Degree of CO_2 reactivity
9. Degree of autoregulation
10. Relationship between CBF and $CMRO_2$

studies of comatose patients with severe head injuries is the wide variability of global CBF in the acute phase after the injury [2-5] with flows ranging from 20 ml/100 g/min to greater than 100 ml/100 g/min. The normal value for mean regional CBF when measured by the intracarotid or intravenous ^{133}Xe technique is approximately 50 ml/100 g/min [6]. There is usually a close coupling between CBF and the cerebral rate for oxygen utilisation ($CMRO_2$), which is the product of CBF and the arteriovenous oxygen difference ($AVDO_2$) across the brain. Meaningful interpretation of CBF measurements after head injury requires simultaneous measurents of CBF and $CMRO_2$ to determine whether CBF is adequate for the metabolic needs of the brain. $CMRO_2$ is consistently depressed after head injuries [7, 8] and therefore both normal and above normal values for CBF may be defined as hyperemic flows with uncoupling of CBF from cerebral metabolism. After cerebral trauma comatose patients generally show reductions in CBF in the acute phase of injury, but flows may be greatly increased with periods of high and low flow existing in the same patient [2, 3, 5, 8, 9] as illustrated in Fig. 1. These variations in flow cannot be predicted from neurological examination. One of the main reasons for the variability is the incidence of hyperemia after severe head injury, but different results have been obtained according to the timing of the measurements of CBF after injury. In 1976 Enelvoldsen et al. studied 23 patients and found evidence of hyperemia at 24 h in all patients with cortical lacerations or severe contusions [4]. In contrast, Overgaard and Tweed studied 43 young patients using intracarotid ^{133}Xe and showed that CBF was elevated in only 17% of patients in the first 24 h after head injury, but in 50% patients studies between the second and seventh day [5]. The hyperemia

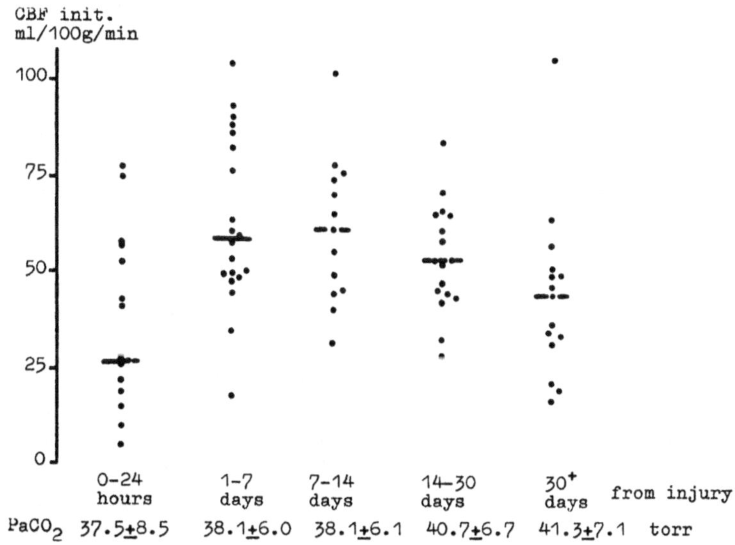

Fig. 1. Mean hemispheric cerebral blood flow (CBF) after severe head injury in 43 patients (intracarotid method, initial slope index). There is a wide variability in CBF especially in the first week. (From [5] with permission)

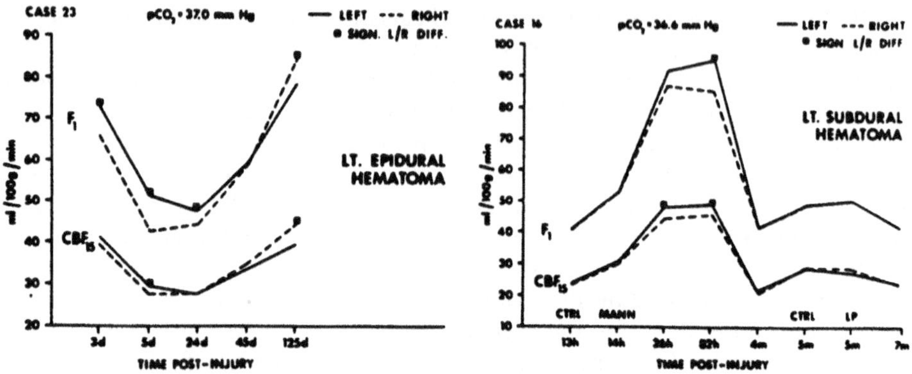

Fig. 2. *Left:* Serial cerebral blood flow (CBF) measurements (intravenous Xe 133 method) plotted against the number of days post injury in a patient with a large epidural hematoma evacuated before the first study. F1 = fast compartment blood flow, CBF_{15} = mean blood flow for fast and slow compartments. An initial hyperemia is followed by a reduction in flow and a return to normal flows as the patient's clinical condition improved. *Right:* Different pattern of CBF after head injury. A delayed hyperemia at 36–82 hours is preceded and followed by a CBF reduction that remained subnormal and was associated with hydrocephalus and dementia. (From [9] with permission)

lasted about two weeks and was supposed to represent a reactive hyperemia after an ischemic episode. Obrist et al. found transient hyperemia lasting on average 3 days in 55% of their patients [9]. Significant reductions of flow which occurred before and after the hyperemic phase were also seen in 37 of their 41 patients with hyperemia. They described two time patterns of hyperemia. In two third of patients, there was an initial hyperemia followed by a reduction in flow that returned to the normal range with recovery. In the other third there was a delayed hyperemia followed by a reduction in flow which remained subnormal and was associated with subsequent neurological impairment (Fig. 2).

These high flows represent a "luxury perfusion" syndrome as proposed by Lassen in 1966 [10]. The term describes focal or regional vasodilation associated with severe brain damage where the blood flow to the tissues is in excess of the metabolic needs. The most likely explanation for the hyperemia is a cerebral metabolic acidosis due to hypoxia. A relationship between CSF lactic acidosis and hyperemia has been shown in head injured patients [4, 5, 11–13]. Although hyperemic flows have been associated with an uncoupling of CBF and $CMRO_2$, results are conflicting regarding the coupling of reduced flows and $CMRO_2$. Obrist et al. found no evidence of ischemia as shown by normal $AVDO_2$'s in patients with reduced flows [9]. Cold however reexamined their three previous studies of CBF and $CMRO_2$ [14–17] and found no coupling between CBF and $CMRO_2$ in patients with reduced flows (< 30 ml/100 g/min) who were examined within 4 days of acute trauma. When 16 patients were studied again several days later, in 44% there was a correlation between CBF and $CMRO_2$ for all values of CBF. These differing results may illustrate some of the difficulties in comparing studies of CBF from different centers. Different techniques for CBF measurement were used (intracarotid versus intravenous ^{133}Xe) and different methods were used to sample jugular bulb blood.

Obrist et al. found a significant association between the occurrence of hyperemia and an intracranial pressure (ICP) greater than 20 mmHg [9]. In this situation where cerebral compliance may already be reduced by congestive brain swelling or an intracranial hematoma, a further increase in cerebral blood volume secondary to hyperemia may greatly increase intracranial hypertension and so decrease CPP. Any impairment of autoregulation exacerbates the situation by allowing capillary hydrostatic pressure to rise and favoring the tendency to cerebral edema.

An age related difference in the response to head injury is also present as the tendency to hyperemia is greater in younger patients [3, 5]. Diffuse cerebral swelling is more common in this age group and Obrist et al showed an association between diffuse swelling on CT-scan, hyperemia and increases in cerebral blood volume [18].

Focal Changes in CBF

Regional differences in CBF may be superimposed on global changes. Patients with hyperemia and localized lesions on CT-scans have been shown to have higher flows on the side of the lesion in contrast to patients with a reduced CBF [18]. Regional hyperemic flows are found in areas of superficial contusion of brain tissue and reduced flows in areas with more severely damage brain tissue and in the arterial boundary zones [19–21]. Focal hyperemia has also been demonstrated after craniotomy and in association with a persisting or evolving mass on CT-scan [4, 18].

Autoregulation

Pressure autoregulation refers to the capacity of the cerebral circulation to maintain a constant CBF over a wide range of cerebral perfusion pressure (CPP = MAP - ICP) changes. Thus CBF remains constant for a CPP of between 50 and 150 mmHg. Below a CPP of 50 mmHg, CBF falls and above 150 mmHg it rises. When autoregulation is impaired adjustments to changes in arterial pressure are slower and less complete;only when it is completely abolished does CBF rise and fall passively with changes in CPP. Ischemic brain damage is found in 55% of patients dying from cerebral trauma [22]. The degree of autoregulation therefore becomes important in the head injured patient. If it is absent the effect of a fall in CPP, for example due to systemic hypotension secondary to hypovolemia or to a rise in ICP secondary to the head injury, will be greatly accentuated, as CBF will fall passively with the decrease in perfusion pressure. Cerebral ischemia may therefore occur at levels of blood pressure that are usually tolerated when autoregulation is intact.

Autoregulation is usually tested by raising or lowering the blood pressure. Angiotensin, which in the normal brain has no direct effect on the cerebral vessels, can be used to raise blood pressure and trimetaphan and/or head up tilt to lower blood pressure.

The effects of head injury on pressure autoregulation have been studied in both animals and man with varying results. Animal studies using a lucite window implanted in the skull have shown prolonged dilatation of the pial vessels after fluid percussion injury [23–25]. This dilatation was attributed to damage caused by the marked elevation in arterial pressure that occurs after experimental head injury, with the release of vasoactive compounds such as various eicosanoids. These compounds produce vasodilation and endothelial damage which result in loss of vascular reactivity. The blood brain barrier was also disrupted in the region of the brain stem allowing proteins to leak into the brain parenchyma. This might cause disturbance of autoregulation by damaging a central regulatory system for CBF. Langfitt et al. described vasodilation and stasis after experimental head injury and used the term vasomotor paralysis to describe the loss of vasomotor reactivity to changes in pressure autoregulation and changes in $PaCO_2$ [26]. Lewelt et al. [27] found generalized impairment of autoregulation which lasted for several hours after fluid percussion injury; this impairment was related to the severity of trauma.

Clinical studies have given conflicting results but demonstrated regional rather than general loss of autoregulation [2, 5, 20]. This may be related to the use of the ^{133}Xe technique to measure CBF as it measures cortical flow rather than deep flow within the cerebral hemispheres. Overgaard and Tweed found an initial impairment of autoregulation, which improved in parallel with the patient's clinical condition [5]. Other workers found no change in autoregulation in the initial period after the injury but later disturbances related to alterations in the clinical condition [3]. Overall the initial variability in the status of autoregulation is too large for it to be a reliable prognostic sign.

CO_2 Reactivity

Acute alterations in arterial CO_2 lead to changes in CBF, which rises or falls in parallel with CO_2 by about 4% per mmHg change in CO_2. The effects of hypercarbia therefore have a profound importance in the head injured patient as CBF doubles it $PaCO_2$ increases from 40 to 60 mmHg causing a marked increase in cerebral blood volume and ICP. The CO_2 reactivity is mediated by changes in pH in the cerebrospinal fluid around and inside the walls of the cerebral arterioles.

Most studies have shown that although the response to changes in arterial CO_2 is impaired [3, 5, 14], complete abolition of the response is rare and is associated with a poor prognosis. The preservation of CO_2 reactivity means that hyperventilation remains effective to decrease cerebral blood volume and ICP. Hyperventilation may also reduce regional variation in blood flow as higher CO_2 reactivity is found in areas of high flow as compared with regions of low flow [15]. Induced hypocapnia therefore may be more effective in decreasing cerebral blood volume in patients with hyperemic flows.

Prognosis

The wide initial variability of CBF values prevents their use in the prognosis of head injuries, but some associations with outcome have been found. Severely reduced flows indicate a poor prognosis. Overgaard and Tweed found the threshold for recovery of communicative brain function to be between 17 and 20 ml/100 g/min. They noted that these flows were most frequently observed in the early hours after injury, but bore no relation to the eventual time of death [5]. There was also a striking fronto-parietal predominance of low flow. Obrist et al. found that CBF flows declined to very low levels in patients who died, but that recovery of consciousness was associated with a return to normal flows in 25 out of 26 patients [1]. Uzell et al. studied neuropsychological outcome within one year of head injury. They found that patients with acute elevations of CBF had a greater overall impairment of intellectual and memory function than those with reduced flow [18].

Evaluation of Therapy

In view of the wide variability in CBF, the altered reactivity and defective autoregulation frequently found after severe head injury must be taken into account in the selection of therapy in each patient. Until recently few studies of CBF have addressed this problem.

In 1986 Messeter et al. measured CBF and ICP in 11 patients with severe head injuries. In 9 patients with an ICP greater than 20 mmHg they used an intravenous infusion of thiopentone in an attempt to control ICP [29]. In 4 patients with normal CO_2 reactivity, barbiturate therapy was accompanied by a 29% decrease in CBF and ICP returned to normal in 3 patients. The decrease in ICP was probably due to a corresponding decrease in cerebral blood volume. By contrast in patients with impaired CO_2 reactivity the response to the thiopentone infusion was variable. In two patients who died CBF markedly increased and in the other two CBF was unchanged or only slightly increased. In a subsequent study where $CMRO_2$ was measured, they confirmed their earlier findings and showed that barbiturate therapy decreased $CMRO_2$ [30]. They concluded that in patients with severe cerebral trauma and increased ICP, CBF and CO_2 reactivity measurements may provide a guide to the barbiturate therapy.

Mannitol is the most common agent administered to decrease ICP in head injured patients. However, Bruce et al. showed that in some patients mannitol infusion resulted in an increase in CBF without a decrease in ICP [2]. This may be a result of the autoregulatory status of the brain. Muizelaar et al. demonstrated that if pressure autoregulation is intact mannitol causes ICP to decrease with only a small change in CBF [31]. In patients with altered pressure regulation the decrease in ICP was much smaller, but CBF increased. They suggested that mannitol lowers ICP by causing cerebral vasoconstriction. This is secondary to an initial increase in CBF induced by a decrease in blood viscosity caused by mannitol and only occurs if autoregulation is intact. Mendelow et al. also showed that mannitol consistently increased CBF in patients whose CPP was below 60 mmHg, the lower threshold for autoregulation [32]. They found that mannitol was most effective in this subset of patients and also in those with focal injuries.

Conclusions

Studies of CBF in severe cerebral trauma have shown an acute derangement of cerebral circulation leading to either reduced flows or luxury perfusion and vasomotor paralysis, with the potential for intracranial hypertension and cerebral edema. Further studies are needed to define more clearly the time course of these events after the initial trauma. The use of positron-emission tomography of nuclear magnetic resonance techniques may clarify the relationship between CBF and $CMRO_2$ after head injury. In view of the disturbances in autoregulation the importance of avoiding hypotension and maintaining CPP must again be emphasized.

Studies are beginning to show that certain subsets of patients will benefit more from different therapies, for example mannitol in patients with preserved autoregulation, or the use of hyperventilation in patients with hyperemia. Future studies must be aimed at showing whether this knowledge can be used to improve prognosis after head trauma.

References

1. Obrist WD, Gennarelli TA, Segawa H, et al (1979) Relation of cerebral blood flow to neurological status and outcome in head-injured patients. J Neurosurg 51:292-300
2. Bruce DA, Langfitt TW, Miller JD, et al (1973) Regional cerebral blood flow, intracranial pressure, and brain metabolism in comatose patients. J Neurosurg 38:131-144
3. Fieschi C, Battistini N, Beduschi A, Boselli L, Rossanda M (1974) Regional cerebral blood flow and intraventricular pressure in acute head injuries. J Neurol Neurosurg Psychiatry 37:1378-1388
4. Enevoldsen EM, Cold G, Jensen FT, et al (1976) Dynamic changes in regional CBF, intraventricular pressure, CSF pH and lactate levels during acute phase of head injury. J Neurosurg 44:191-214
5. Overgaard J, Tweed WA (1974) Cerebral circulation after head injury. Part 1: cerebral blood flow and its regulation after closed head injury with emphasis on clinical correlations. J Neurosurg 41:531-541
6. Obrist WD, Thompson HK Jr, Wang HS, et al (1975) Regional cerebral blood flow estimated by ^{133}Xenon inhalation. Stroke 6:245-256
7. Rappaport ZH, Ransohoff J, Hass WK (1981) Cerebral metabolism in head trauma. Prog Neurol Surg 10:1-13
8. Tabbador K, Bhushan C, Pevsner PH, et al (1972) Prognostic value of cerebral blood flow (CBF) and cerebral metabolic rate of oxygen ($CMRO_2$) in acute head trauma. J Trauma 12:1053-1055
9. Obrist WD, Langfitt TW, Jaggi JL, Crutz J, Gennarelli TA (1984) Cerebral blood flow and metabolism in comatose patients with acute head injury. J Neurosurg 61:241-253
10. Lassen NA (1966) The luxury-perfusion syndrome and its possible relation to acute metabolic acidosis localised within the brain. Lancet 2:1113-1115
11. King LR, McLaurin RL, Knowles HC Jr (1974) Acid-base balance and arterial and CSF lactate levels following human head injury. J Neurosurg 40:617-625

12. Cold GE, Enevoldsen E, Malmros R (1975) Ventricular fluid lactate, pyruvate, bicarbonate and pH in unconscious brain-injured patients subjected to controlled ventilation. Acta Neurol Scand 52:187-195
13. Zupping R (1970) Cerebral acid-base gas metabolism in brain injury. J Neurosurg 33:498-505
14. Cold GE (1986) The relationship between cerebral metabolic rate of oxygen and cerebral blood flow in the acute phase head injury. Acta Anaesthesiol Scand 30:453-457
15. Cold GE, Jensen FT, Malmros R (1977) The cerebrovascular CO_2 reactivity during the acute phase of brain injury. Acta Anaesthesiol Scand 21:222-231
16. Cold GE, Jensen FT, Malmros R (1977) The effects of $PaCO_2$ reduction on regional cerebral blood flow in the acute phase of brain injury. Acta Anaesthesiol Scand 21:359-369
17. Cold GE (1978) Cerebral metabolic rate of oxygen ($CMRO_2$) in the acute phase of brain injury. Acta Anaesthesiol Scand 22:249-256
18. Obrist WD, Dolinskas CA, Gennarelli TA (1979) Relation of cerebral blood flow to CT scan in acute head injury. In: Popp AJ, Bourke RS, Nelson LR (eds) Neutral trauma. Raven Press, New York, pp 40-51
19. Overgaard J, Modsal C, Tweed WA (1981) Cerebral circulation after head injury. Part 3: Does regional cerebral blood flow determine recovery of brain function after blunt head injury? J Neurosurg 55:63-74
20. Enevoldsen EM, Jensen FT (1978) Autoregulation and CO_2 responses of cerebral blood flow in patients with acute severe head injury. J Neurosurg 48:689-703
21. Enevoldsen EM, Jensen FT (1977) Compartmental analysis of regional cerebral blood flow in patients with acute severe head injuries. J Neurosurg 47:699-712
22. Graham DI, Adams JH (1971) Ischaemic brain damage in fatal head injuries. Lancet 1:265-266
23. Wei EP, Dietrich WD, Povlishock JT, Navari RM, Kontos HA (1980) Functional morphological and metabolic abnormalities of the cerebral microcirculation after concussive brain injury in cats. Circ Res 46:37-47
24. Kontos HA, Wei EP, Dietrich WP, et al (1981) Am J Physiol 244:H511-H527
25. Proctor HJ, Palladino GW, Fillipo D (1988) Failure of autoregulation after closed injury: an experimental model. J Trauma 28:347-352
26. Langfitt TW, Weinstein JD, Kassell NF (1965) Cerebral vasomotor paralysis produced by intracranial hypertension. Neurology 15:622-641
27. Lewelt W, Jenkins LW, Miller JD (1980) Autoregulation of cerebral blood flow after experimental fluid percussion injury of the brain. J Neurosurg 53:500-511
28. Uzell BP, Obrist WD, Dolinskas CA, Langfitt TW (1986) Relationship of acute CBF and ICP findings to neuropsychological outcome in severe head injury. J Neurosurg 65:630-635
29. Messeter K, Nordström CH, Sundbärg G, Algotsson L, Ryding E (1986) Cerebral hemodynamics in patients with acute severe head trauma. J Neurosurg 64:231-237
30. Nordström CH, Messeter K, Sundbärg G, Schalen W, Werner M, Ryding E (1988) Cerebral blood flow, vasoreactivity, and oxygen consumption during barbiturate therapy in severe traumatic brain lesions. J Neurosurg 68:424-431
31. Muizelaar JP, Lutz HA, Becker DP (1984) Effect of mannitol on ICP and CBF and correlation with pressure autoregulation in severely head injured patients. J Neurosurg 61:700-706
32. Mendelow AD, Teasdale GM, Russell T, Flood J, Patterson J, Murray GD (1985) Effect of mannitol on cerebral blood flow and cerebral perfusion pressure in human head injury. J Neurosurg 63:43-48

Monitoring Brain Failure Using Evoked Potentials

D. Zegers de Beyl, N. Mavroudakis, and E. Brunko

Introduction

It is 20 years since Brierley et al. reported their experimental work on brain damage induced by profound arterial hypotension in the rhesus monkey [1]. Their data indicate that "a story of the time course of the changes in the primary evoked potentials permits the prediction of the pathological outcome of an episode of hypotension". They were the first to demonstrate that somatosensory evoked potentials (EPs) may be useful in the evaluation of brain damage in humans after severe hypotension and, more specifically, that EPs do reveal information on the functional state of the central nervous system after brain insult earlier that EEG recordings [2]. Since then, many reports have been published dealing with the use of visual, auditory or somatosensory EPs in anesthesia, brain failure or brain death. This review concerns some of the new aspects of EP monitoring in the intensive care unit (ICU). For sake of clarity and conciseness we shall focus our attention predominantly on somatosensory EPs. This modality of EPs is particularly useful in the evaluation of comatose patients because the adequacy of the stimulus is precisely monitored over the peripheral and spinal nervous system. Many experimental studies published over the last 10 years have explored the influence of ischemia and/or hypoxia on the early cortical somatosensory EPs.

What Parameters Can Be Measured with Somatosensory Evoked Potentials?

With stimulation of the median nerve at the wrist the afferent somatosensory volley can easily be recorded over the elbow and the brachial plexus to ensure that the stimulus intensity is adequate and remains constant throughout the recording. A constant stimulus intensity is especially important when brain function is monitored in the operating theater because the amplitude of the cortical EPs are considered to reflect the metabolic state of cortical and subcortical structures [3]; amplitude changes of the cortical waves are significant only if the potentials recorded over the peripheral structures remain identical. The potentials recorded over the elbow and brachial plexus are not influenced by anesthetic drug levels and providing that the temperature of the stimulated limb remains constant, the latency and the amplitude of these potentials remain the same even

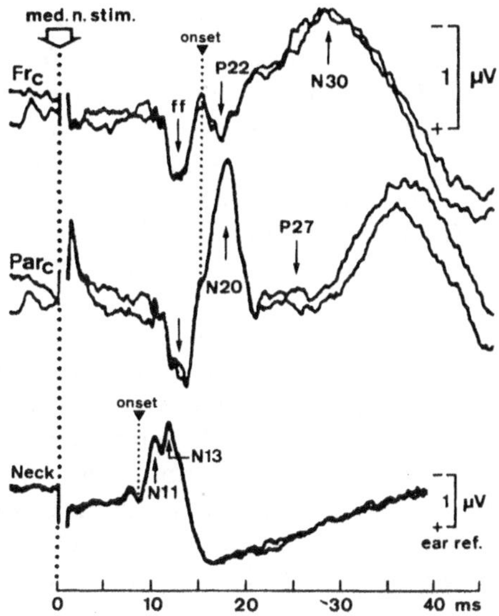

Fig. 1. Two superimposed averages of somatosensory EPs of a normal subject recorded over C6 (Neck) and the contralateral (Parc) and frontal (Frc) scalp. The spinal (N11; N13), cortical (N20; P27; P22; N30) and the P14 far-field (ff) potentials are labeled. The onset of the cortical N20 is indicated (vertical dotted line)

when hypotension or hypoxia occurs. The potentials recorded at the next level of the somatosensory pathways, over the spinous process of C6, have a complex waveform (Fig. 1). The negative potential with an approximate latency of about 11 ms (labeled N11: the actual latency depending on arm length, temperature and afferent conduction velocity) has been shown to reflect the activation of the somatosensory axons travelling through the posterior colums of the spinal cord. The onset point of the N11 defines the beginning of the activation of the central nervous system in the spinal cord [4]. The second negative peak over C6, the N13 potential, is a postsynaptic potential generated in the cervical dorsal horn. The short-latency EPs recorded over the scalp are a mixture of far-field potentials, generated at a distance from the recording electrode, and near-field potentials that originate in cortical structures. The first potential recorded over the scalp (when the reference electrode is over the earlobe and not over the scalp) is a positive far-field potential widely distributed and its onset has been shown to reflect the activation of the medial lemniscus in the lower brainstem [4]. The potentials following the P14 are recorded over the scalp contralateral to the stimulation and are generated by cortical structures. In contrast with the P14, the cortical N20 and P27 recorded over the parietal scalp (behind the central sulcus) and the cortical P22 and N30 recorded over the precentral and frontal scalp (Fig. 1) have a focal distribution [5]. The onset of the N20 potential (over the parietal scalp) coincides with the activation of the parietal cortical structures. There are several arguments that indicate that the parietal N20/P27 and the frontal P22/N30 potentials originate from independent post- and precentral cortical generators [6, 7]. Thus short latency somatosensory EPs reflect the activation of complex networks of neurons from peripheral nerve, plexus, spinal cord, brainstem, thalamus and parietal and precentral generators. The complexity of somatosensory EPs can only be appreciated when the recording conditions are adequate.

The frontal reference electrode, the most commonly used reference in the ICU, is not an appropriate choice: the frontal reference connected to grid II of the amplifier substracts the P14 far-field potential from the potentials recorded at the "active" electrodes over the cervical spine and over the parietal scalp; furthermore, with the frontal reference the postcentral N20/P27 and precentral P22/N30 potentials are mixed and some of the information may be lost [5, 7–9]. When recording conditions are difficult the earlobe reference is appropriate as the P14, the parietal N20/P27 and frontal P22/N30 can be identified easily.

Amplitudes of the cortical N20 or N20-P27 are extremely variable in normal subjects and thus absolute amplitudes are of no use. However, amplitude from one hemisphere can be compared with the other hemisphere. When serial recordings under rapid changing clinical circumstances are performed, percentage changes from control amplitudes are a useful measure reflecting the functional state of the central nervous system. Absolute latencies depend on height, limb temperature and peripheral conduction velocity and clinical interpretation is based on the time between waves (the interpeak latencies). The somatosensory central conduction time is a useful parameter of central nervous function in a variety of clinical conditions and its variability in normal subjects is small. Most clinical neurophysiologists measure the central conduction time from the peak of the N13 (over the spinous process of a cervical vertebra) to the peak of the N20 (over the contralateral parietal scalp). This interval does not include conduction within the posterior columns of the cervical spinal cord and from a physiological point of view it seems appropriate to define the central conduction time from the onset of N11 (over the cervical spine) to the onset of N20 (over the parietal scalp) [10]. When measured from onset latencies (as opposed to peak latencies), the central conduction can be divided in two intervals: from onset N11 to onset P14, a parameter of predominantly spinal conduction, and from onset P14 to onset N20, a parameter of supraspinal conduction (from lower brainstem to parietal cortex). It has been shown that in certain clinical conditions the central conduction time changes only at its supraspinal interval: with isoflurane anesthesia, the slowing of the central conduction with increased end-tidal isoflurane concentrations occurs only at the thalamo-cortical level, whereas the spinal conduction interval (N11-P14) remains stable [3].

Do Evoked Potentials Quantify Neuronal Dysfunction?

Several investigators have relied on serial recordings of short latency somatosensory EPs in animal models of cerebral ischemia to quantify the resulting brain damage: Because of the localisation of cortical somatosensory EP generator structures close to the somatosensory cortex, (the ectosylvian gyrus in animals), the EPs can be correlated with simultaneous measures of local cerebral blood flow in the middle cerebral artery territory. Potentials generated by subcortical structures are more resistant to ischemia than those from the cortex [11]. The amplitude of cortical EPs are correlated with ischemia [11, 13]: after clipping the middle cerebral artery there is a first phase of rapid decline of the EP amplitude and the rapidity of this decline correlates with the local flow after occlusion [13]. After the first rapid decline of EP amplitude there is a steady state. A failure of neuronal function in the cortex occurs when the local blood flow falls below about 16 ml/100 g/min. This failure manifests itself as a progressive reduction in the amplitude of the EPs. The EPs are abolished at flow values of about 12 ml/100 g/min. In the narrow critical range of about 12–16 ml/100 g/min the evoked potential amplitude is critically dependent on flow.

Latency changes in the early cortical EPs appear to be rather different in the various animal models of ischemia. When the middle cerebral artery is clipped in the baboon, the central conduction time is not increased for cortical flow values above 15 ml/100 g/min, but below this level CCT becomes significantly prolonged [14]. There is some suggestion that prolonged latency of cortical somatosensory EPs is more closely associated with white matter (not grey matter) ischemia and metabolism [15]. In the study of Lesnick et al. [15] the first EP change noted was an increase of the conduction time between the thalamus and cortex: this occurred when the blood flow in the white matter (measured with the hydrogen clearance technique in the white matter radiations) was reduced to about 45% of control levels. Amplitude reductions of the control EPs were noted with further reduction in perfusion and the cortical flow values (as opposed to subcortical white matter flow) were less than 45% of control in most animals. These studies indicate that somatosensory EPs provide a non-invasive but adequate method of quantifying ischemia within the brain and that changes of cortical EPs correlate with cerebral blood flow assuming that coupling of cerebral blood flow and metabolism remains intact. McPherson et al. have convincingly shown that changes of somatosensory cortical EPs correlate with cerebral oxygen consumption rather than with cerebral blood flow [16]. In their animal model of cerebral oxygen deprivation without ischemia (hypoxic hypoxia) the changes of cortical somatosensory EPs correlated with the decreased cerebral oxygen consumption and not with the increased blood flow shortly after severe hypoxia, in the recovery phase of their experiment. Their results also confirmed that both cortical wave latency changes and amplitude changes correlate with the cerebral oxygen consumption. However, the magnitude of the amplitude changes (84% decrease) was much greater than the latency changes (11% increase) and amplitude changes thus appear preferable for rapid assessment of oxygen consumption. Thus somatosensory EPs seem related to brain metabolic function, regardless of cerebral blood flow or cerebral oxygen availability. If confirmed these data indicate that monitoring of somatosensory EPs is a more adequate measure of brain function than cerebral blood flow measurements. These promising results based on animal model studies prompted several investigators to monitor human brain function during vascular surgical procedures with serial somatosensory EP recordings [17, 18]. The experience of Gigli et al. of somatosensory EPs monitoring during carotid endarterectomy suggest that there is a link between the rapidity of onset of somatosensory EP abnormality after carotid clamping and the incidence of post-surgical neurological deficits [18]. However, there is no convincing evidence that somatosensory EPs monitoring is preferable to EEG monitoring. The relationship between cerebral blood flow and EEG characteristics is well established [19, 20]. The same range of cerebral blood flow changes that alters the somatosensory EPs causes progressive slowing of the EEG, burst suppression and finally loss of EEG activity. Meaningful somatosensory EP recordings during ischemia are difficult. During brief and rapidly changing periods of ischemia, no more than on brief trial of EPs can be recorded in order to correlate the results with the metabolic state of the brain. The only obvious advantage of somatosensory EPs is their resistance to anesthesia, whereas the EEG is very sensitive to most anesthetic drugs. At the present time, studies dealing with somatosensory EPs in experimental ischemia "tell us as much about EPs as they do about ischemia" [21].

One of the intriguing features of short-latency somatosensory EPs is the contrast between resistance to anesthesia and sensivity to ischemia. Anesthetic drugs (at adequate concentrations) produce coma and greatly decreased cerebral metabolic rate without structural damage. Anesthetics are known to suppress most neurophysiological activities but spare the ability of neurons to respond to an electrical volley. Most, but not all anesthetics, induce a dose related reduction of the amplitude of the early cortical EPs [22–24]. However these data are based on EP recordings with a frontal reference electrode and our experience with isoflurane anesthesia suggests that the situation is complex [3, 25]. Simultaneous recordings of the parietal (N20/P27) and precentral (P22/N30) potentials (with an earlobe reference electrode) show that with end-tidal isoflurane concentrations up to 1%, the amplitude of the parietal N_2O does not change significantly whereas the precentral P22 (Fig. 2) is increased very significantly (mean increase: 100%). At higher concentrations the parietal EPs may disappear whereas the frontal P22 is still recorded. Thus isoflurane appears to have different effects on the post- and precentral generators of early somatosensory EPs. The significance of this observation in relation to the pharmacological effects of anesthetics is still a matter of discussion. Whether similar differences between parietal and frontal somatosensory EPs will be shown with anesthetic drugs other than isoflurane is at present unknown.

Monitoring Comatose Patients with Evoked Potentials

Comatose patients often undergo sudden variations of their homeostasis which can produce additional damage to their central nervous system and lower the probability of meaningful recovery. Assessment of conditions ultimately leading to cerebral death is often difficult. In practice a clinical examination is sometimes limited to corneal and pupillary reflexes, since head trauma and immobilization of the patient frequently hamper or even exclude a full neurological examination. Intravenous barbiturates used to prevent rises in ICP further reduce the value of both clinical and EEG examination. Somatosensory short latency and auditory brainstem EPs have been shown to yield prognostic information in the acute stage of coma and both are resistant to large doses of barbiturates [26] or other commonly used drugs in the ICU.

Comatose patients with gross abnormalities of brainstem auditory EPs invariably have a bad prognosis [27]. Several drugs and anesthetic agents may lengthen the interval between waves I–V but even at high concentrations the first 5 waves

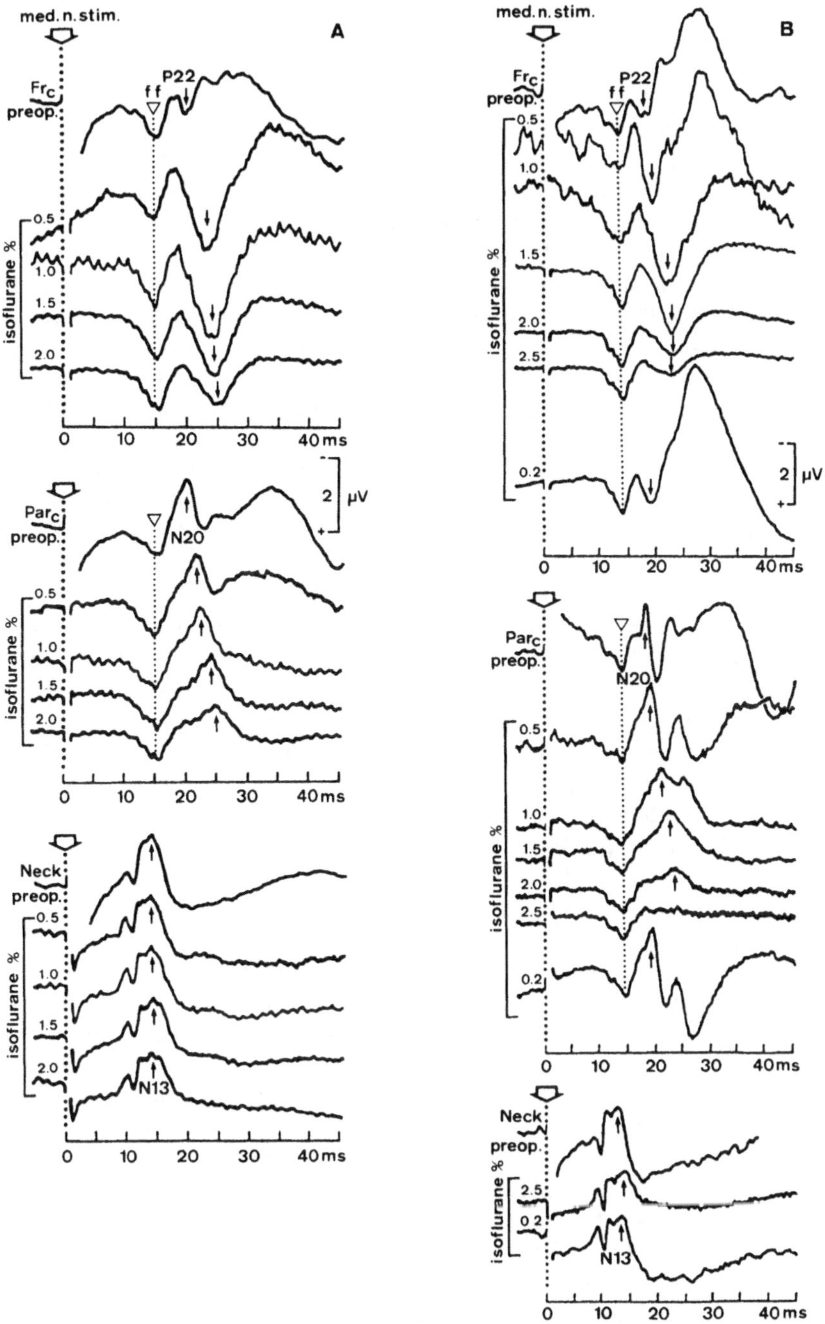

Fig. 2. Somatosensory EPs of a 39-year-old female (A) and a 44-year-old male (B) recorded over C6 (Neck), the contralateral parietal (Parc) and frontal (Frc) scalp. The first trace is recorded before anesthesia (pre-op.), the other traces at various end-tidal concentrations of isoflurane. Note the striking increase of the frontal P22 amplitude at low isoflurane concentrations when the parietal N20 amplitude is not changed. Note the progressive increase of the cortical potentials with increasing isoflurane concentrations

are easily recorded. Bilateral gross abnormalities in patients with coma imply widespread brainstem damage. In patients with brain death, either all auditory brainstem potentials are absent or wave I can be identified and the other waves are not recorded. Recently serial recordings in patients with deep coma have shown that slow preterminal degradation of the auditory brainstem EPs can be seen even when all other parameters such as cerebral perfusion pressure and ICP remain within normal limits [28]. If abnormal brainstem auditory EPs indicate a bad prognosis, normal EPs define the group of patients likely to survive but give no further information on final outcome and the severity of disability. There is some evidence that after a sudden drop in cerebral perfusion pressure (such as when cardiac arrest occurs) the absence of auditory brainstem EPs may be related to anoxic-ischemic damage of the cochlea and not to brainstem damage [29, 30]. In these rare circumstances the absence of the brainstem EPs does not allow any conclusion about the function of the brainstem, as there is no proof that the central nervous system has been activated by the stimulus. This difficulty does not occur when monitoring is performed with somatosensory EPs. The potentials recorded over the spinal cord (N11/N13) are not subject to increased intracranial pressure and are highly resistant to ischemia. Recording of the N11 in deeply comatose patients confirms that the afferent volley has reached the central nervous system. The absence of somatosensory EPs generated more rostrally then becomes highly important. An absent P14 potential over the scalp when the spinal N11/N13 potentials are identified indicates involvement of the brainstem and most comatose patients in whom no P14 is recorded, satisfy the criteria of brain death or have obvious abnormalities of brainstem reflexes [9]. Büchner et al. [8] performed serial somatosensory EP recordings in 35 patients in deep coma who finally developed brain death. Their data show that the N9 (over the brachial plexus) is always recorded as long as artificial ventilation is continued; the N11 (dorsal column activation) is recorded in most whereas the P14 far-field (over the scalp) disappears within a few hours of established brain death.

If the study of developing brain death is of interest to those concerned with the physiology of brain damage, a most fascinating field is the study of recovery of somatosensory cortical EPs after cardiorespiratory arrest in order to predict adequately the recovery of cognition. Whilst clinical examination is rather efficient when used to define these within 48 h, with a hopeless and with a good prognosis, there is an intermediate group of patients in whom prognosis of recovery is more difficult to ascertain on clinical grounds alone. It is in this group that some patients are likely to survive with severely impaired mental function, and the vegetative state more frequently follows hypoxic ischemic brain injury than any other cause of non traumatic coma [31]. Whether a patient with preserved brainstem function, spontaneous eye opening and arousal reactions will recover cognition is difficult to predict within at least two weeks following the onset of coma [32]. A recent work suggests that the prognosis for recovery in the intermediate group can be established at about the 6th day after cardiac arrest by repeated assessment of the Glasgow coma scale [33]; however, Levy et al. [34] emphasize the difficulties of predicting the eventual recovery of cognitive functions in the vegetative state even after two weeks [34]. Despite some experimental studies which suggest that somatosensory EPs allow an estimate of the extent of brain damage early after an ischemic-hypoxic episode there are only sparse data on the prognostic value of somatosensory EPs performed early after cardiorespiratory resuscitation (CPR). We studied prospectively 50 consecutive patients admitted to the ICU in coma after CPR [9]. Patients were included only if other causes of coma were ruled out, if they were in a stable hemodynamic status within 4 h after CPR and if somatosensory EPs were performed within 8 h of coma onset. For the 30 patients without cortical potentials on initial EP recording the outcome was either a vegetative state or death after persistent coma. Sixty percent of patients without cortical potentials had abnormal brainstem reflexes on initial neurologic examination; cortical potentials did not recover when several recordings were performed on successive days. Of the 20 patients in whom cortical potentials were identified on initial EP recording (Fig. 3), 25% recovered a cognitive state; the others died or remained in a chronic vegetative state. Our results indicate that somatosensory EPs recorded a few hours after CPR identify a large group with no chance of meaningful recovery. Some preliminary data suggest that in children after anoxic-ischemic brain damage the absence of short latency cortical somatosensory EPs also excludes recovery of cognition despite

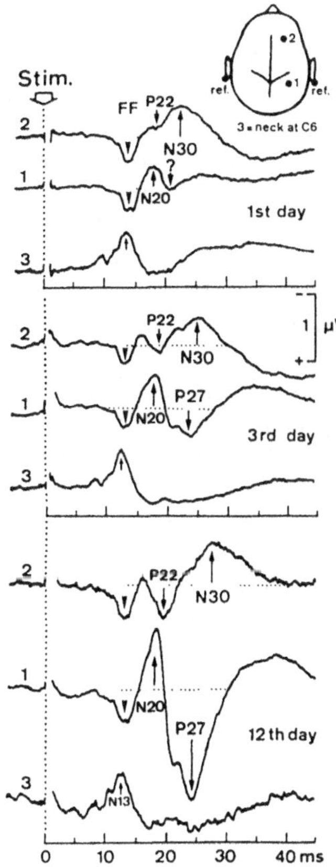

Fig. 3. Somatosensory EPs of a 57-year-old patient in deep coma recorded 6 hours after cardiac arrest (1st day), on the 3rd day and on the 12th day when he had fully recovered. Note the progressive increase of the parietal N20–P27 amplitude whereas the N30 amplitude remains stable

prolonged survival in the chronic vegetative state [35]. Additional studies to confirm and widen these observations are necessary.

If the absence of cortical somatosensory EPs excludes recovery after CPR the same may not be true in coma due to traumatic brain damage. Indeed the distribution of brain damage is quite different after anoxia and after trauma. In anoxic-ischemic coma, the pattern of the brain lesions follow the principle of selective vulnerability which implies that the telencephalic and cerebellar cortex and grey matter are more vulnerable to anoxia than the brainstem structures. In traumatic coma diffuse axonal injury occurs at the moment of impact with widespread damage to axons in the white matter of the brainstem and the hemispheres [36, 37]. Diffuse axonal injury after head trauma frequently involves the medial lemniscus in the pons [36], a structure specifically explored with somatosensory EPs. Absence of cortical somatosensory EPs after trauma may be the consequence of "transient failure of conduction of nerve fibers within the brain" [36] whereas the same finding after anoxic-ischemic damage indicates irreversible damage to the cortex. In patients with traumatic coma somatosensory EPs have been shown to be a reliable prognostic factor [38–42] and the extent of brain damage correlates with the degree of abnormality of the EPs. However, it is unclear whether the absence of cortical somatosensory EPs exclude recovery of cognition after head trauma. Over the last few years we have studied a limited number of deeply comatose (Glasgow coma scale $\leq$ 7) patients after head trauma. None of them had focal brain damage as assessed by a CT-scan performed 72 h after onset of coma. Of 31 patients, 11 had no cortical somatosensory EPs over both hemispheres on initial evaluation; six recovered cognition after prolonged coma (mean duration: 31 days) and were discharged with moderate disability. In this group the initially absent cortical somatosensory EPs reappeared over several weeks whereas in none of the other patients (who did not recover) were the cortical EPs recorded subsequently. Thus our experience indicates that absent somatosensory cortical EPs over both hemispheres after head trauma suggest an unfavorable prognosis, but do not exclude recovery of a cognitive life. Some patients may recover with only moderate final disability. However we studied a highly selected group of traumatic brain injured patients and it is likely that recovery despite absent cortical EPs is a rare event in a non selected large group of patients with traumatic brain damage. The recovery of a cognitive life after CPR when cortical EPs are not identified, has not been reported. Although patients in coma after head injury were usually much younger than the patients studied after CPR, we do believe that the difference in prognosis of patients without cortical potentials in both groups is related to the different pathophysiology of anoxia and head trauma.

Somatosensory EPs are a useful tool to assess prognosis and brain function in comatose patients and prognosis can be accurately predicted if clinical, neurophysiological and pathophysiological data are analyzed with care.

References

1. Brierley JB, Brown AW, Excell BJ, Meldrum BS (1969) Brain damage in the rhesus monkey resulting from profound arterial hypotension. I. Its nature, distribution and general physiological correlates. Brain Res 13:86–100
2. Meldrum BS, Brierley JB (1969) Brain damage in the rhesus monkey resulting from profound arterial hypotension. II. Changes in spontaneous and evoked electrical activity of the neocortex. Brain Res 13:101–118
3. Zegers de Beyl D, Voordecker Ph, Brunko E (1988) Evoked potentials in anesthesia: physiological considerations. Acta Anesth Belg 39 S2:265–269
4. Desmedt JE, Cheron G (1980) Central conduction in man: neural generator and interpeak latencies of the far-field components recorded from neck and right or left scalp and aerlobe. Electroenceph Clin Neurophysiol 50:382–403
5. Desmedt JE, Cheron G (1981) Non-cephalic reference recording of early somatosensory potentials to finger stimulation in adult or aging normal man: differentiation of widespread N18 and contralateral N20 from the prerolandic P22 and N30 components. Electroenceph Clin Neurophysiol 52:553–570
6. Deiber MP, Giard MH, Mauguière F (1986) Separate generators with distinct orientation for N20 and P22 somatosensory evoked potentials to finger stimulation. Electroenceph Clin Neurophysiol 65:321–334
7. Mauguière F, Desmedt JE, Courjon J (1983) Astereognosis and dissociated loss of frontal on parietal components of somatosensory evoked potentials in hemispheric lesions: detailed correlations with clinical signs and computerized tomographic scanning. Brain 106:271–311
8. Büchner H, Ferbert A, Hacke W (1988) Serial recording of median nerve stimulated subcortical somatosensory evoked potentials (SEPs) in developing brain death. Electroenceph Clin Neurophysiol 69:14–23
9. Brunko E, Zegers de Beyl D (1987) Prognostic value of early cortical somatosensory potentials after resuscitation from cardiac arrest. Electroenceph Clin Neurophysiol 66:15–24
10. Zegers de Beyl D, Delberghe X, Herbaut AG, Brunko E (1988) The somatosensory conduction time: physiological considerations and normative date. Electroenceph Clin Neurophysiol 71:17–26
11. Branston NM, Ladds A, Symon L, Wang AD (1984) Comparison of the effects of ischemia in early components of the somatosensory evoked potential in brainstem, thalamus, and cerebral cortex. J Cereb Blood Flow Metabol 4:68–81
12. Meyer KL, Dempsey RJ, Roy MW, Donaldson DL (1985) Somatosensory evoked potentials as a measure of experimental cerebral ischemia. J Neurosurg 62:269–275
13. Branston NM, Symon L, Crockard HA, Pasztor E (1974) Relationship between the cortical evoked potential and local cortical blood flow following acute middle cerebral artery occlusion in the baboon. Exp Neurol 45:195–208
14. Hargadine JR, Branston NM, Symon L (1980) Central conduction time in primate brain ischemia – A study in baboons. Stroke 11:637–642
15. Lesnick JE, Michele JJ, Simeone FA, Defeo S, Welsh FA (1984) Alteration of somatosensory evoked potentials in response to global ischemia. J Neurosurg 60:490–494
16. McPherson RW, Zeger S, Traystman RJ (1986) Relationship of somatosensory evoked potentials and cerebral oxygen consumption during hypoxic hypoxia in dogs. Stroke 17:30–36
17. Symon L, Wang AD, Costa e Silva IE, Gentili F (1984) Perioperative use of somatosensory evoked responses in aneurysm surgery. J Neurosurg 60:269–275
18. Gigli GL, Caramia M, Marciani MG, Zarola F, Lavaroni F, Rossini PM (1987) Monitoring of subcortical and cortical somatosensory evoked potentials during carotid endarterectomy: comparison with stump pressure levels. Electroenceph Clin Neurophysiol 68:424–432
19. Chiappa KH, Burke SR, Young RR (1979) Results of electroencephalographic monitoring during 367 carotid endarterectomies. Use of a dedicated microcomputer. Stroke 10:381–388
20. Sundt TM, Sharbrough FW, Piepgras DG, Kearns DP, Massik JM, O'Fallon WM (1981) Correlation of cerebral blood flow and electroencephalographic changes during carotid endarterectomy. Mayo Clin Proc 56:533–543
21. Ropper AH (1986) Evoked potentials in cerebral ischemia. Stroke 17:3–5

22. Sebel PS, Flynn PJ, Ingram DA (1984) Effects of nitrous oxide on visual, auditory and somatosensory evoked potentials. B J Anaesth 56:1403–1407
23. Pathak KS, Ammadio M, Kalamchi A, Scoles PV, Shaffer JW, Mackay W (1987) Effects of halothane, enflurane and isoflurane on somatosensory evoked potentials during nitrous oxide anesthesia. Anesthesiology 66:735–757
24. Samra SK, Vanderzant CW, Domer PA, Sackellares JC (1987) Differential effects of isoflurane on human median nerve somatosensory evoked potentials. Anesthesiology 66:29–35
25. Nogueira MC, Brunko E, De Rood M, Trempont V, Zegers de Beyl D (1989) Effects of isoflurane on pre- and postrolandic short-latency somatosensory evoked potentials. Neurology (in press)
26. Lundar T, Ganes T, Lindegaard KF (1983) Induced barbiturate coma: methods for evaluation of patients. Crit Care Med 11:559–562
27. Uziel A, Denezeck J (1978) Auditory brain-stem responses in comatose patients: relationship with brain-stem reflexes and levels of coma. Electroenceph Clin Neurophysiol 45:515–524
28. Garcia-Larrea L, Bertrand O, Artru F, Pernier J, Mauguière F (1987) Brain-stem monitoring. II. Preterminal BAEP changes observed until brain death in deeply comatose patients. Electroenceph Clin Neurophysiol 68:446–457
29. Rumpl E, Prugger M, Battista HJ, Badry F, Gerstenbrand F, Dienstl F (1988) Short latency somatensory evoked potentials and brain-stem auditory evoked potentials in coma due to CNS depressed drug poisoning. Preliminary observations 70:482–489
30. Brunko E, Delecluse F, Herbaut AG, Levivier M, Zegers de Beyl D (1985) Unusual pattern of somatosensory and brain-stem auditory evoked potentials after cardio-respiratory arrest. Electroenceph Clin Neurophysiol 62:338–342
31. Levy DE, Bates D, Caronna JJ, et al (1981) Prognosis in nontraumatic coma. Ann Intern Med 94:293–301
32. Dougherty JH, Rawlinson DG, Levy DE, Plum F (1981) Hypoxic-ischemic brain injury and the vegetative state: clinical and neuropathologic correlation. Neurology (Minneap.) 31:991–997
33. Mullie A, Buylaert W, Michem N, et al (1988) Predictive value of Glasgow Coma Score for awakening after out-of-hospital cardiac arrest. Lancet 1:137–140
34. Levy DE, Caronna JJ, Singer BH, Lapinski RH, Frydman H, Plum F (1985) Predicting outcome from hypoxic-ischemic coma. JAMA 253:1420–1426
35. Frank LM, Furgiule TL, Etheridge JE (1985) Prediction of chronic vegetative state in children using evoked potentials. Neurology 35:931–934
36. Adams JH, Mitchell DE, Graham DI, Doyle D (1977) Diffuse brain damage of immediate impact type: its relationship to "primary brain-stem damage" in head injury. Brain 100:489–502
37. Adams JH, Graham DI, Murray LS, Scott G (1982) Diffuse axonal injury due to nonmissile head injury in humans: an analysis of 45 cases. Ann Neurol 12:557–563
38. Greenberg RP, Mayer DJ, Becker DP, Miller JD (1977) Evaluation of brain function in severe human head trauma with multimodality evoked potentials: Part 1; Evoked brain-injury potentials, methods and analysis. J Neurosurg 47:150–162
39. Greenberg RP, Becker DP, Miller JD, Mayer DJ (1977) Evaluation of brain function in severe human head trauma with multimodality evoked potentials: Part 2. Localisation of brain dysfunction and correlation with post-traumatic neurological conditions. J Neurosurg 47:163–177
40. Greenberg RP, Newlon PG, Becker DP (1982) The somatosensory evoked potential in patients with severe head injury: outcome, prediction and monitoring of brain function. Ann NY Acad Sci 388:683–688
41. Anderson DC, Bundlie S, Rockswold GL (1984) Multimodality evoked potentials in closed head trauma. Arch Neurol 41:369–374
42. Cant BR, Hume AN, Judson JA, Shaw NA (1986) The assessment of severe head injury by short-latency somatosensory and brain stem auditory evoked potentials. Electroenceph Clin Neurophysiol 65:188–195

Near Infrared Spectroscopy "In Vivo"

J.-F. Hartmann

Introduction

The brain is exquisitely sensitive to oxygen deprivation. Monitoring of O_2 availability and utilization in the brain tissue has, thus, become a major goal for both physiologists - dealing with experimental conditions - and clinicians responsible for patients with brain insults or potentially at risk of brain oxygen deprivation, such as patients in the operating room or in intensive care unit. Until recently, direct estimation of O_2 availability in the brain tissue relied on invasive measurements obtained through implanted PO_2 electrodes, a procedure only suited for the laboratory.

Introduction of 15_0 positron emission tomography and 31_p NMR spectroscopy in the last decade has made appreciation of brain O_2 and high energy phosphates metabolisms readily available to clinicians. However these two techniques require special facilities, do not easily permit studies in patients linked to modern monitoring and supportive machines and do not provide continuous online informations.

Near infrared (NIR) spectroscopy was first described by Jobsis in 1977 [1] as a new non-invasive technique based on the optical properties of biological tissues in the near infrared spectra, i.e. for wavelengths between 750 and 1100 nanometers. Because the two most abundant chromophores in this spectral region are the heme of hemoglobin and one of the two copper atoms of cytochrome aa3 (cytochrome c oxidase), appropriate selection of wavelengths in the NIR should allow for continuous optical tracking of hemoglobin and cyt. aa3 oxygenation status. In addition, spectral properties of hemoglobin and cyt.aa3 differ according to the presence or absence of O_2: reduced hemoglobin (Hb), oxyhemoglobin (HbO_2) and the level of oxido-reduction of cyt.aa3 can thus be appreciated. Cyt.aa3 is the terminal member of the mitochondria respiratory chain and interacts directly with O_2: 4 electrons are transferred to the O_2 molecule and the rate of transfer is critical for the whole process of oxidative phosphorylation through which most of cellular ATP is obtained. When O_2 becomes insufficient, electrons accumulate and the cyt.aa3 redox level decreases. Effective monitoring of Hb, HbO_2 and cyt.aa3 redex level should thus provide invaluable information regarding the amount of O_2 entering the brain and its availability at the metabolic level.

Of additional interest is the fact that, since all hemoglobin molecules are intravascular, a knowledge of the quantity of hemoglobin in the optical field amounts to information about the blood volume contained in that same field.

Finally, indocyanine green (ICG) also has an absorption peak in the NIR range. The appearance and disappearance of an ICG bolus injected in the circulation can then be recorded in the optical field and mean transit time of the blood entering the field computed. By braking the blood flow into its static and dynamic components – the volume and the transit time – NIR spectroscopy can provide greater insight into the hemodynamic status at the microcirculatory level.

Basis for “In Vivo“ Brain Monitoring with NIR Spectroscopy

The Problem of the Optical Path

When a light beam with an original intensity [10] passes through a cuvette at a perpendicular angle, part of its energy is absorbed by the molecules of the solution contained in the cuvette and part is transmitted as an exiting beam of energy I.

The transmittance T of the solution is defined as:

$$T = I/10 \tag{1}$$

The absorbance A of the solution is related to transmittance

$$A = 2 - \mathrm{Log}\%T \tag{2}$$

Beer’s law relates absorbance, concentration of the molecules in the solution and path length of the beam through the cuvette:

$$A = a \cdot c \cdot l \tag{3}$$

where a is absorptivity, a constant, characteristic of the molecules in solution; c is the concentration; and l is the path length. Once I_0, I, a and l are known, concentration c can easily be computed from equations (1), (2) and (3). This constitutes the fundamental basis of “in vitro” spectroscopy.

Intense scattering of the incident light is a characteristic of biological tissues. As a direct result, the path length of the photons travelling through the biological optical field cannot be equated with the largest diameter of the field: photons may bounce back and forth several times before exiting the field and entering the photodetector. Beer’s law, therefore, cannot be applied unless a mean path length for every detected photon is established. In turn, this means that concentration cannot be measured: only variations from baseline can be recorded and monitored.

Instrumentation

A NIR spectrophotometer includes a light source - incandescent lamp, light emitting diode or laser diode; monochromators if the source produces white light; an optical fiber guiding the incident light over the region of interest; a second fiber, collecting the transmitted/reflected light from the optical field to a photodetector/photomultiplier and electronic circuity. Most instruments are computer operated and offer magnetic storage of the data and digital and analogous outputs.

Two to six different wavelengths are usually used, including one in the 775 nm area - where Hb absorption peaks; one in the 815 nm area - where Hb and HbO_2 spectra share an isobestic point, oxidized cyt.aa3 peaks broadly and ICG gives maximal absorption; and one in the 905 nm area when HbO_2 absorption spectra is maximal. Optical signals obtained at the various wavelengths are processed through an algorithm included in the electronic circuity and converted to electrical signals. More complete details regarding the instrumentation are available in Jöbsis's patients [2–4].

Brain Monitoring - Optical Geometry

Non-invasive brain monitoring by NIR spectroscopy is based on the very low absorption of IR photons by the scalp, the skin and the dura: most of the absorption takes place in the brain tissue and reflects its O_2 availability and utilization.

Brain hemoglobin content has been estimated at 0.5 g/100 g [5] and is localized mostly ($>70\%$) on the venous side. Optical signals for Hb and HbO_2 presumably reflect this unequal distribution between the arterial and the venous side and therefore correlate more with the equilibrium between O_2 demand and supply than with O_2 availability alone.

Two different optical geometry systems are possible depending on the position of the receiving optical fiber in relation with the emitting optical fiber: the receiving fiber may be positioned diametrically away from the source fiber (transmittance spectroscopy) or in its close vicinity (reflectance spectroscopy). The transmittance mode probably minimizes the contribution from non-brain structures [3] but requires a more sensitive photodetector. In addition, it gives a more global picture, whereas the reflectance mode allows selection of a more limited area, an interesting possibility when using two channels instruments, i.e. instruments which offer simultaneous monitoring of two different optical fields.

Results of "In Vivo" Brain Monitoring with NIR Spectroscopy

Data Obtained in Animals

Dogs, cats and rats have been studied by various investigators. Hypoxic hypoxia and acute hemorrhage both induce a reduction in HbO_2 and cyt.aa3 signals and an increase in Hb and total Hb (= cerebral blood volume) in cats and dogs [6, 7]. Increased ICP by mock CSF infusion in cats resulted in similar patterns of the Hb, HbO_2 and cyt.aa3 signals without changes in total Hb [8]. Hyperventilation resulted in ICP reduction but with further reduction in HbO_2 and cyt.aa3. In a similar set of experiments animals with elevated ICP were given 50% O_2 with or without 5% CO_2 [9]: only those receiving CO_2 improved their HbO_2 and cyt.aa3 signals, despite a rise in ICP.

Data Obtained in Humans

NIR recordings were obtained during carotid compression in patients with carotid stenosis prior to carotid endarteriectomy [10]: in patients with EEG slowing upon compression total Hb and HbO_2 decreased during the maneuver, suggesting failure of compensatory mechanisms.

In the newborn, effects of hypoxia, hypertension, bradycardia, O_2 supplementation and head tilting as well as regular nursing procedures have been reported by several groups [11–14]: observed spectral trends of Hb, HbO_2 and cyt.aa3 matched the variations predicted by independent assessement of oxygenation through transcutaneous monitoring or pulse oximeter.

Derivative Near Infrared Spectroscopy (DNIRS)

Because IR photon mean path length remains unknown, absolute measurements of the chromophores of the optical field cannot be obtained: as stated earlier, only percent variations from baseline are expressed. This forms only a small disadvantage when baseline conditions can be assumed to be in the physiological range, as in healthy animals or neonates. However, it makes interpretation of the signal trends difficult when the assumption about a physiological baseline is no longer valid, as would be the case in patients with brain failure.

In order to overcome part of this problem, DNIRS has been developed. DNIRS is a secondary measurement method which is calibrated to a primary conventional analytical method [15]. By using derivative spectra, scattering and non-specific absorption are minimized while selection of wavelengths for the algorithm is optimized. Applying DNIRS, non-invasive determination of cerebral venous saturation was achieved in a dog model, using measured $S\bar{v}O_2$ on sagittal sinus samples as the calibrating analytical method [16].

Unanswered Questions Regarding "In Vivo" Use of NIR Spectroscopy

Several questions remain unanswered and suggest caution in interpreting available data.

Regarding cytochrome aa3 oxido-reduction level – a key parameter in interpreting O_2 transfer from the red cells to the mitochondria – spectral data in the IR range were obtained "in vitro" [17] and suggested from "in vivo" studies in cat brain [1]. Confirmation of an "in vivo" broad peak for cytochrome aa3 in the 800–850 nm range was achieved in fluorocarbon substituted rats [18]. However, the large decrease in absorption in the 800–850 nm range with ongoing substitution strongly suggests that absorption at those wavelengths are dependent on the hemoglobin content and saturation of the optical field. Attribution of spectral changes in this region to cytochrome aa3 in animals and patients with normal hemoglobin levels should thus be done with great caution.

It is assumed that the optical field stays constant under varying experimental conditions and this is an unproven, though probable, hypothesis. Constancy of the optical field is critical in order to interpret variations in the signal trends as modifications of oxygenation and microcirculatory conditions.

Contributions of bone and dura to the absorption process are usually considered minimal. Because internal and external carotid circulations behave differently under various conditions, a substantial contribution from bone and dura could lead to opposite conclusions regarding brain O_2 availability and utilization. A significant contribution by external carotid perfused structure was observed in a dog model, using sympathic superior cervical ganglion stimulation and intracarotid norepinephrine infusions (Hartmann, unpublished data).

The depth of brain parenchyma monitored with NIR spectroscopy is also unclear: "Several millimeters" are usually assumed, such that both grey and white matters contribute to brain tissue absorption. This assumption is supported by data obtained on post-mortem specimen of brain and meninges [19, 20]. Interestingly, penetration depth is 2–3 times higher in neonatal brain [19], a fact probably related to its lower myelin content.

Conclusion

Near infrared spectrophotometry offers the non-invasive capacities for monitoring brain oxygen availability and utilization. It may thus bridge the present gap between bedside functional studies of brain activity and sophisticated investigations of brain metabolism available only under restrictive conditions.

Promising results have been obtained in different animal models and in newborn and adult patients.

However, current uncertainties regarding the quantification and the spatial localization of the signals call for caution in interpreting available data and for additional independent validation through experimental procedures. Derivative NIR spectroscopy [16] and modelization of light transport in tissues [21] may provide greater reliability to the NIR spectroscopy technique in the near future.

References

1. Jöbsis FF (1977) Non-invasive, infrared monitoring of cerebral and myocardial oxygen sufficiency and circulatory parameters. Science 198:1264–1266
2. Jöbsis FF (1981) An apparatus for monitoring metabolism in body organs. VS Patent N 4, 281:645
3. Jöbsis FF (1982) Apparatus for monitoring metabolism in body organs. VS Patent N 4, 321:930
4. Jöbsis FF (1983) Apparatus for monitoring metabolism in body organs. VS Patent N 4, 380:240
5. Carta F, Ferrari M, Giannini I (1987) Inside a quantitative analysis of *in vivo* near infrared monitoring. In: Oxygen transport to tissue X. Plenum Press, New York, pp 275–282
6. Piantadosi CA, Hemstreet TM, Jöbsis FF (1986) Near infrared spectrophotometric monitoring of oxygen distribution to intact brain and skeletal muscle tissues. Crit Care Med 14:698–771
7. Ferrari M, Wilson DA, Hartmann JF, et al (1987) Effects of graded hemorragic hypotension on cerebral blood flow, blood volume and mean transit time in dogs (Abstract). Congress of the American Society of Anesthesiology
8. Proctor HJ, Cairns C, Fillipo D, et al (1984) Brain metabolism during increased intracranial pressure as assessed by niroscopy. Surgery 96:273–277
9. Cairns CB, Fillipo D, Palladino GW, et al (1986) Increased intracranial pressure: potential therapeutic vistas. J Trauma 26:863–867
10. Ferrari M, Zanette E, Sideri G, et al (1987) Effects of carotid compression as assessed by near infrared spectroscopy upon cerebral blood volume and haemoglobin oxygen saturation. J Royal Soc Med 30
11. Ferrari M, De Marchis C, Giannini I, et al (1985) Cerebral blood volume and hemoglobin oxygen saturation monitoring in neonatal brain by near IR spectroscopy. In: Oxygen transport to tissue IX. Plenum Press, New York, pp 203–211
12. Brazy JE, Lewis DV, Mitnick MH, et al (1985) Non-invasive monitoring of cerebral oxygenation in preterm infants: preliminary observations. Pediatrics 75:217–219
13. Brazy JE, Lewis DN (1986) Changes in cerebral blood volume and cytochrome aa3 during hypertensive peaks in preterm infants. J Pediatr 108:983–986
14. Wyatt JS, Delpy DT, Cope M, et al (1986) Quantification of cerebral oxygenation and haemodynamics in sick newborn infants by near infrared spectrophotometry. Lancet 2:1063
15. Williams P, Norris K (1987) Near infrared technology in the agricultural and food industries. American Association of Cereal Chemists, Saint Paul
16. Ferrari M, Wilson DA, Hanley DF, et al (1988) Determination of cerebral venous hemoglobin saturation by derivative near infrared spectroscopy. In: Oxygen transport to tissue XI. Plenum Press, New York
17. Chance B, Leigh JS (1977) Oxygen intermediates and mixed valence stade of cytochrome oxydase: infrared absorption difference spectra of compounds A, B and C of cytochrome oxydase and oxygen. Proc Natl Acad Sci (USA) 74:4777–4779
18. Ferrari M, Giannini I, Carpi A, et al (1983) Non-invasive near infrared spectroscopy of brain in fluorocarbon exchange – transfused rats. Physiol Chem Phys 15:107–109
19. Svaasand IO, Ellingsen R (1983) Optical properties of human brain. Photochem Photobiol 38:293–298
20. Eggert HR, Blazek V (1987) Optical properties of human brain tissue, meninges and brain tumors in the spectral range of 200 to 900 nm. Neurosurg 21:459–462
21. Van der Zee P, Delpy DT (1987) Simulation of the point spread function for light in tissue by a Monte Carlo method. In: Oxygen transport to tissue X. Plenum Press, New York, pp 179–191

Intracranial Pressure Monitoring

J. D. Miller

Introduction

The practice of continuous monitoring of the intracranial pressure (ICP), developed over the last 25 years, has played a major part in establishing neurological critical care as a distinct form of intensive care. Raised ICP is a frequent occurrence in patients with a wide range of disorders of the central nervous system – traumatic, vascular, neoplastic, infective and developmental – particularly when the level of consciousness is depressed.

Intracranial hypertension is not only a marker of brain damage or dysfunction, it can be a source of further dysfunction and damage by limiting cerebral blood flow and inducing brain ischemia. If this process continues unchecked, it leads to cerebral circulatory arrest and brain death. This is the mode of death in almost all fatal cases of subarachnoid hemorrhage and half of all fatal cases of head injury, and is the reason that patients with these disorders from the majority of candidates for organ donation for transplant.

While raised ICP is a frequent complication of primary cerebral disorders, it also complicates a number of systemic disorders. These include post-hypoxic states, near-downing, hepatic failure, diabetic coma and Reye's syndrome. It is therefore important that the general intensive care specialist is familiar with the pathophysiology and management of raised ICP.

Pathophysiology of Intracranial Hypertension

The normal ICP ranges between 0 and 10 mmHg (1.3 kPa), but is somewhat lower in children under 5 years. The pressure waveform exhibits both slow respiratory and rapid vascular pulsations. The steady state level of ICP can be derived from the equation:

$$ICP = If \cdot Ro + Pv$$

where If is the rate of CSF formation, Ro the cerebro-spinal fluid (CSF) outflow resistance and Pv the cerebral venous pressure [1].

The rate of CSF formation is constant over a wide range of CSF pressure, falling only when ICP is increased to the point that cerebral blood flow is reduced. CSF outflow resistance, on the other hand, falls as the level of ICP rises.

The cerebral venous pressure rises in parallel with ICP, remaining 2 to 4 mmHg higher for as long as the cerebral circulation is preserved [2]. Marmarou has calculated that vascular factors account for at least 70% of the increased ICP seen in severeley head injured patients [3]. In contrast, Kosteljanetz, studying patients suffering from the after-effects of subarachnoid hemorrhage, concluded that CSF outflow resistance was the most important factor in causing raised ICP [4].

These studies are important because they show that in different pathological conditions the predominant cause of raised ICP may be different, and that it is possible to make such determinations in individual patients. This points the way from empirical to rational, individual therapy for intracranial hypertension.

The classical approach to describing the genesis of raised ICP is derived from the Monro-Kellie doctrine stating that the contents of the craniospinal axis are incompressible and any addition to or increase in any one component must be made at the expense of the others or ICP must rise [5]. This doctrine and the concept of spatial compensation imply that an addition to the craniospinal contents in the form of a mass lesion (hematoma, tumor, abscess) or in the volume of blood, CSF or brain water will cause a rise in ICP when it exceeds the dis-

Table 1. Factors that increase cerebral blood volume

Hypercapnia	(any increase in PCO_2)
Hypoxemia	(PaO_2 <50 mmHg)
Pyrexia	(any increase in body temperature)
Arousal	(by pain or other stimuli)
Rapid eye movement sleep (ICP increased more often at night)	
Volatile anesthetic agents (e. g. halothane, ethrane)	
Ketamine	
Epileptic seizures (even during full muscular paralysis)	
Venous outflow obstruction (sinus thrombosis)	

Table 2. Types of brain edema (increased brain water content)

Type of edema	Location of fluid	Clinical circumstance	Made worse by
Vasogenic	White matter, extra-cellular, protein-rich	Around tumours, abscess, hematoma, contusion	Increased BP, CO_2, T^0
Hydrostatic	White matter, extracellular protein-poor	After sudden brain decompression	Same
Cytotoxic	Grey matter, intracellular	Ischemia/hypoxia, certain toxins	Hyper-glycemia
Osmotic	Grey and white	Hyponatremia	Water overload
Interstitial	White matter, extracellular	High pressure hydrocephalus	

placeable volume of venous blood or CSF in the cranial cavity. Displacement of fluid takes some time to achieve, so that rapidly expanding lesions such as hematomas will produce intracranial hypertension earlier and at a smaller volume than slowly progressive lesions such as tumors. Common causes of increased cerebral blood volume and brain water content are shown in Tables 1 and 2, respectively. Causes of raised ICP are frequently multiple, acting together. Examples include a brain tumor surrounded by perifocal edema or obstructing the CSF pathway to cause hydrocephalus.

When the volume of the mass first increases, ICP does not rise significantly during the "compensation phase" and there are no symptoms to indicate that anything is amiss. When ICP does begin to increase, it does so slowly at first, then more rapidly as the displaceable volume of blood and CSF are exhausted, reaching an asymptote at the level of the arterial pressure. Clinical deterioration associated with raised ICP may be very rapid, giving rise to the suspicion that a sudden hemorrhage into the tumor bed must have occurred, but the rapidity of deterioration may be due entirely to the steep rise in ICP that can be produced by a modest increase in intracranial volume once compensation has been exhausted. The rapidity with which a critical state may be reached means that treatment must be equally rapidly applied if it is to be effective.

The extent to which ICP will rise following a given volume addition is therefore a function of the time over which the volume increase occurs (the faster the increase the greater the rise in ICP) and status of the intracranial pressure/volume relationship at that time as described by the lumped elastance (the inverse of compliance) of the contents of the craniospinal axis and their covering membranes [6]. The relationship is exponential and predictable, so that the effect of large volume increases on ICP can be extrapolated from the result of smaller experimental increases in volume.

While the level of ICP is very important, it must always be considered in relation to the level of the arterial pressure. Because the cerebral venous pressure is so close to ICP, the difference between the arterial and the intracranial pressures is a very good estimate of the cerebral perfusion pressure, the pressure differential that drives the cerebral blood circulation [7]. Under conditions of normally preserved cerebral autoregulation, the cerebral blood flow (CBF) can be maintained at nutritive levels until cerebral perfusion pressure (CPP) falls to 40–50 mmHg. Further reductions in CPP will cause a sharp fall in CBF. Brain electrical activity ceases as CBF falls to 40% of control levels and membrane pump function begins to fail as CBF falls to 20% of normal. This results in an intracellular brain edema of cytotoxic type, efflux of potassium from the affected cells and an influx of calcium through receptor gated channels, leading in turn to physical destruction of parts of the cells and the conversion of reversible loss of brain function to an irreversible lesion [8, 9].

Unfortunately, most of the conditions in which ICP tends to increase, such as head injury, cerebral hemorrhage and ischemia, brain tumors and the post-hypoxic states are also associated with focal or generalized impairment of autoregulation of CBF [10]. Under these circumstances there is no longer such effective preservation of CBF when ICP increases or arterial pressure falls. In some cases a degree of hyperemia is also present, so that the effects of raised ICP on

CBF are somewhat mitigated, but if not, even small rises in ICP or falls in blood pressure can have a catastrophic effect upon CBF [11]. If ischemia is produced and edema of the cytotoxic type is formed, this serves to increase ICP further and to complete the pathogenetic circle of raised ICP, reduced CPP, brain ischemia, brain edema and raised ICP.

The ill-effects of increased ICP are not, however, limited to its adverse influence on CBF. When the source of the increase in ICP is a focal expanding lesion such as a hematoma, tumor, abscess of swollen infarct, the adjacent brain will be distorted and shifted to accommodate the mass. Because brain tissue cannot be compressed, this local distortion is reflected more distally in shift and herniation of brain tissue that follows a more stereotyped pattern [12]. The cingulate gyrus herniates under the free edge of the falx above the corpus callosum, and in doing so may entrap branches of the anterior cerebral artery. The hippocampal gyrus and uncus, forming the most medial part of the temporal lobe, herniate down between the free edge of the tentorium and the mid-brain, compressing it and entrapping the oculomotor nerve and the posterior cerebral artery, and may cause occipital lobe infarction. The cerebellar tonsils herniate through the foramen magnum and compress the medulla oblongata. Finally, when brain compression is severe the entire brain stem is forced downward toward the skull base, stretching the vital perforating branches of the basilar-artery and causing secondary brain stem ischemia and hemorrhage. Many of the symptoms and signs ascribed to raised ICP, such as headache, vomiting, oculomotor palsy, loss of consciousness, bradycardia, paroxysmal arterial hypertension and apnea are more often due to these shifts and herniations of brain tissue or the resulting local brain ischemia. There is, however, a strong association between brain shift and raised ICP.

When brain tissue shifts to occupy the tentorial hiatus or the foramen magnum, the normal free communication of pressure within the CSF space of the craniospinal axis is interrupted and a pressure gradient can develop between the supratentorial and infratentorial or spinal compartments. Any factor that would normally produce a gernal increase in ICP will now cause a much greater rise in pressure above the tentorium than below it. This transtentorial gradient of pressure serves to drive the process of herniation further, towards irreversible brain stem dysfunction [13].

Measuring Intracranial Pressure

In 1951, Guillaume and Janny reported their first results of continuous monitoring of ICP, measured from a catheter placed in the lateral ventricle of neurosurgical patients [14]. Nils Lundberg, a Swedish neurosurgeon, refined their method, applied it widely to the care of a large number of neurosurgical patients, and in 1960 published a monograph detailing his extensive experience with the method of intraventricular pressure monitoring [15]. This monograph, a model of clarity, established the value of the continuous measurement of ICP and intriduced it into clinical practice where, slowly at first, it gained widespread, although never universal, acceptance and was gradually incorporated into the emerging entity of neurosurgical critical care, contributing largely to the identity of that subspecialty.

With the refinement and miniaturization of strain-guage pressure transducers and other pressure-recording systems, and recognition that in a number of patients with raised ICP the lateral ventricles are too compressed to locate safely with a cannula, a fairly large number of other pressure monitoring systems have been introducted and tried. These induce the insertion of bolts or screws into the skull, coupled to external pressure transducers recording from the epidural or the subdural space, insertion of catheters into the subdural space or insertion of miniature transducers into the epidural or subdural space or even directly into the substance of the brain [16–18]. The very number of such alternative systems suggests immediately that none of them is perfect. Recordings from the subdural space by bolt or catheter are the most popular alternatives to intraventricular pressure recording, but when ICP exceeds 30 mmHg these systems tend to obstruct and show an increasing tendency to underread the true pressure [19]. The newer miniature pressure transducers provide accurate high-quality pressure recording regardless of their intracranial site, but are expensive and still show a disturbingly high rate of technical failure. The original Lundberg method of monitoring ICP remains the "gold standard" against which other methods have to be evaluated, having the outstanding merit that at regular intervals, while the monitoring period is in progress, the entire system can be re-zeroed and recalibrated to ensure accuracy.

Indications for Monitoring Intracranial Pressure

No matter which of the currently available systems are used, this is an invasive measurement that carries with it a degree of risk to the patient, of intracranial infection (2–10%), of intracranial hemorrhage (1–2%) or of epilepsy (less than 5%). The indications to institute ICP monitoring are therefore to be considered on an individual patient basis, and the need to continue monitoring should be discussed daily for each patient.

The most common disorders in which ICP is monitored are head injury, subarachnoid hemorrhage, particularly when coma has supervened, other conditions in which consciousness is depressed such as post-hypoxia, severe meningitis and encephalitits, Reye's syndrome and certain cases of hydrocephalus in which shunt malfunction and/or raised ICP is suspected. More specific indications are shown in Table 3. Computed tomography (CT) can be very helpful in indicating states associated with increased ICP. Midline shift and enlargement of the lateral ventricle opposite a mass lesion is a strong indication that ICP will be high. In diffuse brain injury or swelling loss of the image of the third ventricle and the perimesencephalic CSF cisterns on CT is also strongly predictive of increased ICP [20].

If ICP is to be monitored, this should never be done in isolation. Other variables must always be measured, and most important among these is the intraarterial pressure [11]. Successful therapy for raised ICP must not only reduce the ICP, it must increase, or at least preserve CPP. Body temperature must always be

Table 3. Indications for ICP monitoring

Head injury	- after evacuation of hematoma in comatose patient - patient in deep coma (GCS <6) - CT showing loss of 3rd ventricle and perimesencephalic cisterns - combined head and other injury requiring artificial ventilation
Subarachnoid hemorrhage	- patient in coma (GCS <8) - progressive ventricle enlargement on CT
Hydrocephalus	- symptoms of increased ICP - suspect shunt malfunction - progressive ventricle enlargement on CT
Brain tumor	- certain posterior fossa tumours
Meningitis	- conscious level depressed (GCS <10) - progressive ventricle enlargement on CT
General/metabolic	- coma due to hypoxia, hepatic failure - Reye's syndrome with conscious level depression

measured, preferably both core and peripheral temperature. Regular measurements must also be made of arterial blood gases and serum electrolytes, particularly sodium.

In trying to determine the cause of raised ICP and its effect on brain function, it is helpful to obtain a measure of brain electrical activity, and of the cerebral circulation. If a jugular bulb catheter is inserted, then measurements of cerebral arteriovenous oxygen content difference can be obtained.

Management of Increased Intracranial Pressure: General Measures

The first consideration should be the threshold of increased ICP at which action will be taken. The normal ICP ranges between 0 and 15 mmHg, but with coughing or straining the pressure may rise to 50 or even 80 mmHg, but only for a few seconds. A pressure of 20 mmHg or more that is sustained for more than 2 min is definitely abnormal, but the patients in whom ICP is being monitored all have abnormal brain function. The question is to decide when the abnormality has reached the point where treatment is indicated. Inevitably, a degree of empiricism has to be exercised, and most departments start to treat when ICP exceeds 25 mmHg for more than 5 minutes. Some authorities claim that if treatment is started at a lower threshold, 20 or even 15 mmHg, ICP can be more easily controlled and severe intracranial hypertension avoided. This has never been proved, however, and therapy to control ICP does itself carry some risk to the patient.

When raised ICP is found, the position of the head and neck should be checked to ensure that there is not an excessive degree of flexion or rotation as these may increase ICP. The airway should also be checked for obstruction and the patient observed to ensure that he is not making respiratory efforts or straining against the ventilator. Next, the measuring system should be checked to ensure that the measurement is correct. The body temperature should not be above normal, if it is, efforts should immediately be made to return it to normal. Blood gases or other assessments of the adequacy of ventilation should be done and any abnormality corrected. The sedation/analgesia regimen should be checked to ensure that it is sufficient and the patient is not experiencing pain. The possibility of epilepsy causing raised ICP in a fully paralyzed patient should be considered. In such cases the pupils become dilated and unreactive. If there is doubt, an EEG should be obtained. The serum sodium should be checked to ensure that hyponatremia is not the cause of the intracranial hypertension.

If meticulous attention is paid to detecting and correcting these problems, a relatively small proportion of patients will require specific medical treatment for raised ICP. If such treatment is required, it is important that the most appropriate therapy is applied first time. Because of the rapidity with which ICP can increase to critical levels, the therapeutic window is narrow. Before discussing the way in which this problem can be approached, two general measures often used in managing intracranial hypertension, hyperventilation and steroid therapy, will be reviewed.

Hyperventilation for Control of Raised ICP

When comatose patients are artificially ventilated, arterial PCO_2 lies usually between 4 and 5 kPa (30–37.5 mmHg). This degree of hypocapnia will cause a certain amount of cerebral vasoconstriction, resulting in some reduction in cerebral blood flow and blood volume, and hence in ICP. Provided that cerebral blood vessels have retained their reactivity to carbon dioxide, and in many brain disorders this may not be so, further reduction in arterial PCO_2 will produce more vasoconstriction and greater reduction in ICP. However there are drawbacks. Any reduction in ICP will be at the expense of a certain degree of cerebral ischemia, and while this may not be critical in relatively normal brain, in brain tissue that is already at the threshold of ischemia it may create a problem. It has been claimed that when regional differences in CO_2 reactivity exist then the induction of generalized ischemia may be beneficial since blood will be diverted to the more abnormal and therefore less vasoconstricted area of the brain, the phenomenon of "inverse steal". It is still uncertain whether this happens very often in practice. Induction of severe hyperventilation can cause an increase in the cerebral $AVDO_2$ into the "ischemic range", above 9 ml O_2/dl. The other drawback of relying upon hyperventilation to reduce ICP is that the effects are at best only temporary. Cerebral vessels subjected to constant hypocapnia show progressive relaxation of the vasoconstriction, returning to the normocapnic caliber within 24 h of inducing hypocapnia [21]. For this reason, induced hypocapnia to PCO_2 levels below 4 kPa should be used only as a temporary measure for reducing ICP, to "buy time" before a more effective therapy is applied.

Steroid Therapy for Control of Raised Intracranial Pressure

One of the major advances in neurosurgery during the early 1960s was the introduction of glucocorticoid therapy in the management of chronically raised ICP, notably patients with brain tumors. In cases of chronic perifocal brain edema, related to brain tumor or abscess, the administration of dexamethasone, betamethasone or methylprednisolone produces within 12 h relief from headache, improvement in the level of consciousness and in some of the abnormal neurological signs [22, 23]. There is an increase in brain compliance and loss of waves of increased ICP in 24 h, then a gradual reduction in the baseline ICP over the next 24 to 48 h [24, 25].

Inevitably, the striking successes of steroid therapy led to widespread efforts to increase the indications for its use, and to apply it to cases of acute head injury, stroke and posthypoxic brain swelling, ignoring the advice of Lyle French, a pioneer of steroid therapy in neurosurgery, who pointed out that steroids were most effective when cerebral edema was focal and chronic, and least effective when it was acute and diffuse [22].

Despite this advice steroid therapy became "standard therapy" for acute brain injury in many parts of the world. A number of randomized trials of steroids have failed to show any benefit in patients with severe acute head injury, neither reducing the mortality nor the incidence of increased ICP [26–29]. In one clinical trial, reported by Dearden et al. in Leeds, England, patients with raised ICP who were treated with high-dose dexamethasone had a significantly higher mortality than similar patients who received placebo [30]. Similar conclusions have been reached about the use of steroids in acute stroke.

In experimental cerebral ischemia, cell damage in neurons is greater in the presence of hypoglycemia [31]. This is ascribed to the production of greater amounts of lactate, with more acidosis. The administration of steroids, particularly at high dosage, is associated with hyperglycemia, and raised ICP produces incomplete cerebral ischemia. There is, therefore, reason to suspect that steroids may worsen ischemic brain damage in certain head injured patients with raised ICP. In addition, the patient on high dose steroids will be immunosuppressed, a dangerous situation in the environment of the intensive care unit of a major hospital. Fortunately, the use of steroids in neurosurgery is becoming more selective, restricted to patients which the original indications of chronic perifocal brain edema.

Specific Therapy for Raised Intracranial Pressure

If intracranial hypertension persits despite the meticulous application of general measures, and the development or redevelopment of an intracranial mass lesion has been excluded by CT, then more specific therapy is required. This essentially reduces to a choice between osmotic agents, hypnotic drugs and drainage of CSF. Each of these forms of treatment operates by a different mechanism or mechanisms and the rationale for choice of therapy is based on the supposition that in any individual patient at any given time the predominant cause of elevation of ICP will be an increase in brain water content (edema), an increase in cerebral blood volume (vascular brain swelling) or an increase in the CSF outflow resistance, requiring ICP to attain a higher equilibrium value before it can be absorbed across the arachnoid villus system. It is further proposed that osmotherapy will be the most appropriate treatment for brain edema, hypnotic drugs most appropriate for vascular brain swelling and CSF drainage, when CSF outflow resistance is increased. In this section, the possible mechanisms of action of these methods of treatment are reviewed then we consider the possibility of identifying in an individual patient the predominant cause of the increase in ICP, hence of identifying the most appropriate treatment.

Osmotic agents probably reduce ICP by more than one mechanism. By their osmotic effect, they reduce brain water content. Some believe that this effect is most pronounced in relatively normal brain, where barrier mechanisms are preserved, and the mannitol does not enter cells. Other, more recent studies, using magnetic resonance to estimate brain water in vivo from T_1 relaxation times, have shown that the maximum reduction in brain water content following mannitol administration to patients with peritumoral edema was in the tumor and in the peritumoral white matter [32]. Mannitol also induces cerebral vasoconstriction. This effect, which is present only when pressure autoregulation of cerebral blood flow is preserved, is thought to represent a regulatory vascular response to the reduction in blood viscosity that the mannitol produces [33–35]. The vasoconstriction causes a reduction in cerebral blood volume and in ICP. This may explain the rapidity with which mannitol initiates reduction in ICP, within minutes of the start of the infusion. Mannitol is also thought to cause an osmotic withdrawal of fluid from the lateral ventricles across the ependymal membrane [36]. Mannitol is effective only within a range of serum osmolality values. If multiple doses are required and baseline osmolality has been allowed to rise above 330 mOsm/L further administration of mannitol will be not only useless, but also dangerous as renal failure can follow excessive dosage of mannitol [37].

Hypnotic drugs act primarily by depressing the function of excitable cells, reducing the cerebral metabolic rate. This in turn causes a reduction in cerebral blood flow and blood volume, and a corresponding reduction in ICP, the extent of which depends upon the brain compliance, or intracranial volume-pressure relationship. Since the rate of formation of CSF is also related to cerebral metabolic rate, a drop in CSF formation may also contribute to the reduction of ICP by barbiturate or other hypnotic drugs. The general metabolic depressant effect of these drugs tends to depress body temperature in comatose patients, and this may produce additional reduction in CBF and ICP [38].

Barbiturate and other hypnotic drugs have a variable propensity to cause arterial hypotension, more likely if any degree of hypovolemia is present. While this will in itself cause a fall in an elevated level of ICP, this effect is without benefit for the patient, because cerebral perfusion pressure is always reduced, and brain damage patients are in grave danger of suffering cerebral ischemia [11]. The unpredictable effects of hypnotic drugs upon arterial and intracranial pressure are the reason why both pressures must always be measured when treatment for intracranial hypertension is being considered.

Two randomized controlled trials of the effect of barbiturate therapy upon raised ICP and survival after severe head injury have been reported. Although the design and goals of each trial were different, the conclusions were remarkably similar. Schwartz and his colleagues compared pentobarbital with mannitol in patients in whom ICP had risen after severe head injury [39]. It was concluded that mannitol was superior in controlling ICP, that barbiturate treated patients did not have a better outcome, but in these patients the cerebral perfusion pressure during treatment was significantly lower than in mannitol-treated patients. Ward and his associates compared a standard therapy regimen of hyperventilation, CSF drainage and mannitol as required against pentobarbital treatment started as soon as patients were installed in the ITU, to see whether early barbiturate therapy would prevent the development of intracranial hypertension in a group of severely head injured patients in whom ICP was expected to rise above 20 mmHg in 70% of cases [40]. Barbiturate treated patients showed no reduction in the incidence of raised ICP (75% in both groups) nor any reduction in mortality (50% in both groups). The only significant group difference was a 50% incidence of arterial hypotension in the barbiturate treated patients, despite careful monitoring of central vascular pressures using Swan-Ganz catheters in all cases.

Miller applied thiopentone therapy in 12 severely head injured patients in whom all other means of controlling ICP had failed. Not surprisingly, the results were dismal with 10 deaths and 6 patients with arterial hypotension, all of whom died. More recently, Eisenberg and his fellow participants in the NIH Traumatic Coma Data Bank have conducted another trial of barbiturates in severe head injury [41]. While there was no striking benefit on overall mortality, there were indications that barbiturate therapy of value for reducing ICP in selected cases. This supports the view that a selective approach to therapy using hypnotic drugs is likely to be more effective.

Drainage of CSF can be a useful means of controlling ICP, but it must be done continuously, and the pressure should not be reduced too much in case the ventricular system collapses and the drainage (and pressure-measuring) catheter becomes blocked. It is best to drain against a positive pressure of 20 cmH_2O if an external drain is used. The method is only feasible if the ventricular system is enlarged or at least of normal size. Drainage may be external from a catheter introduced via a burrhole into the frontal horn of one lateral ventricle, usually the right one, or from a CSF access device implanted into the lateral ventricle linked to subcutaneous reservoir, access to which is gained by transcutaneous needle puncture. This method is useful when repeated periods of CSF drainage are required. If long term drainage is needed, a permanent centriculoperitoneal shunt is used. In Edinburgh, a CSF access device is always installed as well, so that subsequent access to CSF for measurement of pressure or its constituents can be achieved without having to puncture the shunt system [42]. We believe that this reduces the risk of shunt infection and other forms of shunt failure. CSF drainage is most suitable for cases in which the predominant cause of raised ICP is an increase in CSF outflow resistance.

Identifying the Predominant Cause of Raised ICP

The outflow resistance of the CSF can be estimated by one of two methods. In the steady state infusion method, fluid is run into the lumbar CSF space at different infusion rates. The steady state ICP levels attained are plotted against the corresponding infusion rate, allowing for CSF formation during this time and any CSF overflow that has occurred. The gradient or the straight line plot is a measure of CSF outflow resistance [43]. In the bolus method, a single rapid injection of fluid is made into the CSF space, ICP rises abruptly to an extent that is a measure of the craniospinal compliance, then falls slowly toward the baseline pressure. The rate of fall in pressure over time is partly a measure of the stress yield of the cranial contents to the bolus volume addition, but is mainly determined by the CSF outflow resistance. An equation developed by Marmarou permits calculation of CSF outflow resistance from the baseline and peak CSF pressures, and the pressure at a finite time from the peak pressure [1]. The steady state method provides more accurate data, but is only applicable under stable conditions. The bolus method tends to underestimate the CSF outflow resistance under conditions of normal compliance but is quicker and becomes more accurate as compliance is reduced [44]. By extending his measurements of CSF outflow resistance and estimating CSF formation rate and cerebral venous pressure, Marmarou has been able to estimate the proportion of the actual ICP level that can be ascribed to changes in CSF outflow resistance and that due to vascular changes in the craniospinal space. In head injury, only 30% of the level of ICP is related to CSF outflow resistance, 70% is due to vascular factors.

Miller and Dearden have used a different approach to the same question in head injured patients. We accept that CSF resistance is less important and propose that increased ICP is predominantly due either to an increase in cerebral blood volume or to an increase in brain water content. We further propose that hypnotic drugs will be most effective when increased blood volume is the major cause of raised ICP and mannitol will be better when brain water content is increased. The major problem in the head injured patient is, then, to differentiate between vascular congestion and edema.

Computed tomography is helpful, since vascular congestion shows a diffuse swelling of the brain and elevated ICP can be forecast from the degree of swelling shown. Cerebral edema can be identified around cerebral contusions, or in the brain underlying a compressing hematoma, often after it has been removed. If brain swelling becomes so severe that generalized brain ischemia occurs, congestive vascular swelling will be followed by cytotoxic brain edema, yet the CT appearance may be the same. Thus, CT, in common with the other factors to be described, must be regarded only as a pointer towards a conclusion that the predominant cause of raised ICP in an individual patient is either edema or vascular swelling. No single measure is as yet diagnostic on its own.

Because raised ICP occurs acutely in the intensive care unit, diagnostic measures need to be rapidly applied at the bedside, so that the correct therapy can be offered to the patient without delay. The ingenious methods used by Marmarou and his colleagues in Richmond, Virginia require injection of fluid into the CSF space and are applicable only to patients in whom ICP is being measured from a catheter inserted into the lateral ventricle of the brain.

A number of investigators are now examining the ICP waveform by subjecting the individual vascular pulsations to Fourier analysis to obtain the frequency spectrum of the compound wave in the form of a series of four to six waves of differing frequency and amplitude [45, 46]. Bray and his colleagues in Houston, Texas have declared that if the frequency spectrum of the ICP waveform is divided into low and high frequency centroids, the former is a reflection of vascular influences upon the ICP waveform, and the latter a measure of compliance that will be influenced by the presence of brain edema [47]. Piper and his coworkers in Edinburgh have studied the effects of altered $PaCO_2$ on the ICP waveform and have reached the same conclusion, that vascular factors predominantly influence the lower frequency components [48]. This approach to establishing the cause of raised ICP in individual patients at the bedside looks promising but as yet remains experimental.

Dearden has suggested a simpler approach to the same question, by comparing the vascular component of the ICP waveform with the slower respiratory component to obtain a pulse: respiratory amplitude ratio [49]. A high value, 1.5 or more, indicated that vascular factors predominate in the ICP level being recorded at that time. A low value, under 0.8, due to increase in the respiratory amplitude or decreased vascular pulsation is an indicant or extravascular factors such as brain edema influencing the ICP waveform. This approach is applicable only when a high quality recording of ICP is obtained, without damping or distortion, ventilatory parameters are standardized and constant and under normovolemic conditions. The same strictures apply to any detailed analysis of ICP waveform.

The most direct approach would be to measure cerebral blood volume. This can be done by positron or single photon emission tomography. These are not bedside estimations and are unavailable to the majority of centers, and will not, therefore, be considered further here. Transcranial Doppler measurements of blood flow velocity in the major cerebral arteries can be made at the bedside, but crucial data on blood vessel caliber are lacking. Nevertheless, by combining velocity data with other information, evidence pointing toward either vascular dilatation or edema as a cause for raised ICP may be strengthened.

A most useful observation related to blood flow had been made by Messeter and Nordström and their colleagues in Lund. In measuring CBF in head injured patients being treated with barbiturates to control raised ICP, they noted that effective lowering of ICP by barbiturates required that the capacity of the cerebral circulation to respond to changes in arterial PCO_2 be retained [50]. Once this had been lost, brabiturates were no longer effective. This might be testable at the intensive care bedside by using transcranial Doppler. A further observation of value has come from Bingham and colleagues in showing that hypnotic drugs fail to reduce ICP unless some brain electrical activity is retained [51]. Bricolo and Glick have also suggested, based upon experimental evidence that when ICP is increased due to an intracranial mass lesion, barbiturate therapy can even produce ischemia in the brain [52].

By combining these various strands of evidence, however incomplete, it is possible to build a theoretical profile of the indications for using barbiturates or other hypnotic agents to control raised ICP and to contrast these with the separate indications for mannitol therapy. Further, examination of the indications for hypnotic therapy may explain the failure of previous trials to demonstrate convincing benefits for barbiturate therapy in the management of raised ICP.

In theory, at least, barbiturate therapy will be most favorable in patients who have diffuse vascular brain swelling suggested by CT, who are young, whose ICP waveform shows a high pulse/respiratory ratio (over 1.5), and a predominance of lower frequency vascular components on spectral analysis, who have preserved brain electrical activity and vascular responsiveness to changes in arterial PCO_2.

In Edinburgh, we are at present engaged in a study aimed at testing this theoretical approach to the selection of therapy for raised ICP. In severely head injured patients in whom stable conditions can be attained in the intensive care unit with respect to ventilatory rate, I/E ratio and inflation pressure, we measure ICP, SAP, CVP and brain electrical activity continuously and obtained arterial and jugular venous samples for gas analysis and calculation of the cerebral $AVDO_2$.

Increase in ICP over 25 mmHg with no obvious correctable cause is treated in randomized order with mannitol (0.5 G/kg) or by hypnotic drugs (thiopentone 5 mg/kg or gammahydroxybutyrate 60 mg/kg). Effective therapy is defined that which reduced ICP to 20 mmHg while preserving or increasing CPP. Seventeen studies have been completed to date, in which mannitol has been superior to hypnotic in 5 cases, hypnotics superior in 3 cases, both effective in 5 patients in neither effective in 4 cases.

In this study, so far, hypnotic have been more effective in younger patients with diffuse brain injury, while mannitol was more effective in cases of focal injury (brain contusion or fater removal of hematoma). Hypnotics were more effective when the pulse/respiratory ratio was increased over 2. When mannitol was the more effective therapy the mean ratio was less than 1. Hypnotics were more effective when brain electrical activity was preserved and the CFM lower border voltage was greater than 5 microvolts. The pre-treatment value of cerebral $AVDO_2$ was not a guide to the more effective treatment, but the changes observed with therapy were informative. Successful therapy that improved CPP produced a reduction in $AVDO_2$ and in two cases unsuccessful treatment that reduced CPP produced an increase of $AVDO_2$ into the ischemic range (over 9 ml/dl). Our experience thus far supports the theoretical indications for mannitol or hypnotic therapy in individual patients with severe head injury.

Conclusions

Raised intracranial pressure and reduced cerebral perfusion pressure continue to present a major challenge in the management of patients with a wide range of disorders of the central nervous system. ICP monitoring should be used more widely in the management of comatose patients in intensive care units. If raised

ICP persists after all remediable causes have been dealt with and the need for further surgical treatment has been excluded by CT, the best approach to the choice of therapy to reduce ICP is a selective one, based upon determination of the predominant cause for the elevation in ICP in that patient at that time. Analysis of the ICP waveform, monitoring of brain electrical activity, tests of cerebrovascular reactivity and measurement of cerebral arteriovenous oxygen content difference all provide information valuable in the selection and evaluation of therapy for management of raised intracranial pressure.

References

1. Marmarou A, Shulman K, Lamorgese J (1975) Compartmental analysis of compliance and outflow resistance of the cerebrospinal fluid outflow system. J Neurosurg 43:523-534
2. Johnson IH, Rowan JD (1974) Raised intracranial pressure and cerebral blood flow 3: Venous outflow tract pressures and vascular resistance in experimental intracranial hypertension. J Neurol Neurosurg Psychiatry 37:392-402
3. Marmarou A, Masel AL, Ward JD, et al (1987) Contribution of CSF and vascular factors to elevation of ICP in severely head injured patients. J Neurosurg 66:883-890
4. Kosteljanetz M (1984) CSF dynamics in patients with subarachnoid and/or intraventricular hemorrhage. J Neurosurg 60:940-946
5. Langfitt TW (1969) Increased intracranial pressure. Clin Neurosurg 16:436-471
6. Miller JD (1975) Volume and pressure in the craniospinal axis. Clin Neurosurg 22:76-105
7. Miller JD, Stanek AE, Langfitt TW (1972) Concept of cerebral perfusion pressure and vascular compression during intracranial hypertension. In: Meyer JS, Schade JP (eds) Progress in brain research, vol 35: Cerebral blood flow. Elsevier, Amsterdam, pp 411-432
8. Astrup J (1982) Energy-requried cell functions in the ischemic brain. J Neurosurg 56:482-497
9. Bell BA, Symon L, Branston NM (1985) CBF and time thresholds for the formation of ischemic cerebral edema and effect of reperfusion in baboons. J Neurosurg 62:31-41
10. Lewelt W, Jenkins LW, Miller JD (1980) Autoregulation of cerebral blood flow after experimental fluid percussion injury of the brain. J Neurosurg 53:500-511
11. Miller JD (1985) Head injury and brain ischaemia - implications for therapy. Br J Anaesth 57:120-129
12. Miller JD, Adams JH (1984) The pathophysiology of raised intracranial pressure. In: Hume Adams J, Corsellis JAN, Duchen LW (eds) Greenfield's neuropathology, 4th edn. Arnold, London, pp 53-84
13. Fitch W, McDowall DG (1971) Effect of halothane on intracranial pressure gradients in the presence of intracranial space-occupying lesions. Br J Anaesth 43:904-912
14. Guillaume J, Janny P (1951) Manometrie intracranienne continue intérêt de la méthode et premiers résultats. Rev Neurol 84:131-142
15. Lundberg N (1960) Continuous recording and control of ventricular fluid pressure in neurosurgical practice. Acta Psychiatr Neurol Scand 36 (Suppl 149):1-193
16. Miller JD (1987) ICP monitoring: present position and future directions. Acta Neurochir 85:80-86
17. North B, Reilly P (1986) Comparison among three methods of intracranial pressure recording. Neurosurgery 18:730-732
18. Ostrup RC, Luersson TG, Marshall LF, Zornow MH (1987) Continuous monitoring of intracranial pressure with a miniaturized fiberoptic device. J Neurosurg 62:206-209
19. Barlow P, Mendelow AD, Lawrence AE, Barlow M, Rowan JO (1985) Clinical evaluation of two methods of subdural pressure monitoring. J Neurosurg 63:578-582
20. Teasdale E, Cardoso E, Galbraith S, Teasdale G (1984) CT scan in severe diffuse head injury: physiological and clinical correlation. J Neurol Neurosurg Psychiatry 47:600-603

21. Muizelaar JP, Van Der Poel HG, Li Z, Kontos HA, Levasseur JE (1988) Pial arteriolar vessel diameter and CO_2 reactivity during prolonged hyperventilation in the rabbit. J Neurosurg 69:923–927
22. Maxwell RE, Long DM, French LA (1972) The clinical effects of a synthetic glucocorticoid used for brain edema in the practice of neurosurgery. In: Reulen HJ, Schurmann K (eds) Steroids and brain edema. Springer, Berlin Heidelberg New York, pp 219–232
23. Brock M, Wiegand H, Zillig C, Zywietz C, Mock P, Dietz H (1976) The effect of dexamethasone on intracranial pressure in patients with supratertorial tumors. In: Pappius HM, Feindel W (eds) Dynamics of brain edema. Springer, Berlin Heidelberg New York, pp 330–336
24. Miller JD, Leech PJ (1975) Assessing the effects of mannitol and steroid therapy on intracranial volume/pressure relationships. J Neurosurg 42:274–281
25. Miller JD, Sakalas R, Ward JD, Adams WE, Vries JK, Becker DP (1977) Methylprednisolone treatment in patients with brain tumors. Neurosurgery 1:114–117
26. Cooper PR, Moody S, Clark WK (1979) Dexamethasone and severe head injury. A prospective double-blind study. J Neurosurg 51:307–316
27. Pitts LH, Kaktis JV (1980) Effect of megadose steroids on ICP in traumatic coma. In: Shulman K, Marmarou A, Miller JD, Becker DP, Hochwald GM, Brock M (eds) Intracranial pressure IV. Springer, Berlin Heidelberg New York, pp 638–642
28. Saul TG, Ducker TB, Salcman M (1981) Steroids in severe head injury. A prospective randomised clinical trial. J Neurosurg 54:596–600
29. Braakman R, Schouten HJA, Blaauw-van Dishoeck M, Minderhoud JM (1983) Megadose steroids in severe head injury: results of a prospective double-blind clinical trial. J Neurosurg 58:326–330
30. Dearden JP, Gibson JS, McDowall DG, Gibson RM, Cameron MM (1986) Effect of high dose dexamethasone on outcome from severe head injury. J Neurosurg 64:81–88
31. Ginsberg MD, Welsh FA, Budd WN (1980) Deleterious effect of glucose pre-treatment on recovery from diffuse cerebral ischemia in the cat. Stroke 11:347–354
32. Bell BA, Smith MA, Kean DM, et al (1987) Brain water measured by magnetic resonance imaging: correlation with direct estimation and change following mannitol and dexamethasone. Lancet 1:66–69
33. Muizelaar JP, Wei EP, Kontos HA, Becker DP (1983) Mannitol causes compensatory cerebral vasoconstriction and vasodilation to blood viscosity changes. J Neurosurg 59:822–828
34. Muizelaar JP, Lutz HA, Becker DP (1984) Effect of mannitol on ICP and CBF and correlation with pressure autoregulation in severely head impairment patients. J Neurosurg 61:700–706
35. Rosner MJ, Coley I (1987) Cerebral perfusion pressure: a hemodynamic mechanism of mannitol and the post-mannitol hemogram. Neurosurgery 21:147–156
36. Takagi H, Saito T, Kitahara T, Morii S, Ohwada T, Yada K (1983) The mechanism of the ICP reducing effect of mannitol. In: Ishii S, Nagai H, Brock M (eds) Intracranial pressure V. Springer, Berlin Heidelberg New York, pp 729–733
37. Becker DP, Vries JK (1972) The alleviation of increased intracranial pressure by the chronic administration of osmotic agents. In: Brock M, Diet H (eds) Intracranial pressure: experimental and clinical aspects. Springer, Berlin Heidelberg New York, pp 309–315
38. Miller JD (1979) Barbiturates and raised intracranial pressure. Ann Neurol 6:189–193
39. Schwartz ML, Tator CH, Rowed DW, et al (1984) The University of Toronto Head Injury Treatment Study: a prospective randomised comparison of pentobarbital and mannitol. Can J Neurol Sci 11:434–440
40. Ward JD, Becker DP, Miller JD, et al (1985) Failure of prophylactic barbiturate coma in the treatment of severe head injury. J Neurosurg 62:383–388
41. Eisenberg HM, Frankowski RF, Contant CF, Marshall LF, Walker MD (1988) High dose barbiturate control of elevated intracranial pressure in patients with severe head injury. J Neurosurg 69:15–23
42. Leggate JRS, Baxter P, Minns RA, et al (1988) The role of a separate subcutaneous cerebrospinal fluid reservoir in the management of hydrocephalus. Br J Neurosurg 2:327–337
43. Borgesen SE, Gjerris F (1987) Relationship between intracranial pressure, ventricular size and resistance to CSF outflow. J Neurosurg 67:535–539

44. Takizawa H, Gabra-Sanders T, Miller JD (1985) Validity of measurements of CSF outflow resistance estimated by the bolus injection method. Neurosurgery 17:63–66
45. Portnoy HD, Chopp M, Branch C, Shannon MB (1982) Cerebrospinal fluid pulse wave form as an indication of cerebral autoregulation. J Neurosurg 56:666–678
46. Takizawa H, Gabra-Sanders T, Miller JD (1987) Changes in the CSF pulse-wave spectrum associated with raised intracranial pressure. Neurosurgery 20:355–361
47. Bray RS, Sherwood AM, Halter JA, Robertson C, Grossman RG (1986) Development of a clinical monitoring system by means of ICP waveform analysis. In: Miller JD, Teasdale GM, Rowan JO, Galbraith SL, Mendelow AD (eds) Intracranial pressure VI. Springer, Berlin Heidelberg New York Tokyo, pp 260–264
48. Piper IR, Dearden NM, Miller JD: Can waveform analysis of ICP separate vascular from non-vascular causes of intracranial hypertension? In: Hoff J (ed) Intracranial pressure VII. Springer, Berlin Heidelberg New York Tokyo (in press)
49. Dearden NM (1985) Intracranial pressure monitoring. Care of the Critically Ill 1:8–13
50. Nordström CH, Messeter K, Sundbarg G, Schalen W, Werner M, Ryding E (1988) Cerebral blood flow, vasoreactivity and oxygen consumption during barbiturate therapy in severe traumatic brain lesions. J Neurosurg 68:424–431
51. Bingham RM, Procaccio F, Prior PF, Hinds CJ (1985) Cerebral electrical activity influences the effects of etomidate on cerebral perfusion pressure in traumatic coma. Br J Anaesth 57:843–848
52. Bricolo AP, Glick RP (1981) Barbiturate effects on acute experimental intracranial hypertension. J Neurosurg 55:397–406

Surgical Management of Head Injury

D. P. Becker

Introduction

Close to 50% of adults and 25% of children with severe brain trauma house an intracranial hematoma at admission to hospital which the prudent neurosurgeon will judge appropriate for evacuation [1, 2]. The primary reason why surgical evacuation is indicated is to help bring the intracranial pressure (ICP) down and prevent brain ischemia. Without evacuation of the large masses, in most cases the intracranial pressure will progressively rise to levels that cause severe brain ischemia, brain infarction and, in many cases, death.

The majority of patients who develop major intracranial mass lesions following trauma develop high intracranial pressure [3], (Fig. 1). Intracranial hematomas which cause a significant shift of the midline and/or exceed 75 to 100 cc in volume can be associated with very high intracranial pressures which may reach levels as high as 50 to 70 mm Hg (Fig. 2). Elevated ICP is dangerous for head injured victims as it ultimately can cause brain ischemia by reducing cerebral blood flow. Elevated ICP is even more problematic in acute brain injury since cerebrovascular autoregulation is usually impaired. In the normal state, just as

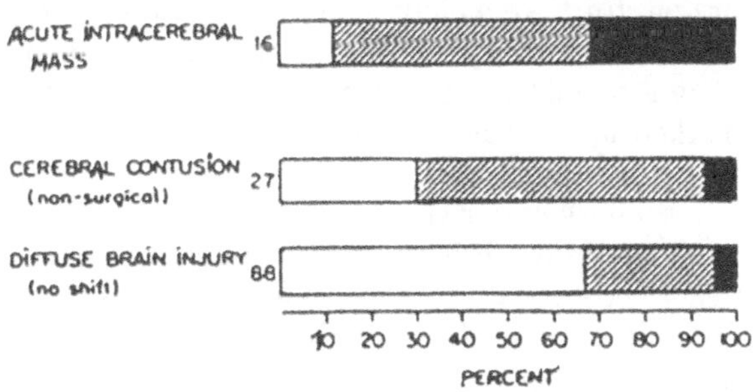

Fig. 1. Most patients who have intracranial mass lesions seen on CT-scan have high intracranial pressure during their hospitalization

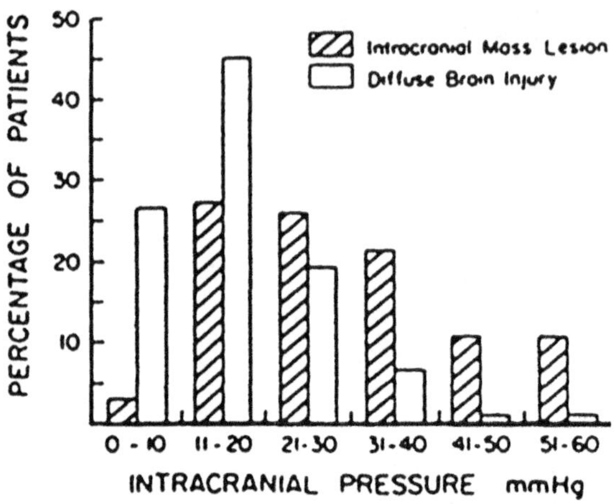

Fig. 2. ICP measurements in over 160 consecutive patients with severe brain trauma. The measurements were made by ventricular tap in the emergency room in the pre CT-scan era

cerebral autoregulation results in arteriolar dilation from a fall in arterial blood pressure, it also results in arteriolar dilation from a *rise* in ICP (which threatens to reduce cerebral perfusion). Thus elevated ICP in the patient with impaired autoregulation can reduce cerebral blood flow at levels of ICP that normally would be well tolerated. This explains observations where patients show significant deterioration in neurological function when pressures rise to 25 to 40 mm Hg, levels normally tolerated by the healthy brain with an intact cerebrovascular regulatory system [4, 5].

Speed in Making the Diagnosis Is Essential

There are clear and well documented reasons why immediate response, quick transfer to a full service hospital and prompt hospital diagnosis is imperative. One of the most compelling is the evidence that speed in evacuation of a subdural hematoma can make a spectacular difference in outcome. With acute subdural hematoma the overall *mortality* rate in published series averages 75% with a range of 60 to 90% [6–8]. This exceedingly high death rate has led many neurosurgeons to assume a pessimistic stance and some to even question the propriety of surgical evacuation and intensive medical treatment. A commonly raised theory put forth to explain the high death rate is that since a subdural hematoma is often caused by tearing of a bridging vein or a cortical laceration, a great amount of intracranial brain movement had to take place to cause the bleeding. This marked brain movement caused a major underlying brain injury. Thus the devastating state the patient is in and the reason for the poor outcome is the extensive primary underlying brain pathology, and evacuation of the subdural hematoma would do little to improve outcome. While it is indeed true that most patients with acute subdural hematoma have a major underlying primary brain injury, the theory is wrong in its assumption that removal of the subdural clot will not significantly improve outcome.

One reported study documented that patients who have their subdural clot removed in *less than 4 h from the time of the accident* will have a mortality rate of only 35%. If the delay from accident to opening of dura and relief of increased ICP exceeds 4 h, the mortality jumps to over 90% [9], (Fig. 3). The explanation for this remarkable difference is the elevated ICP that increases in the few hours after injury in a situation where there exists a traumatized brain more vulnerable to a second insult of ischemia *and* an impaired cerebrovascular autoregulatory system that does not respond appropriately with vasodilation to increasing intracranial pressure.

The presumed reason why 4 h is the golden time period is that the brain can tolerate schemic blood flows only for a limited time before irreversible infarction occurs. In the normal state, ischemic levels of blood flow at or just below 20 cc/100 gm/min can be tolerated for up to 3 to 4 h before irreversible infarction takes place. When flows drop to 10 cc/100 gm/min a period of just 2 to 3 h may be tolerated (Fig. 4), [10–12].

Flows in these low ranges are not uncommon in the early hours after severe brain injury, particularly when the ICP is elevated [13]. Blood flow in these situations is best increased by lowering ICP, most efficiently accomplished by removing the offending hematoma mass.

If there are clinical indications that a patient is developing or harboring a large intracranial hematoma then a large dose of mannitol should be promptly

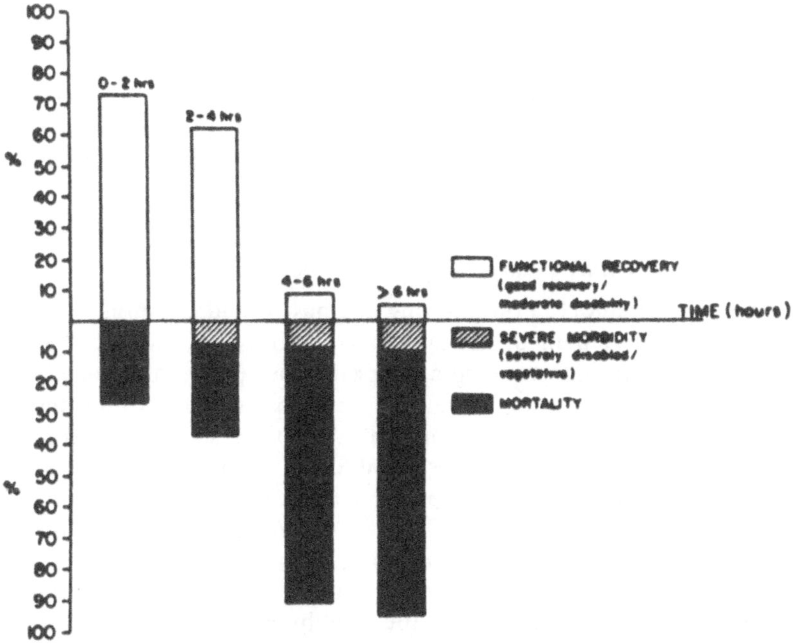

Fig. 3. The mortality rate following evacuation of subdural hematomas is dependent upon the time interval from injury to clot evacuation. When accomplished in under 4 h the mortality rate is in the range of 35%

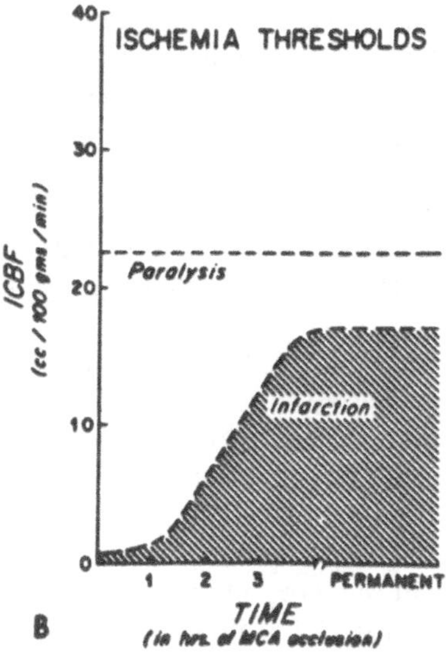

Fig. 4. The relationship between degree of ischemia and ultimate brain infarction depends on the duration of low blood flow

administered (>1 gm/kg). After arrival at hospital a computerized tomographic brain scan should be done promptly after stabilization and control of the airway and arterial blood pressure are obtained. If a large mass is seen on CT brain scan then mannitol should be given immediately (>1 gm/kg). While the patient is being transferred to the operating room and being prepared for surgery. The ICP will continue to rise if agents to raise serum osmolarity are not given. Often the greatest surge in intracranial pressure occurs *after* anesthesia induction and *before* the dura is open. It is during this period that additional brain injury from ischemia can occur and serves to explain the patient who emerges from anesthesia with a worsened neurological condition despite a perfect technical operation and hematoma evacuation.

Intraparenchymal Hemorrhage and Blood Toxicity

The CT-scan and ICP monitoring era has provided ample evidence that progressive enlargement of contusions commonly occurs [14]. Additionally, virtually all contusions develop a temporary but potentially dangerous surrounding edema [15–17]. It is for these reasons that surface contusions larger than 2 cm in diameter should be removed *when observed* at craniotomy for trauma. Larger contusions that are responsible for a midline shift noted on CT-scan should also be considered a primary indication for evacuation because there will be associated progressive increase in intracranial mass and pressure. With patients who are awake and following commands and in patients with smaller contusions, the neurosurgeon must watch the patient particularly closely, often with ICP monitoring, because the likelihood of neurological deterioration is high; in the range of 30%.

The phenomenon of brain swelling around a contusion-hemorrhage and contusion enlargement may well relate to the toxic effects of blood upon brain parenchyma. That blood in the CSF is irritating to blood vessels is accepted and the toxic effects of intraparenchymal blood on muscle tissue is well known. The fact that blood is damaging to surrounding brain tissue as the blood break down products diffuse into adjacent brain is only recently finding recognition as an important pathological problem. A clinical example comparing two patients with traumatic intraparenchymal hemorrhage highlights these points. The first patient had delayed evacuation of his contusions and suffered neurological deterioration and a poor outcome. The second patient had prompt evacuation of his contusion, emerged from coma and went on to an excellent outcome.

Patient 1: This man in his early twenties fell backward off a golf cart and struck the back of his head on the pavement. He was temporarily dazed, but felt ill and complained of headache. At a local emergency room he was lethargic, but easily arousable to an alert state, and he was well oriented. A CT-scan revealed bifrontal contusions with no midline shift and the presence of defined basal cisterns. He was admitted to a general floor for observation. Over the next 18 h he showed progressively increasing restlessness, developed incontinence and then suddenly he became bilaterally decerebrate and his pupils became small and non-reactive. A repeat CT-scan showed enlargement of the contusions, enlargement of the surrounding edema volume and disappearance of the basal cisterns. Contusion evacuation was then performed and the patient ended up in a severely disabled state (Fig. 5).

Patient 2: This 19-year-old college sophomore fell from his fraternity house 2nd floor balcony and landed on his forehead. He was immediately unconscious and was promptly transported to the University Medical Center across the street

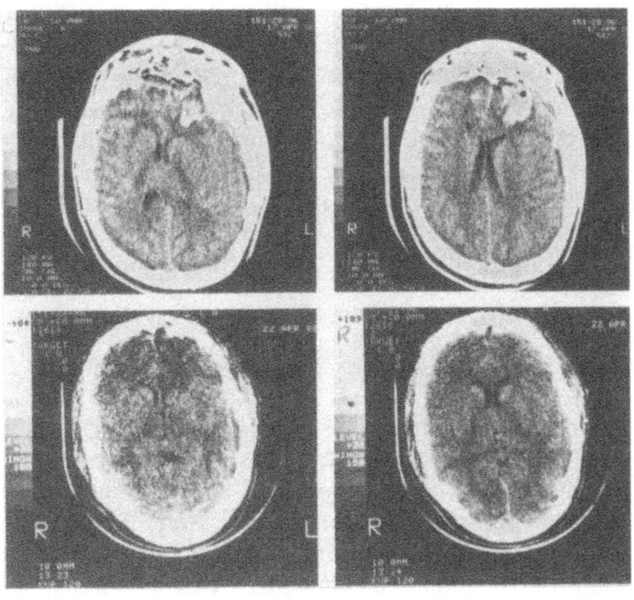

Fig. 5. CT of 19-year-old U.C.L.A. football player who sustained a bifrontal skull fracture and hemorrhagic contusion after a fall. Patient was confused with intermittent lethargy but without focal deficit. He underwent craniotomy with complete resection of hematoma and contused tissue. Scan 5 days postoperatively shows mild edema but no evidence of hematoma or hemorrhagic tissue. Clinically patient did well, returning to school 6 weeks after surgery. His only deficit was anosmia

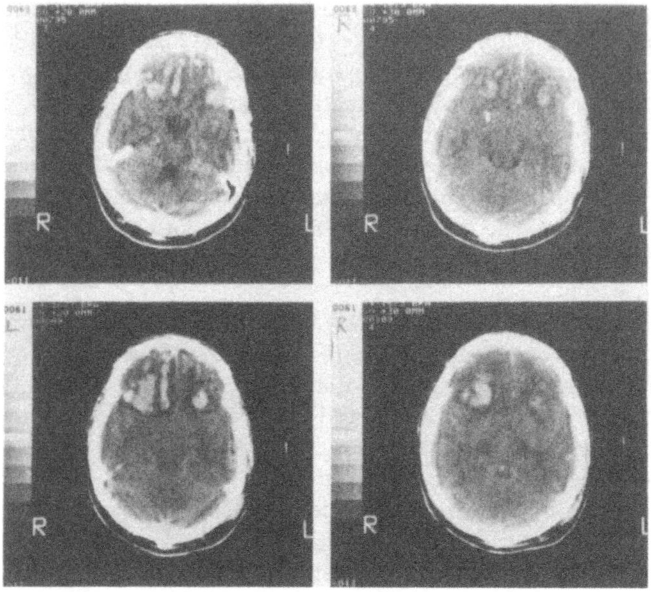

Fig. 6. A 23-year-old male struck in the occipital region with resultant bilateral contrecoup lesions. Upon presentation the patient was conversant but had deteriorated within 36 hours, becoming obtunded and posturing intermittently. CT showed consolidation and enlargement of hemorrhagic tissue. Management elsewhere included hyperventilation and steroids without surgery. Shortly after the second scan patient herniated and expired

where he was responding only to noxious stimuli with normal withdrawal, his eyes remained closed and there was no verbalization. He was intubated and a CT-scan showed a left frontal bone depressed skull fracture with intracranial air and a sizable left frontal contusion with an associated midline shift to the right. He was immediately given mannitol (1 g/kg) and taken to the operating room where the contused purple necrotic hemorrhagic tissue in the left frontal lobe was removed. On day 5 following admission his CT-scan was remarkably improved with absence of midline shift. The young man slowly improved, was discharged from hospital still mentally impaired, but 1 year later returned to college where he has been maintaining his pre-morbid scholastic performance and is attempting to return to NCAA football competition (Fig. 6).

When Should Operative Treatment Be Withheld?

Prognostic indications have been actively sought by clinical researchers [18]. The reasons are threefold. First, to define the expected outcome with standard therapy so that one could determine if a new treatment was effective in improving outcome. Second, to be able to advise families and social agencies how to prepare for the future long term care of the brain damaged victim. Third, to avoid inappropriate intensive and expensive treatment in a patient destined to die or at very best end up a vegetative organism. Efforts to define prognostic indicators in the early hours after injury and *after* restoration of an adequate arterial blood pressure and stabilization of the airway with normoxemia have provided helpful guidelines when deciding whether to treat intensively or to withhold treatment.

In patients with major mass lesions associated with a midline shift after cardio-respiratory stabilization, those who remain flaccid with no motor movement despite intense noxious stimuli, are not expected to recover. Of course associated alcohol or other drug overdosage can cloud this conclusion, and this must be ruled out along with a spinal cord injury as the neurological damage causing motor paralysis.

On the other hand, patients who show all three adverse signs of brain trauma; motor posturing, impaired oculocephalic or oculovestibular responses, and impaired pupillary response (but not cadaverically fixed pupils) can sometimes make a good recovery if they are harboring a major mass lesion that is quickly evacuated. In one study, 10% of patients with this picture ended up in a good recovery category [19] while the remaining 90% subsequently died or were vegetative or severely disabled. It is difficult to withhold treatment because predictors in this situation cannot yet tell who will end up with a good recovery or moderate disability and who will have a poor outcome (Table 1). The reason why some patients do well is because their neurological deficit is related to the mass lesion, brain shift and compression and resulting elevated ICP with associated brain ischemia. The ischemia has not yet resulted in brain infarction. When the mass lesion is relieved and blood flow thus returns to adequate levels, neurological improvement occurs. In those who do poorly, there has been either extensive irreversible primary brain injury, irreversible brain infarction, or the neurological picture represents a combination of these phenomenon. Here reduction of ICP with subsequent restoration of blood flow cannot improve neurological function.

Similarly, the patient who remains with the three adverse neurological signs after resuscitation and who has no intracranial hemorrhagic mass lesion, can be expected to do very poorly [19]. Such patients have usually sustained a diffuse and extensive primary brain injury affecting both the cerebral hemispheres and the brain stem. Some presenting with this picture have had a serious diffuse

Table 1. Outcome of patients with TANS* following head injury

Outcome	Cases	
	No.	[%]
Functional recovery (good recovery/moderate disability)	6	10
Severe morbidity (severely disabled/vegetative)	6	10
Deaths	49	80
Total	61	100

* TANS = three adverse neurological signs.
The three adverse neurological signs are motor posturing, impaired eye movements and impaired pupillary responses.

brain injury compounded by a severe second insult of hypoxia or hypotension and it is the dual insult which creates the devastating neurological picture seen at hospital admission. Modern therapy, as yet, has no effective treatment to provide a good recovery for these patients.

Early Diagnosis and Management

A prompt and orderly analysis of the nature and magnitude of all damage sustained by patients with head injury is necessary for appropriate and definitive emergency management. The most immediate requirement is to determine the intracranial damage. The surgeon must define the presence or absence of intracranial hematomas, contusions, and major zones of diffuse or focal edema. The urgency of a given situation can be quickly determined by testing the ability of the patient to follow a simple stage command, which serves as a measure of a considerable degree of neurological function. Although inability to follow such a command is not necessarily associated with impending neurological deterioration, should deterioration occur in such a patient, he will immediately be in a critical neurological state. For this reason loss of this ability should indicate prompt diagnostic testing. This principle must be adhered to in all patients, since successful therapy must take place before herniation syndromes occur or are permitted to progress.

Clinical Status As an Indication for Operation

A patient who progressively deteriorates from being able to talk to showing signs of tentorial herniation should have prompt operate therapy. Progressively diminishing responsiveness, development of unilateral pupillary dilation, associated flexor or extensor posturing, and increasing arterial hypertension and bradycardia associated with periodic breathing indicate third nerve and brainstem compression from tentorial herniation. While such clinical pictures will inevitably occur and require immediate operation, progressive deterioration should ideally be recognized earlier and the masses should be evacuated. It is incumbent, then, upon nurses and physicians evaluating such patients to be able to recognize the more subtle changes that develop while ICP is rising and brain shift is occurring. Even in fine neurosurgical units, early subtle signs of deterioration may escape recognition, and signs of brain compression and shift are discovered too late for reasonable salvage of the patient [20, 21].

Computed Tomographic Indication of a Mass Requiring Operative Treatment

In unresponsive patients with acute head injury, five variations of lesions seen in the CT-scan are considered as potential operative mass lesions:

Extra-axial mass with a definite shift of the midline: If there is a clearly identifiable extra-axial lesion of increased or decreased density and the midline shift is seen with the naked eye on a standard size CT-scan, the lesion should be evacuated. Any shift of the midline evident on computed tomography (1 mm on the print is roughly equivalent approximately to a 4 mm true shift seen on ventriculography), correspond to lesions almost always associated with high ICP in the early state after injury [22]. If a small extra-axial lesion is seen, but there is no midline shift and no contralateral balancing lesion, the patient may be managed initially without operation.

Midline shift with no extra or intra-axial clot seen on CT-scan: If the midline is clearly shifted in an amount consistent with an actual shift of 5 mm or more and one ventricle is compressed, the patient should have an early follow-up scan if no high density masses are seen on the CT-scan. Often, the delayed scan will demonstrate that the patient has an acute subdural hematoma. Even if the shift is not due to an acute extra-axial clot, then a contusion will usually be discovered in the frontal or temporal lobe that was not seen in the CT-scan. More often, a small extra-axial or intracerebral dense lesion is seen on the scan, with a large midline shift, and at operation one finds that the extra-axial mass is much larger than expected from the CT-scan.

Intra-axial mass with midline shift: The same principles hold true here, and if there is a supratentorial intracerebral dense lesion with midline shift equivalent to 5 mm or more true shift, then the patient should have the contusion and hematoma evacuated. This is particularly important with intracerebral lesions because they almost always develop more surrounding edema and increased mass effect over several days, and if an initial midline shift of 5 mm or more is seen, any further brain swelling can be devastating. Even if the lesion is in the anterior portion of the dominant hemisphere, operative evacuation should be done if the mass or the shift or both are large. Without operation death will almost certainly occur, and with operative evacuation of the mass an occasional good result can be obtained, depending on the location and extent of the irreversible damage. The indications for operation when there is less than 5 mm of midline shift are not clear. In these situations, it is best to individualize treatment on the basis of the patient's clinical course and ICP.

Multiple intra-axial lesions with midline shift: Even when multiple unilateral or bilateral intracerebral lesions are present, if there is a major shift of the midline, the major shift-producing lesion or lesions should be evacuated. It is not advisable to extend the operation across the midline except very rarely for large bifrontal contusions. Bilateral temporal lobe operation for intracerebral contusion and hematoma is also not advisable. If there is no shift of the midline, the patients can often be managed successfully without operative intervention. But ICP monitoring and frequent neurological examinations must be performed in order to guide therapy and determine whether operative mass evacuation is ultimately required.

Bilateral extra-axial dense lesions without shift: Small bilateral extra-axial hematomas may often be managed satisfactorily without operation. Large lesions, especially if they are causing clear brain compression with ventricular impingement, should be evacuated. While even the larger lesions may occasionally disappear without operation, the evidence of brain compression on computed tomography suggests the possibility of real or potential secondary brain injury, and this is best handled by evacuating the mass.

Preparations for Operation and Anesthesia

Once operative therapy is decided upon, the surgeon should proceed with dispatch. Blood should be sent for cross-matching, and two units brought to the operating room as soon as available. Prior to anesthesia, the patient should virtually always be given intravenous mannitol in a dose that will elevate serum osmolarity by 10 to 12 mOsm. This requires at least 1 gm/kg; in an adult 500 ml of a 20% solution will suffice. Smaller amounts should not be used in this preoperative situation. The ICP is already dangerously high in almost all patients with large mass lesions, and serious further brain injury can occur in 15 to 30 min prior to evacuation of the mass lesion. Even if the patient appears reasonably stable on the way to the operation, mannitol should be given before or during endotracheal intubation and induction of anesthesia, as during these maneuvers the brain may be further insulted by increasing brain shift or increase in ICP, and some time will elapse before the dura can be opened [23].

Volatile anesthetics such as halothane should not be used because of their well known cerebral vasodilator effect. This will cause increased intracranial blood volume and, in a patient with a mass lesion, a dangerous rise in ICP toward blood pressure levels together with a reduction in blood pressure. Various combinations of nitrous oxide, barbiturates, narcotics, and tranquillizers are favored because of their minimal effect on ICP. Blood gases should be measured during the operation and arterial oxygen tension maintained above 80 mm Hg. Arterial carbon dioxide tension should be quickly brought to levels between 25 and 30 mm Hg. Intraoperative hyperventilation should be accomplished with a large tidal volume and a slow to normal respiratory rate, rather than by increasing ventilatory rate much above normal levels, to allow time for good venous return [24, 25].

Positioning of the Patient

The patient is generally placed in a mildly flexed position. All pressure points are padded and anesthesia personnel should have access to the patient. In addition, there should be sufficient room for the surgical team. If the CT has shown that the lesion is unilateral, then the head can be placed in a donut and turned in the appropriate position. If there is evidence of bilateral lesions or involvement of the midline structures or if there is any doubt as to extent of the lesion, then provisions should be made to gain access to both sides of the head. We accomplish this by the use of the subdural headrest and the Mayfield head holder. This

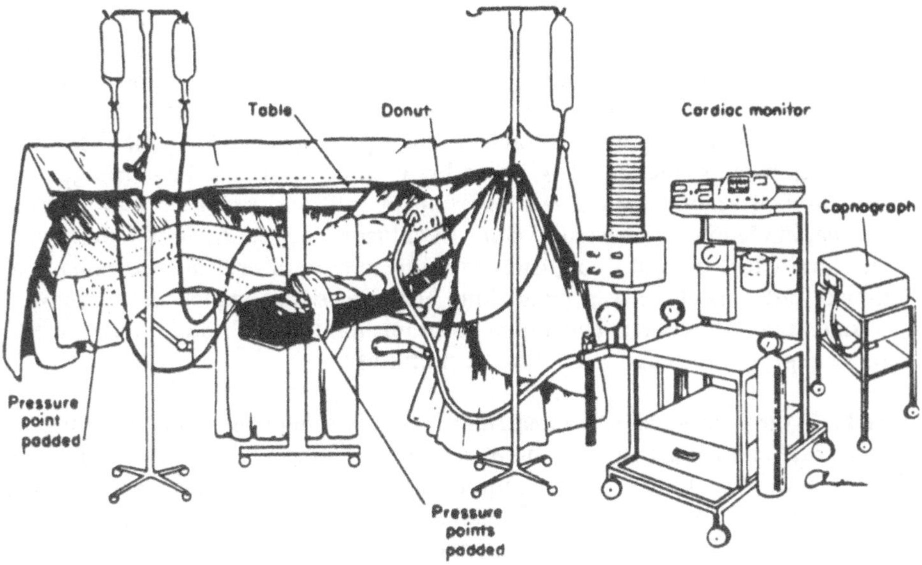

Fig. 7. Positioning of the patient from anesthesia viewpoint. Note that there is good access to the patient and his airway and that all pressure points are padded

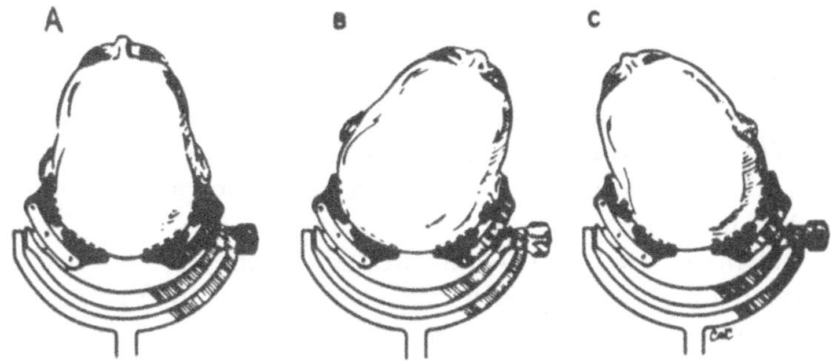

Fig. 8. Position of head in Mayfield head holder to gain access to both sides of head

enables one to do either unilateral or bilateral scalp and skull flaps and to reposition the head during surgery if necessary [26], (Figs. 7 and 8).

Operative Technique for Traumatic Intracranial Mass Lesions

Because most patients with acute subdural hematomas also have an underlying brain contusion, the two entities must be considered together in any discussion of the operation. The most skillful operative technique and the best surgical judgment should be brought to bear on traumatic intracranial mass lesions. Just as neurosurgeons accept that superior surgical skill and judgment will yield improved results in aneurysm, arteriovenous malformation, and benign brain tumor operations, these same efforts will also improve results in the operative treatment of trauma. In performing the "decompression", gentle handling of the brain is imperative, and firm brain retraction should not be done, as acutely injured brain tissue is quite vulnerable to this type of insult. The immediate goals of operation are reduction of ICP and brain shift, control of hemorrhage, and prevention of secondary delayed elevation in ICP and brain shift from brain swelling, inadequately evacuated clot of contusion, or recurrent clot. Judgment regarding extent of brain contusion excision may be a critical determinant of ultimate outcome. Likewise, meticulous hemostasis and maneuvers to prevent postoperative intracranial hematoma or brain herniation through bony defects can be expected to reduce the ultimate morbidity.

The basic large craniotomy trauma flap: There is a high incidence of temporal and frontal contusions and tearing of midline bridging veins in severe brain injury associated with mass lesions requiring operation. The frontal and temporal contusions may not be demonstrable on angiography, and will of course not be seen on ventriculography. Likewise, smaller multifocal contusions may not be seen on computed tomography, particularly soon after injury, before progressive edema develops around the contusion. Since adequate decompressive operations may require debridement of these lesions, the frontal and temporal poles should be accessible in the field of exposure. While the temporal tip and pole are the sites usually involved in temporal lobe contusion, the frontal lesions commonly begin at the tips and extend over the inferior surface, involving the orbital gyri and inferior frontal lobe. Thus, the inferior frontal lobe should be accessible down the floor of the anterior fossa.

With severe rotational brain injuries, one or more midline bridging veins may have been torn. This is a common cause of the acute subdural hematoma, and when the hematoma is evacuated, major intraoperative hemorrhage can occur from these vessels when the pressure tamponade is released [27, 28]. Severe bleeding from these midline vessels may develop after the internal decompression, and if only a limited temporal craniotomy is done for temporal lobe swelling and contusion, great difficulty can be encountered in controlling the hemorrhage that is coming from a distance away from the bone flap [29]. To anticipate this potential problem, the craniotomy flap should also expose the area close to the midline. The basic craniotomy flap, therefore, should be generous enough and placed so as to permit one to deal quickly with the most frequently found disorder without further operative extension for additional exposure [30]. The exposure should provide adequate access to decompress the epidural and subdural space; to debride contused cerebral tissue (anterior temporal and frontal lobes and orbital gyri) and remove associated intracerebral hematomas as necessary; to control hemorrhage from avulsed bridging veins to the sagittal sinus and from temporal lobe to transverse sinus and petrosal sinuses; to control hemorrhage from the skull base, to pack sinuses as necessary, and to repair potential cerebrospinal fluid fistulae; and to explore and manage lesions of vascular and neural elements at the base as necessary.

Technique of basic large trauma craniotomy: Scalp incision. The skin incision is outlined as shown in Fig. 9. It is begun 1 cm anterior to the tragus at the temporal portion of the zygomatic arch, carried superiorly and posteriorly over the ear, posteriorly around the parietal bone to the midline, where it is brought anteriorly on the midline down to the midforehead. The forehead incision, which comes below the hairline, can be closed by using plastic surgical techniques, and the minimal visible scar is small sacrifice for the added exposure of the frontal lobe gained by this flap.

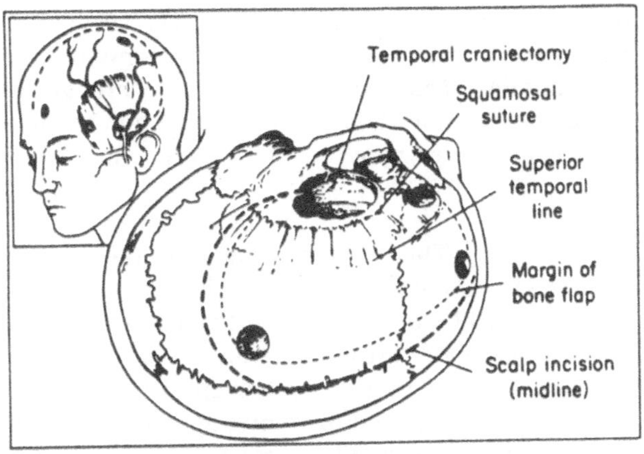

Fig. 9. Outline of the standard craniotomy flap recommended for evacuation of acute epidural, subdural and intracerebral hemotomas and contusions. This exposure will provide access to the critical areas commonly injured in acute acceleration or deceleration "rotational" injuries. Through this flap the surgeon will be able to decompress the epidural and subdural spaces, debride contused anterior temporal and frontal lobes and orbital gyri and control hemorrhage from midline avulsed bridging veins or the basal dural or skull areas

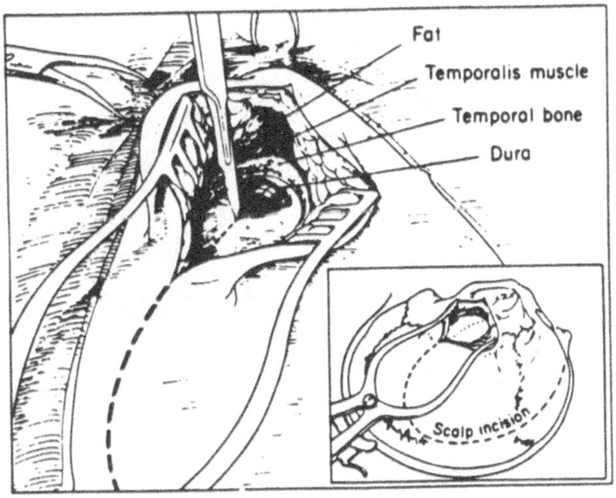

Fig. 10. If the patient has been deteriorating prior to operation or if the intracranial pressure is known to be very high and there is a major shift, an initial quick subtemporal decompression should be done. One should then proceed with the formal craniotomy

Immediate temporal decompression: If the patient has been deteriorating rapidly prior to operation, a quick decompression is the immediate goal. In this situation the portion of the incision just anterior to and above the ear should be opened first down through the temporalis muscle to bone (Fig. 10). A burr hole and small craniectomy should be accomplished quickly, and the dura opened in cruciate fashion. Most often this maneuver will afford some immediate relief of elevated ICP when a small amount of extra-axial clot or contused temporal lobe herniates out through the craniectomy site. One should then proceed to perform the formal craniotomy, and not be satisfied with this small decompression [29–33].

Bone flap: Either a free bone flap or one based on the temporalis muscle can be raised. The medial portion of the craniotomy should be approximately 2 to 3 cm from midline. The bone flap should be brought low across the frontal bone, across the sphenoid wing, below the pterion to the temporal bone. The opening is further enlarged by resection of the lateral portion of the sphenoid wing (Fig. 11).

Dural opening: The incision is begun in the temporal region, a continuation of the dural temporal opening if an initial temporal craniectomy and dural incision have been made, or the anterior frontal region (Fig. 12). With this approach, if the brain herniates through the dura because of mass effect, the herniated cerebral tissue will be part of a relatively silent lobe. This herniation usually occurs only when the temporal or frontal tip is severely contused. The remainder of the dural opening can then be completed with little further herniation of tissue. If intact cortex begins to herniate, further maneuvers to reduce brain swelling should be instituted immediately: additonal mannitol, increased hyperventilation, barbiturates, and perhaps even transient reduction of arterial blood pres-

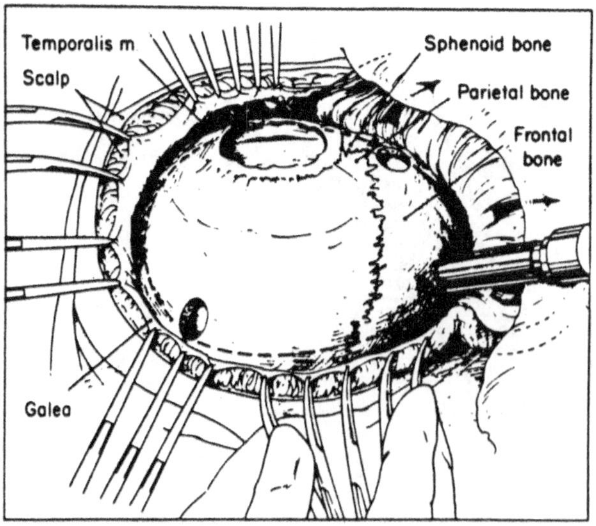

Fig. 11. Either a free bone flap or one based on the temporal muscle can be raised. The medial portion of the bone flap should be 2 to 3 cm from the midline. Far anterior placement of the forward holes permits easy access to anterior temporal lobe and orbital gyri

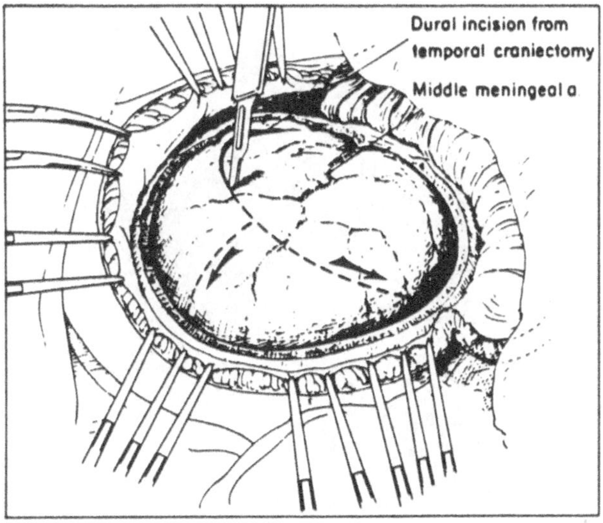

Fig. 12. The dural opening shown here provides safe access to basal, midline, and anterior regions

sure to reduce and relieve cerebrovascular engorgement. The dural opening should be curved gently as it is carried anteriorly up to the anterior medial border of the bone flap. An incision from the center of this dural flap, directed posteriomedially, will complete the opening. This dural opening provides access to the frontal and temporal lobes and the anterior and middle fossae.

The vast majority of unilateral intracranial hemorrhages and contusions can now be dealt with. The lateral parietal and occipital cortex may be inspected, but is not fully exposed. The orbital gyri are readily accessible, as are the inferior temporal gyrus and more basal structures. Inspection of the basal structures can be accomplished, if necessary. Hemorrhage from the middle meningeal artery is readily controlled, even down to the foramen spinosum. The intracranial surface of the sagittal sinus is exposed and hemorrhage from avulsed emissary cortical veins can be controlled without further bone resection or undue retraction on the brain.

The Acute Subdural Hematoma

Acute subdural hematoma should always be dealt with via the large craniotomy, never through burr holes or a limited temporal craniectomy [34, 35]. In fact, a rule to follow in all subdural hematomas, regardless of the age of the lesion, is that if any clotted blood is present, a craniotomy flap should be turned down [36]. Once the dura is opened, the clot should be gently removed from the cortical surface (Fig. 13). Removal of the clot is best done with a combination of irrigation, cup forceps evacuation, and gentle suction. Large fragments of clot that are over the occipital lobe or on the floor of the anterior or middle fossae can be gently washed and teased out. These large fragments can be exposed by placing a brain retractor over the appropriate lobe and allowing the colt to ex-

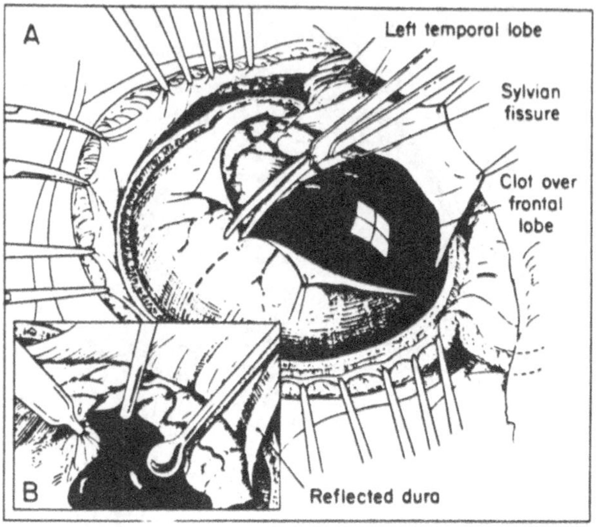

Fig. 13. A) A typical acute subdural hematoma is shown here. B) After the dura is open, the clot should be gently removed by means of irrigation, forceps extraction, and careful suctioning

trude slowly to be extracted with forceps. Tiny bits of clot under the dura and bone should not be vigorously pursued.

A bleeding major surface artery or vein will often be identified after the clot is removed [29]. It can usually be sealed by bipolar coagulation. If the bleeding is coming from a midline bridging vein, a middle fossa vessel, or a vessel that is located under the intact dura and bone, great care must be taken in exposing and controlling the bleeding vessel. In the management of an avulsed bridging vein, the cortical open end is usually easily controlled with bipolar coagulation. The sinus side of the vessel may be troublesome, and if bipolar coagulation or Gelfoam or operative packing fails, a small piece of beaten muscle carefully placed directly over the venous opening will usually produce satisfactory hemostasis (Fig. 14).

Cerebral Contusion in Association with the Acute Subdural Hematoma

Contusions usually appear on the surface of the anterior and inferior frontal lobes and the temporal lobes (Fig. 15). They are composed of necrotic brain tissue that is infiltrated with blood. The brain tissue in a confluent contusion is irreversibly and irreparably destroyed and not only serves as a primary mass lesion but may go on to cause further major brain swelling in and around itself; for this reason necrotic contusions should be removed when exposed at operation. Surface contusions larger than 2 cm in diameter should be removed. Often a surface contusion 2 cm in diameter will extend several centimeters or more deep into the hemisphere, and the cortical edge of the contusion is only the "tip of the iceberg".

Once the contusion is exposed it should be gently sucked out. The soft, friable, wet, purple-blue necrotic tissue can be easily aspirated. Suction should continue

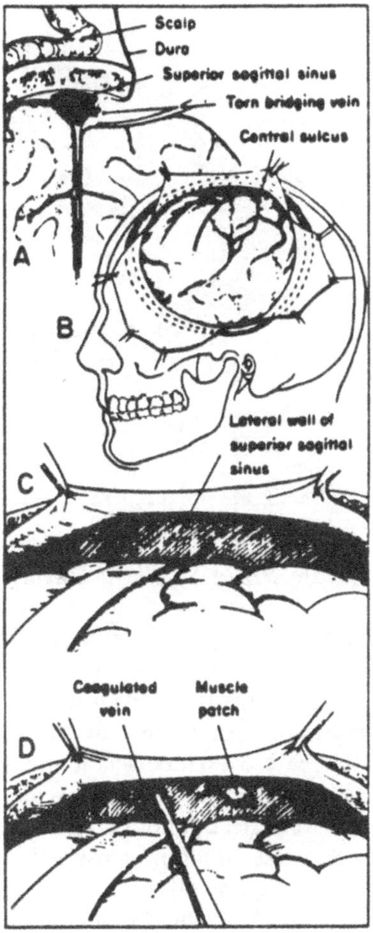

Fig. 14. A) Bleeding from avulsed midline bridging veins commonly occurs after evacuation of the hematoma or contusion. B,C,D) Simple coagulation will often suffice, but a patch of beaten muscle is still the finest hemostatic agent when sinus bleeding from an avulsed draining vein is not easily controlled with coagulation or synthetic hemostatic agents

until a circumferential margin of healthy brain tissue is reached. One should not hesitate to aspirate all necrotic tissue, even in multiple sites, over the anterior temporal and frontal lobes. Contusions over the more posterior superior temporal lobe, or in the region of the central sulcus or the parietal or occipital lobes, should be carefully evaluated, and if they are clearly large necrotic contusions, they should also be removed. Removing contusions in these areas will not increase the neurological deficit if one works entirely within the contusion, and ultimate postoperative neurological function may be surprisingly good even when contusions are removed from areas near the primary motor cortex and surface speech centers. The secondary brain edema that occurs around the contusions can be reduced by operative removal and the postoperative clinical status and ultimate result may be improved [28, 37].

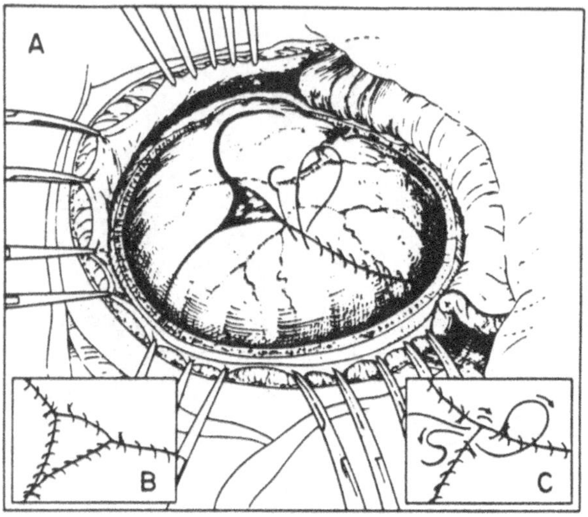

Fig. 15. A) Complete closure of the dura, using a graft if necessary, is recommended for a number of reasons, the most important being that this will help keep the brain from herniating through the craniotomy site over bony edges. The bone flap is also replaced, if at all possible, and fixed in place with non-metallic sutures. B) The graft. C) Detail of suture pattern

Acute Brain Swelling During Operation

Occassionally, sudden and rapid massive brain swelling will occur during an operation. The swelling may occur immediately after dural opening, or sometimes moments or even many minutes after a large clot or contusion has been excised. A probable cause is defective cerebral autoregulation. With the sudden decrease of extravascular pressure that occurs at dural opening or mass lesion evacuation, the cerebrovascular bed distends passively from the arterial blood pressure head, and a sizable increase in cerebral blood volume results [38]. The other less common cause is from new acute intraoperative hemorrhage and the rapid accumulation of a clot contralateral to the craniotomy or in an ipsilateral area hidden from the operative exposure. True brain edema occurring as rapidly as this is only rarely the cause of such intraoperative swelling, and even then is probably associated with cerebral vasodilation.

Intraoperative brain swelling must be dealt with promptly and aggressively. Thiopental (500 mg in an adult) will often produce dramatic detumescence of the swollen brain and permit brain relocation [39]. The barbiturate reduces cerebral blood flow, blood volume and often arterial blood pressure. Reduction of systolic arterial blood pressure to 60 to 90 mm Hg will almost always permit the brain to return to its normal position. Simultaneously the anesthesiologist should rapidly administer even more mannitol and increase the tidal volume to further lower the arterial carbon dioxide tension. After 2 to 4 min the blood pressure should be allowed to seek its own level naturally again. Often, this combination of maneuvers will capture and reverse the acute swelling. The induced hypotension must be avoided or severe brain ischemia will ensue.

If the preceding maneuvers fail to relocate the brain within the skull, a frontal or temporal lobectomy may be necessary for internal decompression. An internal decompression by a frontal or temporal lobectomy should ordinarily be done only if one of these lobes shows some evidence of contusion or hemorrhage. All reasonable maneuvers should be considered to get the brain back into place to permit bone flap replacement [40].

Closure of the craniotomy flap: Complete closure of the dura and replacement of the bone flap should always be done, if possible, and may require a periosteal graft (Fig. 15). Dural closure is recommended because postoperative extradural bleeding is kept out of the subarachnoid space; cortical adhesions to soft tissues are less likely; cerebrospinal fluid wound leak or fistulae may be reduced; any wound infection that may occur will more likely be isolated to the extradural space; and dural closure, even with a graft, helps keep the brain from herniating through the craniectomy site across the bony edges.

Unless brain swelling is massive and cannot be controlled, the bone flap should be replaced and fixed in place with suture material. Brain that herniates through a bony defect usually undergoes infarction and dies, and large craniectomies have not reduced the mortality rate or morbidity [40–43].

In fact, this "herniated" brain that extends out over bony edges tends to develop progressively increasing edema that extends deep into white matter and may go on to involve the entire hemisphere. Brain swelling and elevated ICP in the postoperative period are best managed by medical means in the intensive care unit, and the bone flap should not be left out because the surgeon anticipates delayed brain swelling [23].

Following skin closure the patient should not be extubated but should be taken to the recovery room or intensive care unit and immediately connected to a volume respirator. This prevents early postanesthesia bucking and straining, and permits smooth continuation of controlled ventilation and total care of the helpless patient [25].

References

1. Miller JS, Butterworth JF, Gudeman SK, et al (1981) Further experience in the management of severe head injury. J Neurosurg 54:289–299
2. Langfitt TW (1978) Measuring the outcome from head injuries. J Neurosurg 48:673–678
3. Miller JD, Becker DP, Ward JD, Sullivan HG, Adams WE, Rosner MJ (1977) Significance of intracranial hypertension in severe head injury. J Neurosurg 47:503–516
4. Lewelt W, Jenkins LW, Miller JD (1980) Autoregulation of cerebral blood flow after experimental fluid percussion injury of the brain. J Neurosurg 53:500
5. Lewelt W, Jenkins LW, Miller JD (1982) Effects of experimental fluid percussion injury of the brain on cerebrovascular reactivity to hypoxia and hypercapnia. J Neurosurg 56:332
6. Seelig JM, Becker DP, Miller JD, Greenberg RP, Ward JD, Choi SC (1981) Traumatic acute subdural hematoma: Major mortality reduction in comatose patients treated under four hours. N Engl J Med 304:1511–1518
7. Ransohoff J, Benjamin MV, Gage EL, et al (1971) Hemi-craniectomy in the management of acute subdural hematoma. J Neurosurg 34:70–76
8. Richards T, Hoff J (1974) Factors affecting survival from acute subdural hematoma. Surgery 75:253–258
9. Anderson DC, Cranford RE (1979) Corticosteroids in ischemic stroke. Stroke 10:68–71
10. Marcoux FW, Morawetz RB, Crowell RM, et al (1982) Differential regional vulnerability in transient focal cerebral ischemia. Stroke 13:339–346

11. Branston NM, Strong AJ, Symon L (1977) Extracellular potassium activity, evoked potential and tissue blood flow; Relationship during progressive ischemia in baboon cerebral cortex. J Neurol Sci 32:305–321
12. Muizelaar JP, Becker DP, Lutz HA (1985) Present application and future promise of cerebral blood flow monitoring in head injury. In: Dacey RG, Winn RH, Rimel RW, Jane JA (eds) Trauma of the central nervous system. Raven Press, New York, pp 91–102
13. Roberson FC, Kishore PRS, Miller HD, Lipper MH, Becker DP (1979) The value of serial computerized tomography in the management of severe head injury. Surg Neurol 12:161–167
14. Kishore PRS, Lipper MH, Becker DP, daSilva AA, Narayan RK, Miller HD (1981) The significance of CT in head injury: correlation with intracranial pressure. AJNR 2:307–311
15. Lipper MH, Kishore PRS, Girevendulis AK, Miller JD, Becker DP (1979) Delayed intracranial hematoma in patients with severe head injury. Radiology 133:645–649
16. Gudeman SK, Kishore PRS, Miller JD, Girevendulis AK, Lipper MH, Becker DP (1979) The genesis and significance of delayed traumatic intracerebral hematoma. Neurosurgery
17. Narayan RK, Greenberg RP, Miller HD, et al (1981) Improved confidence of outcome prediction in severe head injury: a comparative analysis of the clinical examination, multimodality evoked potentials, CT and ICP. J Neurosurg 54:751–762
18. Seelig JM, Greenberg RP, Becker DP, Miller JD, Choi SC (1981) Reversible brain stem dysfunction following acute traumatic subdural hematoma: A clinical and electrophysiological study. J Neurosurg 55:516–523
19. Gutterman P, Shenkin HA (1970) Prognostic features in recovery from traumatic decerebration. J Neurosurg 32:330–335
20. Reilly PL, Graham DI, Adams JH, et al (1975) Patients with head injury who talk and die. Lancet 2:375–377
21. Rose J, Valtonen S, Jennett B (1977) Avoidable factors contributing to death after head injury. Br Med J 2:615–618
22. Miller JD, Becker DP, Ward JD, Sullivan HG, Adams WE, Rosner MJ (1977) Significance of intracranial hypertension in severe head injury. J Neurosurg 47:503–506
23. Becker DP, Vries JK, Young HF, et al (1975) Controlled cerebral perfusion pressure and ventilation in mechanical brain injury: Prevention of progressive brain swelling. In: Lundberg N, Ponten U, Brock M (eds) Intracranial pressure II. Springer, Berlin Heidelberg New York, pp 480–484
24. Becker DP, Miller JD, Young HF, et al (1976) The critical importance of intracranial pressure monitoring in head injury. In: Becks JWF, Bosch DA, Brock M (eds) Intracranial pressure III. Springer, Berlin Heidelberg New York, pp 97–100
25. Becker DP, Miller JD, Young HF, et al (1982) Diagnosis and treatment of head injury in adults. In: Youmans JR (ed) Neurological surgery, vol 4. WB Saunders, Philadelphia, pp 1938–2083.
26. Ward JD, Becker DP (1983) Neurosurgery of head injury. In: Ransohoff J (ed) Modern technics in surgery. Futura, New York
27. Gurdjian EA, Thomas LM (1974) Traumatic intracranial hemorrhage. In: Feiring EH (ed) Brock's injuries of the brain and spinal cord and their coverings, 5th edn. Springer, Berlin Heidelberg New York, pp 203–267
28. Becker DP, Miller JD, Sweet RC, Sweet JD, et al (1979) Head injury management. In: Popp AJ, Bourke RS, Nelson LR, Kimelberg HK (eds) Neural trauma, seminars in neurological surgery. Raven Press, New York, pp 313–328
29. Chambers JW (1951) Acute subdural hematoma. J Neurosurg 8:263–268
30. Fell DA, Fitzgerald S, Moiel RH, Caram P (1975) Acute subdural hematomas: a review of 144 cases. J Neurosurg 42:27–42
31. Davis LE (1946) The principles of neurological surgery. Lea & Febiger, Philadelphia
32. Gibbs JR (1960) Middle meningeal hemorrhage. Lancet 2:727–731
33. McKissock W, Richardson A, Bloom WH (1960) Subdural hematoma; a review of 389 cases. Lancet 1:1365–1369
34. Richards T, Hoff J (1974) Factors affecting survival from acute subdural hematoma. Surgery 75:253–258
35. Whaley N (1948) Acute subdural hematoma amenable to surgical treatment. Lancet 1:213–214

36. Bucy PC, Oberhill HR (1968) Subdural hematoma in adults. Arizona Med 25:186–189
37. Heiskanen O, Vapalahti M (1972) Temporal lobe contusion and hematoma. Acta Neurochir (Wien) 27:29–35
38. Kobrine AJ, Timmons E, Rajjoub JK, et al (1977) Demonstration of massive traumatic brain swelling within 20 minutes after injury. J Neurosurg 46:256–258
39. Ward JD, Becker DP, Marmarou A, et al (1985) Failure of prophylactic barbiturate coma in the treatment of severe head injury. J Neurosurg 62:383–388
40. Cooper PR, Rovit RL, Ransohoff J (1976) Hemicraniectomy in the treatment of acute subdural hematoma: a re-appraisal. Surg Neurol 5:25–28
41. Clark K, Nash TM, Hutchinson GC (1968) The failure of circumferential craniotomy in acute traumatic cerebral swelling. J Neurosurg 29:367–371
42. Kjellberg RN, Prieto A Jr (1971) Bifrontal decompressive craniotomy for massive cerebral edema. J Neurosurg 34:488–493
43. Ransohoff J, Benjamin MV, Gage EL Jr, Epstein F (1971) Hemicraniectomy in the management of acute subdural hematoma. J Neurosurg 34:70–76

Prognosis of Brain Failure in the Intensive Care Unit

M. Hemmer

Introduction

Patients with acute brain failure due to traumatic injury, subarachnoid and intracerebral hemorrage, stroke and ischemic-anoxic brain damage are frequently encountered in the Intensive Care Unit. It is a well known and puzzling fact that within the groups of patients with the same etiology of brain failure, there can be a great variability in the recovery from cerebral damage that appears initially to be clinically similar. Therefore, the identification of prognostic factors, in the early stage of brain failure is very important. Early prediction of ultimate disability after brain damage orientates the clinical decision in individual patient, facilitates family counselling and allows the definition of subpopulation of patients with a similar potential for recovery, in whom the efficacy of various prophylactic and therapeutic regimens may be assessed in prospective studies.

The selection of factors with predictive power requires a longlasting prospective collection of numerous variables in computerized data banks and their subsequent statistical analysis in relation to outcome. For this purpose, outcome scales which classify and quantify the ultimate degree of combined mental and neurological deficit and which can be used for both traumatic and non-traumatic brain damage have been devised. Their reliability has been confirmed by a high interobserver agreement rate [1, 2].

The generally adopted assessment of outcome in individual patients is the Glasgow Outcome Scale (GOS) devised by Jennett and Bond in 1975 (Table 1). This five point scale, based more on functional than neurological aspects of recovery, classifies the outcome categories as death, vegetative state, severe disability, moderate disability and good recovery.

Many studies on prognostic factors use for simplification of statistical analysis, a binary assessment of outcome (survival/death) or a three point contracted

Table 1. Glasgow Outcome Scale

Dead	
Vegetative state	(nonscient survival)
Severe disability	(conscious but dependent)
Moderate disability	(independent but disabled)
Good recovery	(able to participate in normal social life)

scale where "good outcome" corresponds to both the categories of good recovery and moderate disability, "bad outcome" corresponds to severe disability and the third category encompasses death and vegetative state. On the other hand, when the rate and the degree of recovery have to be analyzed in more detail, an extended scale is sometimes used which stratifies the degree of the disability in the three upper categories into a better and a worse grade; then the outcome scale is divided into eight categories. However, the use of the more extended scale diminishes the rate of interobserver agreement in the determination of the outcome categories and decreases the accuracy of prediction [3].

Neuropsychological outcome, - the assessment of intellectual and behavioral function of survivors from brain damage-, may be evaluated by a battery of standard neuropsychological tests examining higher cognitive function, new problem solving skills, focused attention, concentration and memory.

The assessment of outcome from traumatic head injury, has been particularly well studied. Trumatic brain injury is a complex and dynamic pathology which combines the features of the primary impact and the secondary ischemic/anoxic brain damage and exhibits the presence of both diffuse and focal cerebral lesions. Therefore the prognostic factors which are predictive in traumatic brain injury and reflect the severity of general cerebral dysfunction are also valid in non traumatic causes of brain failure, such as intracerebral hemorrhage, subarachnoidal hemorrhage, stroke or ischemic/anoxic brain damage.

Prognosis in Brain Failure After Severe Head Trauma

Several studies have shown that the severity of the initial injury is the major determinant of prognosis after severe head trauma [4, 5]. The severity of the initial injury may be evaluated by the level of impaired consciousness (categorized by standard assessment scales), the degree of impairment of brain stem reflexes, radiological diagnosis (CT and MRI classification of the injury patterns) and electrophysiological findings (abnormalities in multimodal evoked potentials) [6-10]. An assessment based on biochemical evaluation has also been proposed as biochemical markers can indicate the magnitude of the stress response, the degree of impairment of cellular metabolism and the extent of cellular destruction [11-14].

Age is a major independent factor affecting the outcome in the head injury [15-19]. The clinical course of the disease, including the duration of coma and of posttraumatic amnesia (PTA) is also important [20].

Poot outcome has been associated with the development of secondary ischemic/hypoxic brain damage, which is related to alterations in cerebral hemodynamics, and may be due to several intracranial and extracranial factors (intracranial hypertension, systemic hypotension, hypoxia and anemia..) [21-25]. The management of head injured patients, including pre-hospital care, initial resuscitation, surgical treatment, ventilatory and hemodynamic support, treatment of incranial hypertension, cerebral metabolic protection and nutritional support may also influence outcome.

The Predictive Value of Standard Assessment Scales

Several assessment scales have been suggested to evaluate the degree of acute brain dysfunction, and predict outcome [26]. In order to be widely accepted, such scales should be reliable, practical and validated by a high interobserver agreement rate [2].

The Glasgow Coma Scale (GCS) was originally designed as a system of three separate scores for assessing arousal (E = eye opening), awareness (V = verbal response) and motor ability (M = motor response) of the head-injured patient during the acute stages [6] (Table 2). Later, the GCS score (E + M + V) was proposed to compare groups of patients with similar degrees of impaired responsiveness and was extended to brain failure of other etiologies [27–29]. The GCS definition of coma (no eye opening, no spoken word and inability to obey commands = GCS score $\leqslant$ 8) and the subdivision of head injury into severe (GCS 3–8), moderate (GCS 9–12) and minor (GCS 13–15) injury are commonly used [26]. It has been demonstrated that GCS score is well correlated with outcome in the patients with head trauma or other acute brain disorders [1, 29].

However, many difficulties occur in assessing the GCS score in the clinical situation: sedation, eye swelling and intubation render the E and V scores less reliable. In many studies the assessment of patients' responsiveness and its relationship to outcome are based on the 6 points of the motor scale alone, or on the practice of pseudoscoring, i.e. the adoption of an estimated value of 1 for untestable response. Although the evaluation of the motor score may be influenced by the patients' body posture during testing and the site of stimulation [30], a global agreement rate of 73% for the motor response was reported by Born et al. [31]. Jagger et al has recently suggested that the motor score alone yields a better prediction of outcome than the sum of the three GCS scores [32].

Because of these difficulties in the assessment of the GCS, a more simple scale has been proposed which provides basically the same information with a better interobserver agreement, especially in the categories corresponding to the middle ranges of GCS [33]. Nevertheless the GCS remains the most widely used scale in patients with acute brain disorder. A recent survey of the neurosurgical literature reported that the majority of studies using this scoring system made no reference to methodological problems [26]. The authors suggest that the use of the GCS should be standardized regarding time of the patients' assessment, def-

Table 2. Glasgow Coma Scale (GCS)

Eye opening	Score	Verbal response	Score	Motor response	Score
Spontaneously	4	Orientated	5	Obeys	6
To speech	3	Confused	4	Localizes	5
To pain	2	Inappropriate	3	Withdraws	4
No response	1	Incomprehensive	2	Abnormal flexion	3
		No response	1	Extension	2
				No response	1

Table 3. Glasgow-Liège Scale (GLS)

Eye opening	Score	Verbal response	Score	Motor response	Score	Brain stem reflexes	Score
Spontaneously	4	Orientated	5	Obeys	6	Fronto-orbicular	5
To speech	3	Confused	4	Localizes	5	Vertical oculovestibular	4
To pain	2	Inappropriate	3	Withdraws	4	Pupillary light	3
No response	1	Incomprehensive	2	Abnormal flexion	3	Horizontal oculovestibular	2
		No response	1	Extension	2	Oculo-cardiac	1
				No response	1	No response	0

inition of coma, pseudoscoring and use of combined scores. After this, further studies of the reliability of the CGS may be necessary.

The best early GCS score obtained, after initial resuscitation, accurately predicts prognosis in about 60% of patients. The accuracy is much better for low scores related to bad outcome and higher (> 6) scores related to meaningful survival than for the intermediate scores [3–6, 33, 34].

A GCS score of 5 appears to be a critical level where patients outcome is most difficult to predict [31, 33, 35].

The confidence of prediction can be increased when the evaluation of pupillary light reflexes and spontaneous and reflex eye movements are combined with the GCS [7].

The Glasgow – Liege Coma Scale provides in addition to the classical EMV score, a scoring system based on the order of disappearance of brain stem reflexes due to the rostrocaudal spread of the injury. This scale has a better predictive value than the GCS alone especially for the patients with a GCS score of 5 (Table 3). Born et al. have recently reported that the combination of the motor response score together with the brain-stem reflexes score permits a correct prediction of the three categories of outcome in 74% of the patients [31, 35].

The Influence of Age

Several reports suggest that outcome from brain injury is better in children than in adults. This relationship might be dependent of the patient selection, the injury mechanism, the therapeutic modalities, and the lower incidence of surgical mass lesions in children [15–19].

A recent prospective multicenter study compared pediatric and adult patients, treated with the same protocol in the same institutions. Mechanism and severity of brain injury, presence of associated traumatic lesions and presence of subdural or epidural hematomas were correlated with posttraumatic mortality [18]. Pediatric patients had a significantly lower mortality rate through all ranges of severity of head injury except those who had a subdural hematoma or who were profoundly hypotensive at admission. In contrast to adults, the mortality in the pediatric groups declines with age, the lowest rate being at the age of 12 years.

Alberico et al. also demonstrated after severe head injury a better outcome in pediatric than in adult patients with the exception of the very young (0 to 4 years of age) children with surgical mass lesion and those with increased ICP [17].

Both studies have shown that the more favorable outcome in children cannot be explained only by a lower incidence of surgical mass lesions and that age itself is a major independent prognostic factor in brain injury. In both studies, patients over 40 years of age had higher mortality rates and poorer outcome than young adults.

Development of a Model for Prediction Based on Clinical Variables

An early specific prediction model of outcome expressed in four categories (good recovery, moderate disability, severe disability and vegetative state/death) has recently been developed by Choi et al. [36]. The authors based their model on data prospectively collected from 523 severe head trauma patients. They analyzed 21 variables, recorded after initial cardiopulmonary stabilization. Several factors (the three separate scores of GCS, age, oculocephalic reflexes, midline shift, pupillary size and response, hematocrit, cardiac and respiratory rate and time from injury to admission) had some prognostic value when used alone, but the combination of the three factors of age, motor score and pupillary response yielded a highly predictive model of outcome. This model correctly predicted the outcome into four categories in 78% of cases and allowed "grossly accurate predictions" (predictions into an outcome category adjacent to the actual outcome were accepted) in 90% of cases.

CT and MRI Injury Patterns

Computed tomography (CT) imaging on admission reveals rapidly and noninvasively brain abnormalities related to trauma and indicates the severity of the initial lesions. In 1982, Generelli et al proposed various categories of CT patterns of injury and showed that CT classification could be used together with the clinical evaluation of the severity of injury by GCS to predict prognosis [8]. In 1983 Lobato classified the CT findings into eight distinctive patterns related to outcome [9]. Three of these patterns, i.e. extracerebral hematoma with acute hemispheric swelling (pattern 2), multiple unilateral brain contusion with or without subdural hematoma (pattern 4) and diffuse axonal injury (pattern 7), were related very significantly to a poor outcome. Multiple bilateral brain contusions (pattern 5) and a normal CT (pattern 8) yielded both good and bad outcome scores. The best prognosis was in patients with pure extracerebral hematoma (pattern 1), general brain swelling without focal injury (pattern 6) and single brain contusion (pattern 3).

More recent studies have demonstrated the importance of midline shift, the degree of obliteration of cerebrospinal fluid spaces and the volume of mixed high and low density lesions in the prediction of the development of elevated ICP. The combination of the two CT features-midline shift and the status of the

mesencephalic cisterns is the best predictor of mortality [21, 23, 25]. It has also been reported that non-lateralized diffuse swelling on CT is frequently associated with early posttraumatic hypoxia and that a rapidly developing massive swelling of a single cerebral hemisphere is associated with the high incidence of arterial hypotension and/or hypoxemia at admission [21, 25]. Although the initial CT patterns are highly indicative of the severity of injury, CT imaging alone does not produce an absolute prognosis. Repetitive neurological assessment and results of ICP monitoring evaluated together with serial CT scanning may improve the predictive value.

Early magnetic resonance imaging (MRI) is more sensitive than CT in visualizing cortical, subcortical and deep white matter lesions. It may be particularly useful in patients with normal CT-scan and with CT patterns suggestive of diffuse anoxal injury. However, a MRI examination is time consuming and the technical restrictions due to the application of a high powered magnetic field make its use difficult in the acute situation [37, 38].

Late MRI findings are particularly useful to visualize residual posttraumatic brain lesions and especially to detect functionally significant deep intracerebral abnormalities and ventricular enlargement, which are associated with poor neuropsychological outcome in brain injured patients [37, 38].

Multimodality Evoked Potentials

Multimodality evoked potentials are good indicators of outcome in brain injury [10]. It has been demonstrated that mild abnormalities recorded after injury are indicative of a favorable outcome, while severe deficits are rarely compatible with survival or recovery of consciousness with the exception of a focal abnormality. (see chapter on somatosensory evoked responses)

Biochemical and Metabolic Markers of Brain Injury

Biochemical markers of severe head injury are a direct consequence of the neurological lesion and their concentration in CSF reflects the extent of structural brain damage. The principal markers are glycolytic and mitochondrial enzymes such as creatine kinase (CK), lactate dehydrogenase (LDH) and neuron specific enolase (NSE) released from the membranes of dead cells. CSF CK-BB seems to provide the best correlation with the impairment of consciousness (assessed by Glasgow-Liege Coma Scale) and prognosis [12].

Early posttraumatic elevation of CK-BB has a high predictive value as an indicator of poor outcome and reflects the severity of initial lesion. Delayed elevations in the CK-BB, also associated with a poor outcome, may reflect secondary brain damage.

Traumatic brain injury activates the sympathetic nervous system, induces a massive release of catecholamines and initiates a cascade of deleterious events which result in severe metabolic and systemic disturbances. Woolf et al. have recently demonstrated that the postinjury levels of norepinephrine, epinephrine

and dopamine reflect the severity of the neurological insult and enhance the reliability of GCS in assessing the severity of injury. Circulating norepinephrine levels may be used as independent predictors of outcome in both the acute and chronic phases of traumatic brain injury [13].

Brain tissue acidosis, due to cellular hypoxia or impaired metabolism, is considered to play an important role in the clinical course of severe head injury [39]. A high CSF lactate concentration is observed early after trauma and its decrease to normal value in the following 48 hours is a reliable sign of improvement. Lactate levels remaining elevated or increasing over time indicate neurological deterioration. Monitoring of CSF lactate levels via a ventricular catheter has been proposed to evaluate prognosis [14].

However a recent study of Inao et al. has suggested that the post-injury CSF lactate elevation is due to both the systemic and cerebral response to trauma, and recommended caution in interpreting elevated CSF lactate levels following head injury [40].

Intracranial Pressure, Cerebral Blood Flow, and Cerebral Metabolic Rate

There is overwhelming evidence that increased intracranial pressure (ICP) is associated with poor prognosis in head injury. Several studies have shown an inverse correlation between the elevated ICP and outcome [22, 24, 25, 41]. In ICP above 20 Torr is related to an increase in mortality and an ICP above 50–60 Torr, is almost universally fatal, irrespective of any other features.

Recent studies have shown that not only are the absolute value and duration of an elevated ICP important in prediction of outcome but also the agressiveness of therapy to control ICP. In some patients the intracranial hypertension is a secondary manifestation and a physiological marker of irreversible brain swelling due to a progressive lesion of the neurons and the endothelial cells, set in motion either by the initial traumatic insult or by secondary ischemic/anoxic brain damage. In this setting a temporary decrease in ICP with very agressive treatement does not improve the prognosis.

The values of cerebral perfusion pressure (CPP) representing the difference between mean arterial pressure (MAP) and ICP have also been used in prediction of outcome. Changaris et al. have postulated that the average CPP is a better predictor than ICP or MAP alone and have also suggested that its optimal value should be greater than 80 mmHg. A "critical" level of CPP lower than 40 mmHg seems to be of particular importance in the development of secondary ischemic brain damage [34].

Several studies have shown that posttraumatic brain failure is associated with cerebral blood flows (CBF) ranging from reduced to hyperhemic. Different CBF patterns are also observed in patients with different types of injury. Because of these large variations of early posttraumatic measurements the initial CBF values are not predictive of outcome [42].

Cerebral metabolic rates ($CMRO_2$) are uniformely low in patients with a poor outcome. They have a better predictive value than CBF [42]. When serial measurement of CBF and $CMRO_2$ are performed, CBF declines to very low levels in

all patients who die while both CBF and $CMRO_2$ increase in patients who survive [42]. Recently, Uzell et al. showed that the presence of early hyperemia, especially when related to intracranial hypertension, may influence the neuropsychological outcome in conscious survivors of severe head injury, assessed one year after trauma [43]. Early hyperemia appeared to be associated with an overall intellectual and memory impairment whereas intracranial hypertension was associated with both general and specific memory deficits.

Influence of Pre-hospital Care and Impact of Associated Lesions

Improved pre-hospital care and rapid transport has been shown to decrease the mortality rate in head injury [44]. High quality pre-hospital care is important for patients with acute respiratory disturbances and systemic hypotension following injury as the deleterious role of hypoxia has been well shown [22, 25, 45].

A recent study demonstrated that both early posttraumatic hypotension and hypertension were associated with higher mortality rates in adults, but only hypotension was related to a poor outcome in children [18]. The presence of associated traumatic injuries other than spinal trauma significantly increased mortality both in adults and children. This effect was most pronounced for chest and abdominal injuries [18].

Kraus et al. have shown that in severe head trauma patients who survive the first 24 hours, 52% of subsequent deaths are due to irreversible brain failure and 48% to associated systemic causes such as respiratory failure, pulmonary infection, sepsis, peritonitis and cardiac disorders [46].

Influence of Therapy

In the late seventies, several reports emerged claiming that a standardized aggressive treatment protocol which included early detection and removal of mass lesions, routine mechanical ventilation and routine use of therapeutic regimens to lower the ICP and to provide cerebral protection may improve the outcome in brain injured patients. Undoubtedly, surgical decompression within four hours improves the prognosis of acute subdural hematoma which usually carries the highest mortality rate of all traumatic lesions [47]. A standard management protocol including prophylactic hyperventilation, CSF drainage, osmotherapy and prophylactic administration of hypnotic agents has been recommended for cerebral protection and lowering ICP [48].

However, each component of this prophylactic regimen has a different mechanism of action, and their individual effect on brain homeostasis is influenced by cerebral hemodynamics and metabolism. Several randomized trials have failed to show any improvement in outcome with the prophylactic use of "blanket" therapies such as steroids [49], barbiturates [50], and hyperventilation [51]. A more selective choice of treatment for cerebral protection, based on bedside evaluation of the cerebral metabolism and circulation, and guided by continuous monitoring of ICP, CPP and cerebral electrical activity is nowadays advocated.

New randomized trials in carefully selected homogenous groups of head injured patients are necessary to demonstrate the net effect of these therapies on outcome.

Patients with severe brain injury are hypercatabolic and exhibit the systemic post-injury acute phase response which may complicate recovery. For these reasons it has been agreed that they should be provided with early nutritional support. However, disturbances of gastrointestinal motility and intolerance to enteral feeding are frequently observed in the early posttraumatic period. Young et al. have recently demonstrated that the administration of total parenteral nutrition, which permits the earlier delivery of more proteins and calories, was related to a better outcome at 3 months, than the use of enteral nutrition, but the final outcome at 1 year was similar [52].

Neuropsychological Outcome

Neuropsychological outcome and residual deficits in conscious survivors of head trauma are significantly related to the severity of brain injury and the pre-injury IQ of the patient [53]. The majority (about 80%) of brain injured patients have even in the good outcome categories some residual neuropsychological deficit.

Recently, Uzell et al. have investigated the relationship between the severity of injury determined by the GCS and the quality of survival. Although severely head injured patients (GCS $\leq$ 8) had more neuropsychological impairment in areas of intelligence, attention, memory, oculomotor speed and motor skills than those with moderate and mild (GCS $>$ 8) injuries, both groups were below normal in areas of learning, memory and oculomotor speed. An effect of age on neuropsychological outcome does appear important in minor head injuries. However, unemployment increases after both severe and minor brain injury [54].

Severe brain injury carries a mortality rate of 30% to 50%. It remains the most common cause of death under the age of fourty years in industrialized countries. Ten to 20% of brain injured patients become severely disabled or permanently vegetative and require constant institutional care. The majority of survivors classified into good outcome categories present with intellectual, behavioral and emotional difficulties and need prolonged rehabilitation programs and psychological counselling for themselves and their families.

Prognosis in Brain Failure Due to Cerebrovascular Disease

Acute ischemic stroke (embolic or thrombotic), intracerebral hemorrage (ICH) and subarachnoid hemorrage (SAH) are the most frequent manifestations of cerebrovascular disease in ICU patients.

Prognosis in Stroke

Acute ischemic stroke is one of the most common causes of death in Western industrialized countries and a leading cause of permanent disability. Hypertension, diabetes mellitus, cardiac disease with arrhythmias, obesity and cigarette smoking have been recognized as important risk factors.

A quantitative assessment of the neurological deficit following stroke may be obtained by the GCS or any other scoring system. The Mathew scale has been most frequently used although a recent Dutch study demonstrated a considerable interobserver disagreement for this assessment scale [55]. The ideal classification system should differentiate the various subcategories of stroke and provide a severity score. Ideally it would include initial clinical evaluation, natural history, CT and MRI neuroimaging, determination of the vascular anatomy by noninvasive studies and angiography, together with functional studies such as single photon emission computed tomography (SPECT), positron emission tomography (PET) and xenon cerebral blood flow [56]. Such a classification could be used to predict outcome in well selected subgroups of stroke patients with similar etiologic features and also for the evaluation of efficacy of randomized therapeutic trials. However, most recent studies on outcome from stroke have centered on clinical and CT findings only or employ a very general WHO definition of stroke.

Age, presence of coma and severity of motor deficit at the onset of stroke have been shown to be the most important factors predicting mortality [57, 58]. A recent Australian, community based study, in unselected stroke patients demonstrated that the combined factors of age, state of consciousness and place of residence (home versus institutional care; which may reflect the degree of prestroke independence) were the strongest early predictors of mortality at 3 years. The survival rate of people living at home at the onset of stroke and remaining conscious, was 58% compared with 5% in those who were in institutional care and became comatose. Marital status, ethnic group and history of recurrent stroke were also predictors of mortality [58].

Prognosis in Hypertensive Intracerebral Hematoma

Intracerebral hematoma (ICH) is a potentially lethal manifestation of cerebrovascular disease. Prediction of outcome of ICH of nontraumatic and traumatic origin has been investigated [59–61]. A prognostic model based on multivariate discrimination analysis with stepwise logistic regression has been recently proposed by Portenoy et al. The combination of three variables: severity of coma (evaluated by GCS score), ICH size (on CT) and intraventricular extension of blood, was most predictive of outcome. The location of an hematoma was not a prognostic factor by itself but interacted with ICH size and thus may have influenced the prognosis. Acute hypertension, abnormal pupillary reactivity and ataxic respiration were also associated with a bad prognosis. Poor outcome was observed in 63% of patients (death in 58%; severe disability or vegetative state in 5%) and functional independence in 37% [59].

The surgical indication for ICH is still controversial [61]. Prompt surgical removal is recommended in lesions that may rapidly lead to brain stem compression (cerebellar, temporal and temporo-parietal hematoma). However, no significant difference in long-term outcome has been demonstrated between the series of patients submitted to surgical or conservative management [60, 61].

Prognosis in Subarachnoid Hemorrhage

Subarachnoid hemorrhage (SAH) is most frequently caused by the rupture of a cerebral vascular aneurysm. Other causes are: intracranial and intraspinal arteriovenous malformations, hypertensive hemorrhage, bleeding from intracranial vascular tumors and blood dyscrasias. SAH is also a common finding in head trauma. The presently available neuroimaging techniques permit the localization of 80 to 98% of sources of the SAH but 2 to 18% of SAH remain of unknown origin. Recently, the Framingham study has confirmed that preexisting arterial hypertension and heavy cigarette smoking, especially in women, are important risk factors for SAH [62].

The severity of brain failure due to the primary bleeding is the most important prognostic factor [62–64]. An episode of rebleeding or an arterial vasospasm may all cause further brain damage and unfavorably influence outcome [62–66]. Nevertheless, the age of the patient does not seem to be an important independent prognostic factor [62].

Several grading systems for the evaluation of the severity of SAH has been developed. The most frequently used is the Hunt and Hess five graded scale, which separates patients who remain conscious and do not exhibit neurological deficits (grade I and II) from those who present with altered consciousness and focal neurological signs (grade III, IV and V) [67]. However, this system does not provide a well defined assessment of coma. Lindsey et al. have shown that the GCS is more reliable in SAH than the Hunt and Hess scale [28]. Recently a new neurological grading scale combining the features of the previously used systems, has been proposed by the World Federation of Neurosurgical Surgeons (WFNS) (Table 4). This new scale should be used for the estimation of the patients'prognosis, day-to-day assessment of neurological changes and for thera-

Table 4. Proposed WFNS SAH Scale*

WFNS grade	GCS score	Motor deficit
I	15	Absent
II	14–13	Absent
III	14–13	Present
IV	12–7	Present or absent
V	6–3	Present or absent

* *WFNS* = World Federation of Neurological Surgeons; *SAH* = subarachnoid hemorrhage; *GCS* = Glasgow Coma Scale.

peutic trials [68]. It is based on the assumption that the level of consciousness is the most important predictive factor for both death and disability in SAH whereas the presence of hemiparesis and aphasia is important only for disability but has no effect on mortality. According to the WFNS recommendations this new scale, together with the Glasgow Outcome Scale should be generally used for the classification and the assessment of outcome in SAH patients.

Several early studies reported catastrophically high mortality and morbidity rates from SAH and very high rebleeding rates from non-operated ruptured aneurysms [69]. More recent studies have demonstrated that less than half of the patients surviving to reach hospital will have a good outcome and that the rate of delayed complications was very high even in the initially good risk patients with aneurysmal SAH and treated by surgery [63–66]. It has been also shown that many of the patients with an apparently satisfactory neurosurgical outcome will suffer from a diffuse encephalopathy causing emotional and intellectual disturbances, similar to those encountered in head trauma patients [66].

Since the therapeutic management of SAH may influence the incidence of the secondary brain lesion due to hemorragic and ischemic complications, early agressive treatment of SAH patients has been proposed. Early operation may prevent rebleeding and reduce the incidence of vasospasm because of the removal of subarachnoid blood. Prophylaxis and more effective management of delayed ischemia with the administration of the calcium entry blocker nimodipine and intravascular volume expansion may decrease the incidence of delayed ischemic deficits [63, 70, 71]. These therapeutic modalities are nowadays tested in controlled trials. The recent reports suggest that the timing of surgery is still controversial, especially in high risk patients, but the prophylactic administration of nimodipine seems to decrease the incidence of delayed mortality and neurological deficits [64, 70, 71].

Prognosis in Hypoxic/Ischemic Encephalopathy

ICU patients can present with ischemic/anoxic encephalopathy which is due neither to head trauma nor to cerebrovascular disease, but results from extracranial causes such as cardiac arrest, severe hypotension, or severe hypoxia of various origins. Several studies have shown that the early neurological findings and the duration of coma are important predictors of outcome in these patients [29, 72].

Recently, Levy et al. prospectively studied a large group of patients with ischemic/hypoxic coma and developed simple algorithms, based on the state of pupillary eye reflexes and the degree of impairment of spontaneous eye movements and motor response. This permits a confident prediction of outcome at the initial examination and at days 1, 3, 7, and 14 after the insult. In this series 77% of patients died or became vegetative, 10% remained severely disabled and 26% recovered independent function. Age, sex, site of the initial insult and the cause of coma were not significantly related to outcome [72]. A multicenter Belgian study evaluated the prospective value of the GCS for regaining consciousness from coma due to out-of-hospital cardiac arrest. The neurological outcome could be correctly predicted 48 hours after the insult in 80% of patients with a GCS of 10 or above, or 4 or below as cutoff points. For patients with a best GCS of 5 to 9 the outcome could only be predicted late. A best GCS of 8 during the first 6 days was a cut off point, but only when the subset of patients with GCS 8 who died of non-neurological causes were excluded from statistical analysis [29].

Conclusion

Brain failure in ICU patients carries very high mortality and morbidity rates, essentially related to the severity of the primary insult and the occurrence of the secondary ischemic/anoxic events. Early prediction of functional and neuropsychological outcome in brain failure is necessary for clinical decision-making, family counselling and the establishment of health-care strategies. The identification of various risk factors for different forms of brain failure permits the development of preventive programs.

In all forms of brain failure the clinical assessment of the severity of coma and the degree of impairment of brain stem reflexes have an important prognostic value. A better methodology of assessment with a more general use of standard scoring scales and outcome categories is necessary to define the groups of patients with a similar degree of brain failure and similar potential prognosis and to determine the outcome in individual patient.

A better knowledge of the pathogenesis of brain failure based on the recently available techniques should allow a more precise definition of prognostic factors and a better choice and timing of a more specific and efficient therapeutic management.

References

1. Jennett B, Bond M (1975) Assessment of outcome after severe brain damage. A practical scale. Lancet 1:480–484
2. Teasdale G, Knill Jones R, Van der Sande J (1978) Observer variability in assessing impaired consciousness and coma. J Neurol Neurosurg Psychiatr 41:603–610
3. Maas AIR, Braakmann R, Schouten HJA, Minderhoud JM, van Zomeren AH (1983) Agreement between physicians on assessment of outcome following severe head injury. J Neurosurg 58:321–325
4. Langfitt TW (1978) Measuring the outcome from head injuries. J Neurosurg 48:673–678
5. Braakman R, Gelpke GJ, Habbema JDF, et al (1980) Systematic selection of prognostic features in patients with severe head injury. Neurosurgery 6:362–370
6. Teasdale G, Jennett B (1974) Assessment of coma and impaired consciousness: A practical scale. Lancet 2:81–84
7. Plum F, Posner JB (1966) Diagnosis of stupor and coma. Davis, Philadelphia, pp 329–344
8. Genarelli TA, Spielmann GM, Langfitt TW, et al (1982) Influence of the type of intracranial lesion on outcome from severe head injury. J Neurosurg 56:26–32
9. Lobato RD, Cordobes F, Rivas JJ, et al (1983) Outcome from severe head injury related to the type of intracranial lesion. J Neurosurg 59:762–774
10. Greenberg RP, Newlon PG, Hyatt MS, et al (1981) Prognostic implications of early multimodality evoked potentials in severely head injured patients. J Neurosurg 55:227–236

11. Bakay RAE, Ward AA (1983) Enzymatic changes in serum and cerebrospinal fluid in neurological injury. J Neurosurg 58:27-37
12. Hans P, Born JD, Chapelle JP, Milbouw G (1983) Creatine kinaze isoenzymes in severe head injury. J Neurosurg 58:689-692
13. Woolf PP, Hamill RW, Lee LA, et al (1987) The predictive value of catecholamines in assessing outcome in traumatic brain injury. J Neurosurg 66:875-882
14. de Salles AAF, Kontos HA, Becker PD, et al (1986) Prognostic significance of ventricular CSF lactic acidosis in severe head injury. J Neurosurg 65:615-624
15. Bruce DA, Schut L, Bruno LA, et al (1978) Outcome following severe head injuries in children. J Neurosurg 48:679-688
16. Berger MS, Pitts LH, Lovely M, et al (1985) Outcome from severe head injury in children and adolescents. J Neurosurg 62:194-199
17. Alberico AM, Ward JD, Choi SC, Marmarou A, Young HF (1987) Outcome after severe head injury. J Neurosurg 67:648-656
18. Luerssen TG, Klauber MR, Marshall LF (1988) Outcome from head injury related to patient's age. J Neurosurg 68:409-416
19. Wagstyl J, Sutcliffe A, Alpar EK (1987) Early prediction of outcome following head injury in children. J Ped Surg 2,22:127-129
20. Bricolo A, Turazzi S, Feriotti G (1980) Prolonged posttraumatic uncounsciousness. J Neurosurg 52:625-634
21. Lobato RD, Rivas JJ, Cordobes F, et al (1988) Acute epidural hematoma: an analysis of factors influencing the outcome of patients undergoing surgery in coma. J Neurosurg 68:48-57
22. Miller JD, Butterworth JK, Gudeman SK, et al (1981) Further experience in the management of severe head injury. J Neurosurg 54:289-299
23. Eisenberg HM, Jane JA, Marmarow A, et al (1988) CT findings in 595 patients with severe (GCS ⩽ 8) closed head injury: a report from the NIH Traumatic Coma Data Bank. The Seventh International Symposium on Intracranial Pressure and Brain Injury, Ann Arbor, Michigan, June 19-23 Proceedings, Abstract, p 74
24. Langfitt TW, Genarelli TA (1982) Can the outcome from head injury be improved? J Neurosurg 56:19-25
25. Lobato RD, Sarabia R, Cordobes F, et al (1988) Posttraumatic cerebral hemispheric swelling. J Neurosurg 68:417-423
26. Starmark JE, Holmgren E, Stalhammar D (1988) Current reporting of responsiveness in acute cerebral disorders. J Neurosurg 69:692-698
27. Teasdale G, Jennett B, Murray L, et al (1983) Glasgow coma scale: to sum or not to sum. Lancet 2:678
28. Lindsay KW, Teasdale GM, Knill Jones RD (1983) Observer variability in assessing the clinical features of subarachnoid hemorrage. J Neurosurg 58:57-62
29. Mullie A, Verstringe P, Buylaert W, et al (1988) Predictive value of GCS for awakening after out-of-hospital cardiac arrest. Lancet 1:137-140
30. Barolat-Romana G, Larson SJ (1984) Influence of stimulus location and limb position on motor response in comatose patient. J Neurosurg 61:725-728
31. Born JD, Hans P, Albert A, et al (1987) Interobserver agreement in assessment of motor response and brain stem reflexes. Neurosurgery 20:513-517
32. Jagger J, Jane JA, Rimel R (1983) The Glasgow coma scale, to sum or not to sum. Lancet 2:97
33. Starmark JE, Stalhammar D, Holgren E, et al (1988) A comparison of the Glasgow coma scale and the reaction level scale (RLS 85). J Neurosurg 69:699-706
34. Changaris DG, Mc Graw PC, Richardson JD, et al (1987) Correlation of CPP and GCS to outcome. J Trauma 27:1007-1013
35. Born JD, Hans P, Dexters G, Kalangu K, Lenelle J, et al (1982) Evaluation pratique du dysfonctionnement encéphalique chez le traumatisé crânien. Neuro chirurgie 28:1-7
36. Choi SC, Narayan RK, Anderson RL, Ward JD (1988) Enhanced prognosis in severe head injury. J Neurosurg 69:381-385

37. Snow RB, Zimmerman RD, Gandy SE, Deck MDF (1986) Comparison of magnetic resonance imaging and computed tomography in evaluation of head injury. Neurosurgery 18:45-52
38. Wilson JTL, Wiedmann KD, Hadley DM, et al (1988) Early and late MRI and neuropsychological outcome after head injury. J Neurol Neurosurg Psychiatry 51:391-396
39. Rosner MD, Becker DP (1984) Experimental brain injury: successful therapy with the weak base, thromethamine. J Neurosurg 60:961-971
40. Inao S, Marmarou A, Clarke GP, Andersen BJ, et al (1988) Production and clearance of lactate from brain tissue, CSF and serum following experimental brain injury. J Neurosurg 89:736-744
41. Marmarou A, Anderson R, Ward J, et al (1988) The traumatic coma data bank: monitoring of ICP. The Seventh International Symposium on Intracranial Pressure and Brain Injury. Ann Arbor, Michigan, June 19-23, Proceedings, Abstract, p 75
42. Obrist WD, Genarelli TA, Segawa H, et al (1979) Relation of cerebral blood flow to neurological status and outcome in head injured patients. J Neurosurg 51:292-300
43. Uzell BP, Obrist W, Dolinskas CA, Langfitt TW (1986) Relation of acute CBF and ICP findings to neuropsychological outcome in severe head injury. J Neurosurg 65:630-635
44. Klauber MR, Marshall LF, Toole BM, et al (1985) Cause of decline in head injury mortality rate in San Diego County, California. J Neurosurg 62:528-531
45. Frost EAM (1977) Respiratory problems associated with head trauma. Neurosurgery 1:300-305
46. Kraus J, Conroy C, Cox P, et al (1985) Survival times and case-fatality rates of brain-injured persons. J Neurosurg 63:537-543
47. Seelig JM, Becker DP, Miller JD, et al (1981) Traumatic acute subdural hematoma. Major mortality reduction in comatose patients treated within 4 hours. N Engl J Med 304:1511-1518
48. Marshall LF, Smith EW, Shapiro NM (1979) The outcome with aggressive treatment in severe head injuries part I and II. J Neurosurg 50:20-25 and 26-30
49. Dearden NM, Gibson JS, Mc Dowall GD, et al (1986) Effect of high dose dexamethasone on outcome from severe head injury. J Neurosurg 64:81-88
50. Ward JD, Becker DP, Miller DJ, et al (1985) Failure of prophylactic barbiturate coma in the treatment of severe head injury. J Neurosurg 62:383-388
51. Ward JD, Choi S, Marmarou A, et al (1988) Effect of prophylactic hyperventilation on outcome in patients with severe head injury. The Seventh International Symposium on Intracranial Pressure and Brain Injury. Ann Arbor, Michigan, June 19-23, Proccedings, p 98
52. Young B, Ott L, Twyman D, et al (1987) The effect of nutritional support in outcome from severe head injury. J Neurosurg 67:668-670
53. Williams JM, Gomes F, Drudge OW, Kessler M (1984) Predicting outcome from closed head injury by early assessment of trauma severity. J Neurosurg 61:581-585
54. Uzell BP, Langfitt TW, Dolinskas CA (1987) Influence of injury severity on quality of survival after head injury. Surg Neurol 27:419-429
55. Gelmers HJ, Gorter K, de Weerdt CJ, Wiezer HJA (1988) Assessment of interobserver variability in a dutch multicenter study on acute ischemic stroke. Stroke 19,6:709-711
56. Weisberg LA (1988) Diagnostic classification of stroke, especially lacunes. Stroke 19,9:1071-1073
57. Howard G, Walker MD, Becker C, Coull B, et al (1986) Community - hospital based stroke programs. Stroke 17:294-299
58. Bonita R, Ford MA, Stewart AW (1988) Predicting survival after stroke - a three year follow up. Stroke 19,6:699-673
59. Portenoy RK, Lipton RB, Berger AR, et al (1987) Intracerebral hemorrhage: a model for the prediction of outcome. J Neurol Neurosurg Psychiatry 50:976-979
60. Andrews BT, Chiles BW, Olsen WL, Pitts LH (1988) The effect of intracerebral hematoma location on the risk of brain-stem compression and on the clinical outcome. J Neurosurg 69:518-522
61. Kanno T, Sano H, Shinomiya Y, et al (1984) Role of surgery in hypertensive intracerebral hematoma. J Neurosurg 61:1091-1099

62. Sacco RL, Wolf P, Bharucha NE, et al (1984) Subarachnoid and intracerebral hemorrhage. Natural history, prognosis and precursive factors in the Framingham study. Neurology 34:847-853
63. Ljunggren B, Säveland H, Brandt L, Zygmunt S (1985) Early operation and overall outcome in aneurysmal subarachnoid hemorrhage. J Neurosurg 62:547-551
64. Chyatte D, Fode NC, Sundt TM (1988) Early versus late intracranial aneurysm surgery in SAH. J Neurosurg 69:326-331
65. Ropper AH, Zervas NT (1984) Outcome 1 year after SAH from cerebral aneurysm. J Neurosurg 60:909-915
66. Ljunggren B, Sonnesson B, Säveland H, Brand L (1985) Cognitive impairment and adjustment in patients without neurological deficits after aneurysmal SAH and early operation. J Neurosurg 62:673-679
67. Hunt WE, Hess RM (1968) Surgical risk as related to time of intervention in the repair of intracranial aneurysms. J Neurosurg 28:14-20
68. Neurosurgical Forum (1988) Report of world federation of neurological surgeons committee on a universal subarachnoidal hemorrhage grading scale. J Neurosurg 68:985-986
69. Kassel NF, Adams HP Jr, Torner JC, et al (1981) Influence of timing of admission after aneurysmal subarachnoid hemorrhage on overall outcome. Stroke 12:620-623
70. Petruk KC, West M, Mohr G, et al (1988) Nimodipine treatment in poor-grade aneurysm patients. J Neurosurg 68:505-517
71. Ohman J, Heiskanen O (1988) Effect on nimodipine on the outcome of patients after aneurysmal SAH and surgery. J Neurosurg 69:683-686
72. Levy MD, Caronna J, Singer BH, et al (1985) Predicting outcome from hypoxic - ischemic coma. JAMA 253:1420-1426

Subject Index